Advances in Probiotics for Health and Nutrition

Edited by Vasudeo Zambare, Mohd Fadhil Md. Din, Puja Gupta and Bhupendra Gopalbhai Prajapati

Published in London, United Kingdom

Advances in Probiotics for Health and Nutrition
http://dx.doi.org/10.5772/intechopen.104299
Edited by Vasudeo Zambare, Mohd Fadhil Md. Din, Puja Gupta and Bhupendra Gopalbhai Prajapati

Contributors
Meriem Msaad Guerfali, Haytham Hamden, Kamel Charaabi, Salma Fadhl, Amor Mosbah, Ameur Cherif, Arezoo Aghakouchakzadeh, Ahmadreza Mirzaei, Niayesh Daneshvarpour, Sanda Maria Cretoiu, Bogdan Severus Gaspar, Ruxandra Florentina Ionescu, Robert Mihai Enache, Elena Codruta Cozma, Maria Iancu, Matei Mandea, Monica Profir, Oana Alexandra Roşu, Sadegh Sulaimany, Kajal Farahmandi, Alojz Bomba, Martin Haranta, Doina Georgescu, Ana Lascu, Ioana Ionita, Oana-Elena Ancusa, Mihai Ionita, Ciprian Ilie Rosca, Despina Calamar-Popovici, Daniel Lighezan, Mihaela Jurdana, Darja Barlič Maganja, Vasudeo Zambare, Rasika Pawar, Janvi Kadam, Mohd Fadhil Md. Din, David Shih, John Ryan, Shruthi Narasimha, Youssef Ghobrial, Robert Pattison, Rasiq Zackria, Syed Abdul Basit, Christian Stone, Tarek Ammar, Vijay Jayaraman, Akash Kumar, Bhupendra G. Gopalbhai Prajapati, Nandani Goyal, Jhilam Pramanik, Dimple Chauhan

First published in London, United Kingdom, 2024 by IntechOpen
IntechOpen is the global imprint of INTECHOPEN LIMITED, registered in England and Wales, registration number: 11086078, 5 Princes Gate Court, London, SW7 2QJ, United Kingdom

British Library Cataloguing-in-Publication Data
A catalogue record for this book is available from the British Library

Additional hard and PDF copies can be obtained from orders@intechopen.com

Advances in Probiotics for Health and Nutrition
Edited by Vasudeo Zambare, Mohd Fadhil Md. Din, Puja Gupta and Bhupendra Gopalbhai Prajapati
p. cm.
Print ISBN 978-1-83768-610-0
Online ISBN 978-1-83768-611-7
eBook (PDF) ISBN 978-1-83768-612-4

For EU product safety concerns:
IN TECH d.o.o., Prolaz Marije Krucifikse Kozulić 3, 51000 Rijeka, Croatia,
info@intechopen.com or visit our website at intechopen.com.

Meet the editors

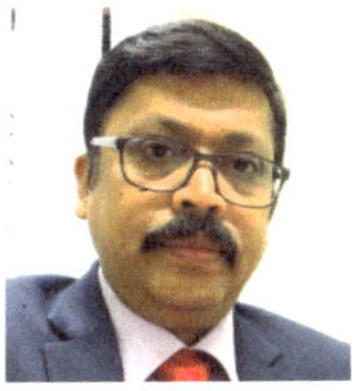

Dr. Vasudeo Zambare is a Head of R&D, Balaji Enzyme and Chemical Pvt Ltd, Mumbai, Maharashtra, India, and a fellow at the Center for Environmental Sustainability and Water Security (IPASA), Universiti Teknologi Malaysia (UTM). Dr. Zambare obtained his Ph.D. in Biochemistry from the Agharkar Research Institute, Pune University, Pune, Maharashtra, India in 2007. He has 3 patents, more than 230 technical and scientific publications, and more than 80 peer-reviewed journal articles to his credit. Dr. Zambare is a multi-skilled researcher with biorefinery industry experience in the United States, Canada, the European Union, India, and Malaysia. He has developed bioprocesses for the leather, textile, paper and pulp, and biofuel industries. He has more than 20 years of achievements in advancing knowledge by devising fermentation processes, assays, and analytical methods to solve complex research problems with potential commercial applications (biofuel, food, and pharmaceuticals). His research expertise includes industrial enzymes, probiotics, extremophiles, biofertilizers, biopesticides, waste management, and leather bioprocessing.

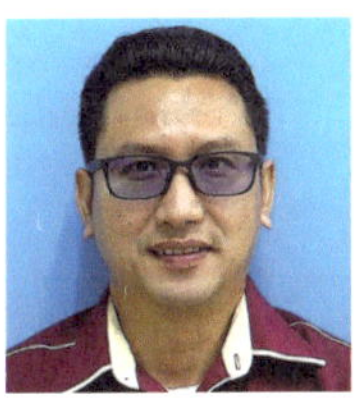

Dr. Mohd Fadhil Md. Din graduated from Universiti Teknologi Malaysia (UTM) in 1999 and obtained an MEng in 2001. He further studied under a double program between UTM and Delft University of Technology, Netherlands. Dr. Din has more than 280 technical and scientific publications to his credit. He is the recipient of several funding grants and prestigious awards. He is a director of campus sustainability, working for an environmental and sustainable operational framework on campus. His expertise is in environmental sciences and application, environmental management systems (EMS), environmental impact assessments (EIA), risk management, and transportation projects (mobility transformational agenda). He is involved in undergraduate and postgraduate courses in environmental science and engineering, specializing in water and wastewater treatment, biotechnology and bioengineering, fundamental chemical sciences, and river rehabilitation, particularly issues related to developing countries. He has received several awards and recognitions at both national and international levels.

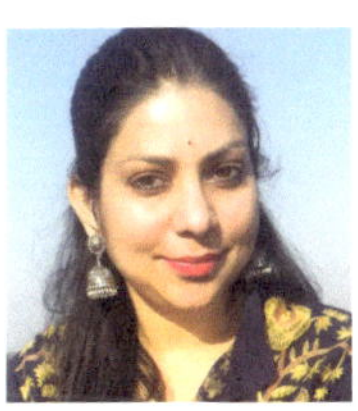

Dr. Puja Gupta is an Associate Professor of Biotechnology at the Regional Institute of Management and Technology (RIMT), Mandi Gobindgarh, Sirhind, Punjab. She is the recipient of various fellowships from the Department of Science and Technology (DST), Government of India and the Council of Scientific & Industrial Research (CSIR), India. She has more than 18 years of academic and research experience and has published more than 20 research and review papers in international and national journals. She has also edited one book and is currently editing two others. She has authored fifteen book chapters and participated in various conferences and workshops. Her research interests include metagenomics, microbiology, microbial genetics, and plant–microbe interactions.

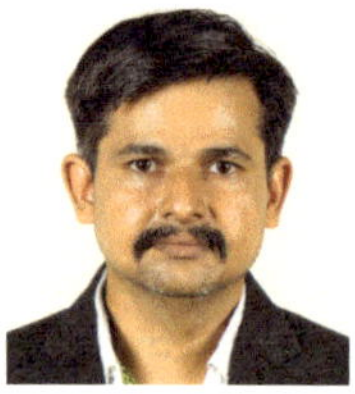

Dr. Bhupendra Gopalbhai Prajapati is a professor in the Department of Pharmaceutics, Shree S.K. Patel College of Pharmaceutical Education and Research, Ganpat University, Gujarat, India. He has more than 21 years of academic and research experience and has published more than 120 research and review papers in international and national journals. He has also edited one book, with six more forthcoming. He has authored forty book chapters on novel drug delivery. He has two Indian patents to his credit and has three applications under evaluation. He is a guest editor, section/topic editor, editorial board member, and reviewer for various scientific journals.

Contents

Preface

Advances in Probiotics for Health and Nutrition examines the exploitation of probiotics from natural habitats for plant, animal, and human health and nutrition. Though the world is experiencing rapid advancements in science and technology, probiotics and probiotic-based products, which have been around since ancient times, are still effective as health and nutritional supplements for plants, animals, and humans. Scientific advancements have led to the creation of new tools and techniques for developing next-generation probiotics from various natural habitats. This book explores novel probiotics and the microbiome and its impact on plants, animals, and humans. Probiotics in agriculture act as biostimulants and plant protectants, whereas probiotics in food and feed act as nutraceutical supplements and immune boosters for the treatment and prevention of various diseases, pathogens, and disorders. This book includes eleven chapters organized into two sections: "Probiotics in Health" and "Probiotics in Nutrition".

Chapter 1, "Translation of Immunomodulatory Effects of Probiotics into Clinical Practice", provides insight into the health benefits of probiotics. It surveys the interaction between probiotics, innate immunity, adaptive immunity, and the host gut microbiome. The introduction of probiotics to the diet greatly influences the microbial composition and type of gut microbiome. These are described to preserve a healthy state with many curative properties. The main highlights of this chapter include the clinical uses of probiotics in human health.

Chapter 2, "Nonalcoholic Fatty Liver Disease, Procalcitonin, and Gut Microbiota: Players in the Same Team", explains the correlations between procalcitonin (PCT) and gut dysbiosis in non-cirrhotic patients with non-alcoholic fatty liver disease (NAFLD). Procalcitonin (PCT) is a peptide whose levels may increase in patients with liver diseases as a response to pro-inflammatory conditions, even without a bacterial infection. The chapter describes that dysbiotic patients with NAFLD exhibit significant elevation of PCT that correlates well to the H-index of stool's microbiota biodiversity, F/B ratio, CRP level, and severity of cytolytic syndrome.

Chapter 3, "Personalized and Targeted Gut Microbiome Modulation in the Prevention and Treatment of Chronic Diseases", examines the role of gut microbiota in health. Distinct shifts in the composition and diversity of gut microbiota have been closely correlated with various chronic diseases. In this chapter, the authors explore the diverse methods available for modulating gut microbiota, including dietary interventions, probiotics, prebiotics, postbiotics, pharmabiotics, and fecal microbiota transplantation. These approaches have the potential to revolutionize the treatment of chronic diseases by reshaping the gut microbiota to promote health and mitigate illness. Furthermore, this chapter offers a concise overview of a multitude of research studies that shed light on the specific alterations in the diversity, composition, and function of the gut microbiota. These investigations provide valuable insights into the intricate relationship between the gut microbiota and chronic diseases, offering a promising path toward personalized and targeted interventions.

Chapter 4, "Probiotic Effects on Disease Prevention and Treatment", explores the profound influence of probiotics on mitigating and preventing various diseases through a range of intricate mechanisms. These mechanisms encompass the direct elimination or inhibition of pathogenic growth, the production of antimicrobial substances, toxin neutralization, competition with target cells, immune system modulation, restoration of microbial balance, reinforcement of intestinal integrity, and heightened mucus production. The chapter highlights that the effectiveness of probiotics depends on the type of utilized strain, duration, dose administration, and whether single or combined strains are used. Probiotics have helped in enhancing resistance to respiratory tract infections, reducing inflammation and oxidative stress in pancreatic cells, preventing the onset of diabetes, and regulating important neurotransmitters. They are also effective in the improvement of mental disorders. Nevertheless, a more extensive body of evidence is necessary to firmly establish the efficacy of probiotic microorganisms in these contexts, which underscores the importance of further randomized clinical trials with various probiotic strains.

Chapter 5, "Adherence of *Candida albicans* on Polymethyl Methacrylate in Probiotics Solution", discusses the role of probiotic solutions in the oral cavity and treatment of candidiasis. *Candida albicans* is a ubiquitous microorganism, typically residing harmlessly in various mucous membranes throughout the body, including the ears, eyes, gastrointestinal tract, mouth, nose, reproductive organs, sinuses, skin, stool, and vagina. The chapter explains that an imbalance in the normal flora causes an overgrowth of *C. albicans* thereby causing candidiasis or thrush. Probiotic solutions can be used to reduce the number of *C. albicans* microorganisms and their adherence thereby treating candidiasis or thrush. The chapter discusses how probiotic solutions can serve as valuable tools for reducing the adherence of *C. albicans*, thereby offering a potential therapeutic approach to managing candidiasis. Comprehending the intricate interactions between probiotics and *C. albicans* can lead to an advanced understanding of innovative solutions for tackling this prevalent oral health concern.

Chapter 6, "Advances on Probiotics Utilization in Poultry Health and Nutrition", explores the profound impact of probiotics on enhancing poultry immunity, optimizing growth performance, improving feed utilization, and maintaining overall health. The poultry industry is experiencing rapid growth, particularly in developing countries. Historically, antibiotics have played a crucial role in ensuring the safety and well-being of poultry flocks. However, the rising concerns about antibiotic resistance have spurred a pressing demand for antibiotic-free poultry production. This chapter presents probiotics as promising alternatives to antibiotics, revolutionizing the poultry farming landscape. It highlights the concept, impact, and mode of action of probiotics in sustainable poultry production. Significant work and studies have proved that probiotics help in maintaining health status in poultry animals, as they improve gut conditions and enhance nutrient absorption, thus improving overall growth performance.

Chapter 7, "Regular Physical Activity Influences Gut Microbiota with Positive Health Effects", explains how the gut microbiota is influenced by physical activity. In this chapter, the authors describe recent animal and human studies that suggest that regular physical activity improves gut health through the modulation of the gut ecosystem. They explain that aerobic exercises may significantly change the composition of the microbiota, depending on the types and intensities of exercise. This chapter also explores recent studies that have shown that probiotics reduce inflammation and improve gut barrier function and the immune system. Through these actions, probiotics may influence the performance of athletes by preventing diseases that can affect exercise. Specific probiotic strains have been associated with improved body composition and lean body mass, faster recovery of muscle from intense exercise, and overall health. The main highlights of this chapter are how physical activity, gut bacteria, and probiotics work together to improve the health, well-being, and performance of athletes.

Chapter 8, "Probiotics in the Management of Diabetes", discusses how probiotics play a crucial role in the management of diabetes through the modulation of the gut microbiome. This chapter provides valuable insight through a discussion of experimental and clinical trials that highlight the significant potential of probiotic strains in the management of diabetes. Since insulin signaling is hindered by lipopolysaccharides, trimethylamine, and imidazole propionate, probiotic administrations enhance the secondary bile acids, short-chain fatty acids (SCFAs), and tryptophan metabolites and improve impaired glucose metabolism. This chapter also reviews the mechanisms through which probiotics alleviate diabetes by addressing the gut microflora from the perspectives of amino acid metabolism, intestinal permeability, immunological responses, oxidative stress, and SCFAs.

Chapter 9, "Probiotics as a Beneficial Modulator of Gut Microbiota and Environmental Stress for Sustainable Mass-Reared *Ceratitis capitata*", explores the transformative potential of probiotics in medfly control, summarizing the evidence and shedding light on symbiotic relationships. Probiotics hold promise not only for medflies but also for insect farming, including edible insects, by enhancing production quality and quantity. The probiotic selection schemes outlined in the chapter can be adapted for other insects' mass-reared for Sterile Insect Technique (SIT) and beyond. This chapter explores the practical application of probiotics for innovative biocontrol tools.

Chapter 10, "Intestinal Microbiomics in Physiological and Pathological Conditions", explores the realm of microbiomics, a pioneering science that explores the entirety of microorganisms within a given community. This chapter focuses on the human microbiome, a significant organ boasting 150 times more genes than the human genome. It explores the associations between intestinal dysbiosis and inflammatory and metabolic diseases, even though the intricate mechanisms are not fully elucidated. As microbiomics parallels human genomics and the microbiome is recognized as a second genome within the human body, this chapter points towards an exciting future in precision medicine. The ongoing development of next-generation sequencing technologies will offer new insights into modulating the microbiome via non-invasive methods such as prebiotics, probiotics, and dietary changes.

This book provides a comprehensive overview of advancements in probiotics research, presenting cutting-edge knowledge and recent trends.

The editors and authors would like to thank Ms. Martina Scerbe, Ms. Ana Cink, and the publishing staff at IntechOpen for their invaluable assistance in writing and publishing this book.

Vasudeo Zambare
R&D Department,
Balaji Enzyme and Chemical Pvt Ltd,
Mumbai, India

Center for Environmental Sustainability and Water Security (IPASA),
Department of Water and Environmental Engineering,
School of Civil Engineering,
Universiti Teknologi Malaysia,
Bahru, Malaysia

Mohd Fadhil Md. Din
Centre for Environmental Sustainability and Water Security (IPASA),
Department of Water and Environmental Engineering,
Universiti Teknologi Malaysia,
Bahru, Malaysia

Puja Gupta
Regional Institute of Management and Technology,
Mandi Gobindgarh, Punjab, India

Bhupendra Gopalbhai Prajapati
Shree S.K. Patel College of Pharmaceutical Education and Research,
Ganpat University,
Mehsana, Gujarat, India

Section 1

Probiotics in Health

Chapter 1

Translation of Immunomodulatory Effects of Probiotics into Clinical Practice

John Ryan, Shruthi Narasimha, Robert Pattison, Rasiq Zackria, Youssef Ghobrial, Syed Abdul Basit, Tarek Ammar, Vijay Jayaraman, Christian Stone and David Shih

Abstract

Probiotics have emerged as an in-demand and highly marketed commodity in the healthcare space. In 2021, the global market valued the probiotic industry at USD 58.17 billion in 2021. It is expected to have a compound annual growth rate of 7.5% yearly from 2021 to 2030. The inclusion of probiotics in various products has become synonymous with health benefits despite limited understanding of mechanism of action or benefit. This chapter will survey the state of our understanding of the interactions between probiotics with the innate immunity, adaptive immunity, and the host gut microbiome. Additionally, we will also highlight the theorized beneficial and possible detrimental immunomodulatory effects of probiotics on human health.

Keywords: probiotics, adaptive immunity, innate immunity, microbiome, clinical use of probiotics

1. Introduction

The word probiotic comes from the Latin word *pro* and the Greek word bios, which when joined together, literally means "for life." The concept of probiotics has evolved over the many millennia but modern scientific theory of it only began in the twentieth century. The term probiotics was first used in 1953 by Werner Kollath, a German scientist who defined it as an "active substance that is essential for a healthy development of life." The definition of the term changed multiple times through the century but the most accepted one comes from the Food and Agriculture Organization of the United Nations and the World Health Organization (FAO/WHO). They define probiotics as "live microorganisms which when administered in adequate amounts confer a health benefit on the host [1–3]."

Although probiotics are believed to confer important health benefits, including amelioration of C. diff colitis, inflammatory bowel disease, metabolic syndrome, etc., the understanding of the mechanisms of action of probiotics is limited. Thus, the aim of the present chapter is to review the immune modulatory effects of probiotics and how it interacts with the host gut microbiome. We will also highlight the practical clinical uses of probiotics on human health and disease. Lastly, we will speculate on the future direction on the use of probiotics.

2. Modulation of innate immunity by probiotics

Innate immunity is one of the major arms in our immune system and consists of a complex complement cascade that acts as a physical and chemical barrier. It works to protect against infectious agents by recognizing conserved features of pathogens that become quickly activated to help destroy microbial invaders and to produce factors such as cytokines to activate adaptive immune response.

The most recognized innate mechanism comes from the concept of a barrier. This intrinsic wall helps evade foreign microbe penetration and prevents all the deleterious effects of colonization. The three major components that have been studied in barrier protection are mucin production, reinforcement of tight junctions in the epithelial layer, and enzyme regulation. Mucin production made by epithelial cells helps deter pathogen attachment. The permeable gel-like layer offers innate immunity by helping release secretory IgA, which prevents invading pathogen adherence. Additionally, the mucin layer helps identify self with nonself and can activate the immune system against invaders. Pathogen-associated molecular patterns are embedded in commensal microbiome organisms and these are recognized by Toll-like receptors to be noninvasive microbiota. The mechanisms of mucin for barrier enforcement are well known but studies now are starting to show how probiotics may help with boosting this barrier production [4]. *In vivo* rat studies have shown that administration of a specific probiotic mixture named VSL#3, which included strains of *Lactobacilli*, *Bifidobacteria*, and *Streptococci*, was associated with increased mucin gene expression and secretion. Increased mucin production theoretically leads to a more robust barrier [5]. The third barrier mechanism includes enzyme activity modification. Foreign microbes can also invade by activating destructive enzymatic processes. Pathogens secrete enzymes like B-glucuronidase that result in toxic metabolites and can be pre-carcinogenic in the intestines. *Bifidobacterium longum* is a probiotic that was used in animal studies and showed a decrease in fecal B-glucuronidase activity and abnormal intestinal crypt structure by about 53% [6].

Tight junctions between epithelial cells help create a firm seal and prevent invasion. *Lactiplantibacillus plantarum* WCFS1, a probiotic, was noted to increase proteins like zonula occludens-1 (ZO-1) and transmembrane occludins near tight junctions, which help promote a good seal and ensure integrity of the epithelial barrier [7]. Another probiotic, *Lactobacillus rhamnosus*, was used to pretreat intestinal epithelial cells of pigs and was later exposed to enterotoxigenic *Escherichia coli* (ETEC). Pretreated cells have less TNF-α inflammatory response, higher ZO-1/occludin levels, and helped deter pathogenic adhesion to the epithelium. TNF-α activity correlates with an inflammatory cytokine response, which can lead to cell injury, so a subdued response helps taper these detrimental events [8]. In addition to the formation of a strong barrier, the components of the epithelial layer also add to its fortitude. Basolateral cells in the intestine have B cells that secrete sIgA, a secretory IgA transporter, which helps build a robust innate immunity. This secretory immunoglobulin works through a process called immune exclusion, which is when sIgA recognizes surface molecules on pathogens and prevents adherence. Probiotics like *Bifidobacterium breve, L. rhamnosus*, and *Lactobacillus casei* have shown to increase the sIgA production and thus prevent colonization [9, 10].

Competitive exclusion is another important innate mechanism used to prevent pathogenic growth. The general concept here is that one microbe outcompetes, through various mechanisms, another and dominates the microbiome. Probiotics take advantage of this principle by creating toxic environments, competitively taking over resources, and producing antimicrobial bacteriocins to overtake pathogens [9].

Another key area of probiotic function comes from the cytokine cascade that leads to immune activity. Several examples exist but to understand their function, a brief review of immune cells and cytokines will help showcase the various mechanisms. Natural killer (NK) cells are lymphocytes that work to kill foreign pathogens with their cytotoxic proteases. Monocytes include macrophages and dendritic cells, which work by phagocytosis and present antigens to adaptive immune cells, respectively. IL-10 and IL-4 are anti-inflammatory interleukins that can prevent cell damage [11]. A plethora of studies exists to showcase how particular strains evoke a complex cytokine pathway. Daily consumption of *Lactobacillus salivarius*, a probiotic from breast milk, increased production of natural killer cells, monocytes, immunoglobulins, and IL-10 [12]. The SETOPROB study showed that probiotics like *L. rhamnosus*, *L. casei*, and *B. breve* increased IL-4, IL-10 and fecal secretory IgA. These cytokine and cell activations lead to downregulation of inflammation and prompt the activation of the adaptive immune system [9].

Finally, probiotics help maintain homeostasis by way of pathogen recognition and T cell regulation. Pattern recognition receptors (PRRs) bind to pathogen-associated molecular patterns (PAMPs), or damage-associated molecular patterns (DAMPs), which are expressed on most pathogens. PRRs are made up of toll-like receptors (TLRs) and NOD-like receptors (NODLRs), which function to activate immune activation and protect the cytoplasm. Additionally, TLR activation by PAMPs or DAMPs on monocytes triggers T cell activation and naïve T cells are prompted to differentiate. Activation of TLRs and NODLRs prompts cytokine cascade activation and the resulting inflammation could facilitate cell damage. Probiotics, however, regulate nuclear factor-κB (NFκB) and dampen the inflammatory response [9, 13–15].

The innate immunity is the body's initial defense mechanism and is made up of a variety of pathways to fortify the barriers and activate immune cascades. Probiotics assist in this pathway in many ways as outlined above. This initial response lends itself to initiate the acquired immunity discussed below, which goes on to form a more long-lasting immune response.

3. Modulation of adaptive immunity by probiotics

Adaptive immunity is responsible for identifying and destroying individual invading microbes in mammalian hosts. The cells that carry out the adaptive immune response are B and T cells, which produce a cascade of immune responses upon recognition of foreign antigens interacting with their specific toll-like receptors (TLRs) [16]. Unlike the innate immune system, which is preprogrammed to react to common broad categories of pathogens, the development of adaptive immune responses to new pathogens is slower. Due to its highly specific antigen receptors, specifically the B cell receptor (BCR) and T cell receptor (TCR), to the pathogen, the body has encountered. Adaptive immunity creates immunological memory after an initial response to a specific pathogen and leads to a robust response to encounter with pathogens in the future. B cells act *via* humoral immunity by secreting antibodies while T cells work *via* T helper cells (CD4+) and cytotoxic T cells (CD8+) to either expand or suppress downstream immune activation [17]. CD4 T cells can be broken down into 5 major subsets: Th1, Th2, Th17, T regulatory (Treg), and follicular T helper (Tfh). This categorization is determined based on the expression of specific cytokines and lineage-specific transcription factors. Th1 cells activate macrophages to help protect against intracellular pathogens such as bacteria and viruses. Th2 cells recruit eosinophils, basophils, and mast cells to sites of infections caused by parasites. Th17 cells aid in the clearance of extracellular bacteria by stimulating continuous neutrophil recruitment and the creation of antimicrobial peptides by epithelial cells. Treg cells contribute to the maintenance of immune tolerance and the prevention of autoimmune diseases. Tfh cells support B cells in the production of antibody formation by aiding in germinal center formation and immunoglobulin class switching [18]. The gastrointestinal tract is the largest immune organ in the human body and comprises the epithelial layer, lamina propria, and mucosal-associated lymphoid tissue (MALT). Adaptive immunity plays a vital role in the development and maintenance of the mucosal immune system (MIS) [16, 19]. Peyer's patches are aggregates of lymphoid follicles found throughout the intestinal mucosal cells [20]. They are the main site for B cell activation and class-switch recombination from IgM to IgA. These cells also aid the immune system in discriminating between pathogenic and commensal bacteria. Their function is imperative to maintaining the integrity of the gut mucosal barrier, protecting the host from infections, and maintaining homeostasis with the native microbiota [21]. At the mucosal level, antigen-presenting cells (APCs) present in Peyer's patches will retrieve immunoglobulin A antigen from mucosal folds and communicate with T cells resulting in different T cell activation, which then ensures mucosal barrier integrity [16, 22].

Numerous studies have demonstrated a variety of molecular pathways where probiotics appear to have influence, such as the production of cytokines, IgA secretion, formation of antibacterial compounds, mucosal cellular integrity, and competition with opportunistic pathogens for enterocyte adherence. A proposed probiotic immunomodulation works by antigenic proteins native to the probiotic microorganism crossing epithelial cells and interacting with the innate and adaptive immune system that resides in Peyer's patches [23]. In turn, this interaction produces a cascading effect resulting in the release of cytokines, such as tumor necrosis factor (TNF), interferons (IFN), interleukins (IL), and chemokines. This interaction between probiotics and the host suggests probiotics play an important role in the production and deployment of a more robust immune response by the host when faced with pathogenic organisms. Cellular wall compounds, such as lipoteichoic acid, which is found in *Bifidobacteria* and *Lactobacilli*, are known to stimulate nitric oxide (NO) synthase. The production of NO is a critical component in the cell death mechanism carried out by macrophages when dealing with pathogen-infected cells [24]. *B. longum* is considered one of the first immune-priming probiotics. Known as the "maternal probiotic", most of the inoculation comes *via* the mode of vaginal birth. Studies have demonstrated that *B. longum* plays a crucial role in immune system priming, Peyer's patch development, and IgA production [25]. Lactic acid bacteria such as *L. casei*, *Lactobacillus acidophilus*, *L. rhamnosus*, *Lactococcus lactis*, and *Streptococcus thermophilus* have been shown to play a role in maintaining the intestinal barrier by stimulating B cells to produce IgA. Lai, Hung-Hsiang, et al. administered *L. casei* and *L. rhamnosus* to children with acute diarrheal illness. When compared to the control group, the children who received the probiotics had higher total fecal IgA levels and significantly lower concentrations of fecal lactoferrin and calprotectin. This study suggests that the probiotics *L. casei* and *L. rhamnosus* may be useful supplements during acute diarrhea to reduce clinical severity and intestinal inflammatory reaction [26].

Additionally, probiotics have been observed to modulate pro−/or anti-inflammatory responses by the adaptive immune system *via* interaction with dendritic, Th1, Th2, and Treg cells at the intestinal mucosal surface [24]. In Celiac disease (CD) patients, dysbiosis is thought to play a primary role in its pathogenesis [27]. Numerous studies have demonstrated a significant difference between intestinal microbial populations in healthy children and children with CD [28]. With a gluten-free diet, many of these microbial differences dissipate, except for persistently reduced levels of *Bifidobacterium* in the CD subjects [29]. This finding is particularly important as *Bifidobacteria* has been shown to protect human intestinal cells from the noxious effects of gliadin peptides by altering their molecular structure. Unmodified gliadin peptides result in an adaptive immune response leading to the development of anti-tissue transglutaminase antibodies (anti-tTG), which cause a local inflammation destroying microvilli responsible for nutrient absorption and disrupting the intestinal mucosal barrier [30]. Current murine model studies suggest that the immunomodulatory effects of probiotics are strain specific. Borruel et al. studied ileal mucosal samples from patients with active Crohn's disease and cultured them with either *Escherichia coli*, *Lactobacillus casei*, *Lactobacillus bulgaricus* or *Lactobacillus crispatus*. The probiotic *Lactobacillus bulgaricus* and *Lactobacillus casei* cultured samples demonstrated a significant reduction in TNF-α, a known proinflammatory cytokine. The most robust effect on the downregulation of TNF-α came from viable bacteria, while heat-killed bacteria did not produce a statistically significant change. This finding suggests that cellular products manufactured by viable bacteria play an important role in the suppression of TNF-α production in inflamed tissue [31]. Livingston et al. explored the immunoregulatory response of bone marrow-derived dendritic cells to *Lactobacillus reuteri* 100–23, as previous studies suggested that this bacterial strain had modulatory effects on proinflammatory cytokines in murine models. They found that exposure to *L. reuteri* increased the production of IL-10 suggesting an induction of a regulatory dendritic cell phenotype. This resulted in lower IL-2 production while increasing TGF-β output [32]. This is important as IL-10 and TGF-β are immunoregulatory cytokines and the overall suppression of the murine immune response directed at *L. reuteri* allows the bacteria to colonize and have a commensalistic relationship with the host. Moreover, various probiotic strains have demonstrated the ability to stimulate immunoglobulin receptors in intestinal epithelial cells [33].

4. Modulation of the gut microbiome by probiotics

Probiotic mechanisms resulting in human gut microbiome alteration include effects on the microbial composition and function of these native organisms. More recent studies have utilized culture-dependent methods and metagenomic sequencing techniques to evaluate probiotic effects on changes in microbiome composition, diversity, and function. Certain strains of probiotics have been shown to release antimicrobial proteins or metabolic waste products that suppress the growth of other bacteria in the local vicinity. Others have been shown to compete with local bacterial populations for receptors and binding sites on the intestinal epithelial cells [34–36]. *Lactobacillus reuteri* is an anaerobic probiotic that converts glycerol into reuterin, a potent antimicrobial compound that inhibits the growth of pathogenic gram-negative and gram-positive bacteria. Agar spot testing has demonstrated these inhibitory effects on enterohemorrhagic *E. coli* (EHEC), enterotoxigenic *E. coli* (ETEC), *Salmonella enterica*, *Shigella sonnei*, and *Vibrio cholerae* [34]. Gut microbiota growth and metabolism are heavily dependent on the supply of dietary carbohydrates. The probiotic *Bifidobacterium* has been observed to contribute to interspecies cross-feeding resulting in an increase in beneficial microorganisms, including *Firmicutes* bacteria. This occurs as *Bifidobacterium* can utilize starch and fructo-oligosaccharides for energy and release lactate as a metabolic byproduct. The lactate is then used by local *Firmicutes* bacteria for energy. This relationship is important for the host as *Firmicutes* bacteria produce butyrate, a beneficial short-chain fatty acid [37, 38]. Interestingly, cross-feeding between different *Bifidobacterial* strains has been shown to upregulate the transcription and expression of various genes resulting in metabolic profile changes, primarily genes that play a role in carbohydrate metabolism [38]. Shifts in metabolic gene expression have also been observed in murine models when supplemented with fermented milk products that harbored a variety of probiotic bacteria. Results of metatranscriptomic analysis on fecal samples revealed a significant change in carbohydrate enzyme gene expression, further strengthening the proposed relationship between probiotic bacteria supplementation and shifts in the metabolic function of the gut microbiome [39].

A study analyzing the fecal microbiota of 6-month-old infants explored the changes in intestinal microbiota communities when supplemented with *L. rhamnosus*. Their results showed an abundance of *L. rhamnosus* and an increased microbial species evenness index suggesting ecological stability and diversity [40]. In murine models, supplementation of *L. reuteri* resulted in an increase in microbial community evenness and diversity when compared to vehicle-treated mice [41]. These findings are notable as maintaining diversity in microbial communities is associated with ecological stability [42]. Interestingly, insults such as infections or antibiotic therapy that result in a decline in microbial diversity have been associated with autoimmune diseases such as Crohn's disease and eczema [43, 44]. These findings suggest that probiotics may induce local changes in the gut microbiota and directly contribute to healthy diversity and stabilization of microbial communities.

5. Clinical uses of probiotics

Probiotics are live bacteria meant to inoculate the gut of the host and incorporate into an already diverse microbiota. Probiotics are broadly used in three categories: immunomodulation, normalization of intestinal microbiota, and metabolic effects [45]. In general, the quality of evidence for use in clinical conditions remains low. The literature to support their use has been most clear in necrotizing enterocolitis (NEC) in neonates and pouchitis in ulcerative colitis (UC) patients. However, the use of probiotics well beyond the gastrointestinal tract is ongoing. We will review the studies about the current state of probiotics used in various disease states in this section (**Table 1**).

5.1 Antibiotic-associated diarrhea

Antibiotic-associated diarrhea (AAD) is a common side-effect of the antibiotics that can affect up to a third of patients receiving antibiotics [58]. Broad-spectrum

Probiotic	Human health condition	Proposed mechanism	References
Saccharomyces cerevisiae variant boulardii	Antibiotic-associated diarrhea	Interference with cell signaling, direct production of bacteriocins, and augmentation of the systemic immune response of the host.	[46]
Lactobacillus GG, E. faecium (SF68 strain) and *S. boulardii*			[47, 48]
S. boulardii	*Clostridioides difficile* infection	Protease that inhibits *Clostridioides difficile* toxin A and B activity.	[1, 49]
Lactobacillus spp.		Inhibit toxin A/B in human enterocytes Caco-2 and HT-29 cells.	[50]
Lactobacillus GG	Inflammatory bowel	To inhibit pro-inflammatory cytokines such as NF-Kb potentially providing anti-inflammatory properties to the host.	[51, 52]
S. boulardii			[46]
Lactobacillus reuteri		Tumor Necrosis Factor (TNF) a common target of biologics often used in IBD treatment was reduced.	[53]
VSL#3 containing *Lactobacillus, Bifidobacterium*, and *Streptococcus*			[54]
Bifidobacterium infantis and *Lactobacillus acidophilus*	Necrotizing enterocolitis	Unclear	[55, 56]
Bifidobacterium spp	Irritable bowel syndrome	Unclear	[57]

Table 1.
Summarization of known effects of probiotics in specific disease states.

antibiotics with activity against anaerobes are associated with higher rates of the AAD [47]. AAD may last two months after the onset of antibiotic therapy resulting in significant morbidity [47]. Several randomized-controlled trials and meta-analyses, including bacterial strain-specific trials, have shown that the use of Lactobacillus and Saccharomyces has shown potential benefits of probiotics in addressing AAD [59, 60]. It is postulated that probiotics could antagonize the pathogenic microorganisms in the human flora when the host has been exposed to antibiotics [61]. The mechanism of their interference involves interference with cell signaling, direct production of bacteriocins, and augmentation of the systemic immune response of the host [62–66]. Most studies in AAD have focused on inpatients who were on intravenous antibiotics at higher concentrations where concurrent administration of probiotics has conferred a protective effect in some instances [67]. Probiotics have also been shown in meta-analyses to have a protective effect in outpatients receiving antibiotics without adverse side effects [68]. However, there remains a dearth of direct comparisons between specific strains and their effectiveness when used in conjunction with specific antibiotics. In addition, in the studies finding evidence of benefit, there are inconsistent definitions of diarrhea, specific infections treated, and the types of antibiotics being used [59]. This makes it challenging for clinicians to target probiotic treatment regiments to specific diseases. Thus, clinicians are not able to make specific recommendations to patients despite the strong interest and high prevalence of AAD.

To date, there is no global consensus on the use of the probiotics for AAD. The World Gastroenterology Organization (WGO) has supported their use of AAD in both adults and pediatrics. The use of *L. rhamnosus* GG and *Saccharomyces boulardii* was recommended by the Canadian Agency for Drugs and Technologies (CADTH) [69]. However, this recommendation is not shared by AGA or the IDSA (Infectious Disease Society of America) [49]. While there are certainly benefits to using probiotics in patients with AAD, the recommendations have not been able to clearly define the most appropriate patient or context.

5.2 Probiotics in *Clostridioides difficile* infections (CDI)

C. difficile is the most prevalent AAD for inpatients and outpatients leading to significant morbidity and mortality [70]. CDI is often associated with exposure to anaerobic coverage and antibiotics such as clindamycin, fluoroquinolones, or cephalosporins. Strategies to prevent *C. difficile* spread have typically involved patient segregation and hygiene measures. However, attempts to alter the host microbiota with fecal transplant or probiotics have become mainstream and shown themselves to be conclusive. In hospitalized patients receiving antibiotics, prophylactic administration of probiotics has been shown to significantly reduce the risk of developing *C. difficile*-associated diarrhea [71–75].

A proposed mechanism of this has been seen in *Saccharomyces boulardii,* which in murine models was shown to make a 54-kDa serine protease that cleaves toxin A and its intestinal receptor [50, 72, 76]. This has also been replicated in humans where toxin A and B cytotoxic effects in the human colon were attenuated when incubated in purified *S. boulardii* protease prior to being placed in the human colon [77]. When used in combination with metronidazole or vancomycin it reduced the number or relapses of diarrhea [78]. Efforts made for targeted primary prevention of CDI have typically focused on a multi-modal approach involving hygiene, antibiotics, and probiotics. A specific formulation of probiotics known as Bio-K+, which includes *L. acidophilus* CL1285, *L. casei* LBC80R, and *L. rhamnosus* CLR2, has been marketed in North America since 1996. Mouse models exposed to Bio-K+ have been found to increase concentrations of *lactobacilli* while decreasing levels of *staphylococci* [1]. The pathology in the human colon arises from toxins A and B of *C. difficile* that affects the colonic epithelium, which results in loss of cellular integrity and disruption of the colon mucosal cell cytoskeleton. Bio-K+ strains have been shown to produce supernatants (extracellular products) that inhibit toxin A/B in human enterocytes Caco-2 and HT-29 cells [1].

The American College of Gastroenterology (ACG), ESCMID (European Society of Clinical Microbiology and Infectious Diseases), and IDSA recommend probiotics for prevention or treatment of primary and recurrent *C. difficile* infections. However, the AGA is in favor of the use of *S. boulardii*, *L. acidophilus* CL1285, and *L. casei* for adults and children who are being treated with antibiotics except in situations of severe illness [79]. The difference among professional organizations comes from lack of clear evidence on the safety profiles and whether there is a true benefit [49]. Given the conclusive evidence on fecal microbiota transplants as a definitive treatment for recurrent CDI, there is no question of the significance that microbiota plays in the development of CDI and the potential manipulating it has in the prophylaxis and treatment of CDI. Furthermore, optimizing probiotic supplementation may have a meaningful role in CDI treatment.

5.3 Inflammatory bowel disease and probiotics

IBD pathophysiology involves a complex interplay between genetics, the host microbiome, environmental conditions, and the individual's immune response [80, 81]. Changes in the intestinal mucosa and microbiota may disrupt homeostasis between the human immune system and the flora [82]. These changes may then trigger a reaction of the human immune system playing a role in development of the IBD. Indeed, specific intestinal microbiota profiles have been associated with active disease [83]. CD and UC patients have been found to have less *Firmicutes* and *Bacteroidetes* and more *Proteobacteria* and *Actinobacteria* when compared to healthy controls [84]. In addition, CD patients have been found to have reduced levels of *Bacteroides*, *Eubacterium*, *Faecalibacterium*, and *Ruminococcus* possibly leading to increased gut permeability [84]. A technology to help distinguish commensal from quiescent pathologic bacteria has been developed known as IgA-SEQ, which combines cell sorting with 16srRNA gene sequencing to quantify the amount of IgA on various taxa of bacteria found in the gastrointestinal tract. By measuring the amount of IgA coating, immunostimulatory and immunoregulatory taxa of the microbiota can be measured more accurately. This can then be used to confer susceptibility to IBD. While IgA itself does not contribute to the inflammatory response in IBD, this technology revealed three potential bacteria, which were associated with disease progression in IBD and three protective taxa. Taxa with relatively low abundance (based on 16S rRNA) were *Erysipelotrichaceae* sp. and *Faecalibacterium prausnitzii*, as well as low IgA coating of *Oscillospira* was associated with less progression to surgery [85]. These studies identify disease-modifying taxa and biomarkers for disease severity and progression. By identifying bacteria taxa as so-called "bad actors" in the human microbiome there may be a framework for the development of more refined biomarkers impacting disease courses and the possibility of microbiome-based therapeutics.

There has also been an association between CD and the colonization of adherent-invasive *Escherichia coli* (AIEC). AIEC is thought to impair mitochondrial function in epithelial cells of the gastrointestinal mucosa by invading the Peyer's patches and the lamina propria *via* M cells [86]. It is thought that AIEC incorporates into macrophages and possibly increases the proinflammatory cytokine TNF-α. Patients with highly expressed CEACAM6 and CHI3L1 receptors, which are often expressed during times of inflammation, have been shown to promote the adhesion of AIEC and consequently bacteria invasion at the ileum [87]. Monocyte-derived macrophages (MDM) taken from patients with CD are unable to restrict AIEC as compared to healthy controls MDM *in vitro* models leading to pathologic immune response [88]. The overall prevalence of AIEC in healthy individuals is about 0–16% in the colon and 6–19% in ileal samples compared to 21–63% in CD patients suggesting that AIEC may be an additive factor in the pathogenesis of CD [51, 89, 90].

The increasing interest in the immune response to the gut microbiome in IBD has been met with interest in probiotic supplementation in this condition for induction and maintenance of remission. Specifically, it is thought that probiotics might be able to impact IBD pathophysiology by improving epithelium integrity, downregulating inflammatory bacterial byproducts, and reducing mucin production [91, 92]. Certain probiotic strains such as *lactobacilli* and *bifidobacteria* produce bacteriocins that act as antimicrobial peptides [54, 93]. *Lactobacillus paracasei* L74 CBA often found in fermented milk products like Kefir has been shown to inhibit pro-inflammatory cytokines such as NF-Kb potentially providing anti-inflammatory properties to the host. In addition, Duary et al. found that TNF-α was reduced by *Lactiplantibacillus plantarum* Lp91. While these findings have not been shown in human-based clinic trials, they provide a potential mechanism by which probiotics may have some clinical value in IBD [94].

The most used formation of probiotics in IBD patients is known as Visbiome®/ VSL #3® (Italian form), which was developed by Sigma-Tau Healthscience/ Alfasigma. The original formulation was changed in 2016 and there is now a U.S. version known as Visbiome® and an Italian version known as (VSL3®). In CD, the data has remained mixed on the efficacy of probiotics to induce or retain remission as an adjuvant or stand-alone therapy. The mechanism of action possibly includes improving tight junction protein function, positive composition of the intestinal microbiota, and regulating immune-related cytokine expression. In regard to CD, there was one randomized control (RCT) that evaluated the ability of VSL#3 to prevent human recurrence after surgery. This study looked at early and the late administration of VSL#3 and found that early VSL#3 administration was associated with later recurrence after surgery. While there have been no statistical differences in endoscopic recurrence rates at day 90 between patients who received VSL#3 and patients who received placebo. Levels of inflammatory cytokines and recurrence rates leading to repeat surgery were lower among patients who received early VSL#3 (for the entire 365 days). This indicated that this probiotic should be further investigated for prevention of Crohn's disease recurrence [94, 95].

While it is understood that there may be a potential for probiotics in UC, there is still no convincing data to constitute a recommendation. In a small cohort of pediatric patients with UC, *Lactobacillus reuteri* was shown to improve clinical and endoscopic disease activity [96, 97]. This has not been replicated in adults. However, in patients with UC who have undergone total proctocolectomy and ileal pouch-anal anastomosis for UC, a definitive connection to gut microbiota has been made. There has been a potential benefit in VSL#3 containing *Lactobacillus*, *Bifidobacterium*, and *Streptococcus* for prevention of the initial episode of acute pouchitis. To date, there have been four clinical trials showing VSL#3 could prevent or maintain remission in patients with chronic pouchitis [98–101]. A potential mechanism suggested is the improvement of the intestinal barrier function (IBF). While VSL#3 has shown efficacy in chronic pouchitis, an open-label trial showed that most patients on chronic antibiotics for pouchitis were not able to use VSL#3 for long-term therapy largely due to disease recurrence [102]. This formulation has been demonstrated in preventing future episodes and improving inflammation [96]. However, according to the AGA, this only constitutes a weak recommendation due to the small size of the patient population in which these studies were done.

The next generation of probiotics in IBD may involve the use of genetically engineered bacteria that could release therapeutically operative molecules in the intestine. This will involve organisms that could sense and respond to intestinal inflammatory cytokines or topically produce molecules to treat the inflammation. Harnessing the power of the biotherapeutics with synthetic biology could provide a future of personalized medicine in the diverse IBD patient population [103].

5.4 Necrotizing enterocolitis

Preterm birth impacts about 10% of newborns born in the US and 15 million pregnancies worldwide. A preterm infant's gut is exposed to colonization of commensal and pathological bacteria. During this time, their innate immune system is sorting through a constant excess of peptidoglycans and liposaccharides [104]. In this delicate time, NEC inflammation can be driven by Toll-like receptor 4. By influencing the innate and adaptive immune systems, probiotics are thought to aid in the balance of these two systems and prevent the pathogenesis of NEC [104, 105]. NEC is associated with bowel necrosis leading to short bowel syndrome and impaired development, and can be fatal in up to 30% of patients [55]. There have been case-control studies identifying an overpopulation or so-called "bloom" of Gammaproteobacteria tending to precede NEC in many preterm infants [56, 106]. In contrast, commensal bacteria such as bifidobacterial are found to be protective of NEC and plentiful in breastfed infants likely due to the breast milk-specific oligosaccharides that this preferentially consumes [107].

A Cochrane review article found probiotics were superior to placebo in reducing the risk of severe necrotizing enterocolitis (RR = 0.43; 95% CI, 0.33–0.56; 20 studies with 5529 infants) and mortality (RR = 0.65; 95% CI, 0.52–0.81; 17 studies with 5112 infants) [108]. Combinations of certain probiotics containing *Bifidobacterium infantis* and *L. acidophilus* have shown strong association with preventing NEC and reducing need for abdominal surgery and all-cause mortality [109, 110].

There are numerous hypotheses on the mechanism of how they might protect against NEC in infants. One such proposition involves the production of butyrate and other short-chain fatty acids that could supply nutrition to the colonocytes thereby lowering the pH and decreasing the oxygen tension within the intestinal lumen. This ultimately is thought to suppress the growth of *Enterobacteriaceae* (phylum *Proteobacteria*), which is well known to be pathologic in NEC [111, 112]. Other proposed mechanisms include supporting the maturation and functions of the infants' bowels by regulating the Th1:Th2 balance [57, 113]. Specifically, it is known that an imbalance of Th2 levels greater than Th1 levels can predispose to autoimmune disease and gut inflammation by lack of regulation of the gut immune response [57]. According to the AGA, in babies less than 37 weeks of gestational age and low-birth-weight infants, it is recommended to use a combination of probiotics containing *Lactobacillus* spp. and *Bifidobacterium* spp. over no probiotics to prevent the development of NEC in this population. This constitutes a conditional recommendation with a moderate to high level of evidence in this population.

5.5 Irritable bowel syndrome

Irritable bowel syndrome (IBS) is classified as a functional gastrointestinal disease [114]. Prevalence rates worldwide are around 11% with impact on younger patients. For this reason, there is a significant economic and sociologic burden associated with this disease. This has amounted to around $20 billion per year in direct and indirect costs to the U.S. Economy [115]. The pathophysiology of IBS involves changes in the gut microbiota, malabsorption of bile acid, and changes to the enteric nervous system. Prior metanalyses have found that probiotics demonstrate improved overall symptom response and pain [116, 117].

One particular strain, *Bifidobacterium bifidum* MIMBb75, was found in a randomized control study by Guglielmetti et al. to cause a significant reduction in global assessment of IBS by −0.88 points (95% CI: −1.07; −0.69) when compared with only −0.16 (95% CI: −0.32; 0.00) points in the placebo group ($P < 0.0001$) with excellent tolerability and no difference in adverse events [118]. Andresen et al. replicated this result using a heat-inactivated *Bifidobacterium bifidum* MIMBb75 (SYN-HI-001) in a high-powered study finding that the beneficial bacterial effects of this strain on IBS were independent of bacteria viability [119].

The metabolites of microbiota often include bile acid (BA), which has been attributed to IBS symptoms. BAs are released in the duodenum after conjugation in the liver, which are then made into secondary BAs by gut bacteria. BAs can have prosecretory effects that can regulate gut motility and impact gut sensitivity [120]. BAs are impacted by bacteria in the gut and impact the gut themselves, thus it is thought they may impact IBS. Patients with IBS have been reported to have changes in their microbial profiles. For example, there has been a significant increase in fecal primary BA and a decrease in secondary BA in patients with IBS-predominant diarrhea. There has also been a direct positive correlation between primary BA and IBS symptoms. In IBS with predominant diarrhea, there has been an observed reduction in bacteria from genera *Ruminococcaceae* and a negative correlation with primary BAs. There seems to be a definite connection between BAs and IBS, which will need to be further investigated [120].

Overall, the quality of the evidence behind the use in IBS remains weak. Indeed, the ACG states that there is very low evidence for the use of probiotics in IBS, which has resulted in a weak recommendation for their use in IBS. The AGA shares this sentiment and makes no recommendation for the use of probiotics in IBS [121]. This weak recommendation is justified given significant heterogeneity between studies, publication bias, and small sample size studies. This being said, the ACG does acknowledge that when probiotics are studied as a group, they improve bloating and the flatulence in IBS patients [121]. While there has been no broad recommendation for the use of probiotics in IBS. There is evidence that they make a difference and are of continued interest among patients and providers.

5.6 Probiotics in the critically ill

There is growing evidence that probiotics may reduce the rate of the ventilator-associated pneumonia (VAP), overall infection rate, nosocomial pneumonia, duration of mechanical ventilation, and antibiotic use for critically ill patients. VAP is considered the second most common nosocomial infection in the U.S. imposing a significant economic burden. While the American Thoracic Society (ATS) makes recommendations on the prophylaxis of the VAP in patients in the ICU typically involving antibiotics, the prospect of probiotics is compelling [122, 123]. Probiotics have also been used in patients with pancreatitis in the ICU. A meta-analysis analyzing 13 studies with N = 1188 found a statistically significant decrease in the length of ICU stay when probiotics were administered [124]. While no study has been able to find any effect on probiotics and length of hospital stay or mortality, there is convincing evidence that the flora may impact the outcomes of the critically ill patients. Like most areas of probiotics research, more detailed research needs to be done on how specific strains impact specific problems experienced by the patient.

6. Safety of probiotics

Probiotics are often perceived as "natural" and safe alternatives to pharmaceuticals. They are routinely marketed as something which restores or aligns the patient back into a state of health rather than treating a specific disease state. In general, probiotics are considered safe provided the user has a competent immune system.

A review by the Agency for Healthcare Research and Quality (AHRQ) looked at 387 studies of which there were 24,615 users and there was no statistically significant increase in the number of adverse events in the probiotic group compared to the control group [125].

Although there have been great strides to incorporate probiotic therapy into modern medicine, researchers have presented concerns about the potential negative effects of probiotic supplementation. Numerous virulent pathways can be expressed and carried out by probiotics that can put the human host at risk as there is a possibility of resistance transfer from the probiotic to pathogenic bacteria. Horizontal gene transfer (HGT) is the movement of genetic code between organisms mediated by transformation, transduction, conjugal transfer, or with specialized gene transfer vehicles such as viruses or other bacteria [126]. Recent literature has suggested the human gut rich in HGT activity and the transfer of genetic code from successfully adapted organisms to recipients provides useful properties resulting in increased fitness and competitiveness in the microbial ecosystem. Examples of HGT among probiotic strains have been documented for *Lactobacillus rhamnosus*, *Lactobacillus gasseri*, *Lactobacillus paracasei, Lactobacillus reuteri*, and *Lactobacillus plantarum*. Some literature suggests there has been a gene flux from Gram-positive cocci for genes encoding for streptogramin resistance [127]. Tetracycline resistance gene transfer has been reported from *L. reuteri* to other bacteria native to the human gut microbiota [128].

The use of probiotics in the processed food industry has increased over the years as some byproducts of these organisms are used as additives. One of the most popular microbial-derived additives is transglutaminase. Interestingly, this catalytic enzyme has been implicated in intestinal tight junction permeability and the increasing incidence of autoimmune diseases [129]. This molecule can be detrimental when crosslinked with gliadin as this complex mimics tissue transglutaminase and is immunogenic in patients with celiac disease [130]. In addition to the potential for immunogenicity, numerous case reports have described systemic infections caused by probiotic strains. Fungemia caused by *Saccharomyces cerevisiae* and *Saccharomyces boulardii* is by the far the most reported single event associated with the consumption of *S. boulardii* [131]. Other complications reported include overt sepsis and endocarditis associated with *S. bouldarii*, *Lactobacillus* GG, *Bacillus subtilis*, *Bifidobacterium* breve, *Lactobacillus*, and *Streptococcus* species [132–137].

The PROPATRIA trial highlighted a concern surrounding probiotic safety in critically ill patients. Researchers explored the ability of multi-strain probiotics to help prevent infectious complications in patients with severe acute pancreatitis. Patients in the experimental arm that received the probiotic were shown to have a much higher mortality rate. The authors of the study suggested that the increase in mortality was associated with bowel ischemia caused by either increased mucosal oxygen demand by the exogenous bacterial metabolic demand in the setting of decreased blood flow or an inflammatory cascade triggered by the probiotic in the setting of decreased capillary blood flow [138]. Other metabolic derangements such as D-lactic acidemia and acidosis in humans have been associated with *Lactobacillus* and *Bifidobacterium* species. Interestingly, these species of bacteria are among the most used in probiotic formulations. D-lactic acidosis has been associated with abdominal bloating, chronic fatigue syndrome, and neurocognitive symptoms such as brain fogginess [139–142]. These findings have also been implicated in the literature surrounding small bowel intestinal overgrowth (SIBO). The resolution of symptoms after antibiotic therapy, in this population, reinforces the proposed causative association [143]. In general, the current medical literature cautions against the use of probiotic supplementation in patients with immunocompromised states such as those undergoing chemotherapy or immunosuppressive therapy, HIV/AIDS, post-organ transplant, pregnancy, neutropenia, antibiotic-induced diarrhea, and inflammatory bowel disease [144–146].

To date, there is no data on long-term safety of probiotic usage. This makes meaningful safety recommendations on such a diverse array of bacterial strains and dosages within probiotic formulations a nearly impossible task. For this reason, probiotics tend to fall under the unregulated form of other supplements.

7. Future research and directions

As mentioned earlier, probiotics are living nonpathogenic bacteria or yeast that can potentially be beneficial by restoring the microbial balance in the gut; however, only some probiotic products are backed by evidence-based trials [147–150]. Probiotics have been extensively utilized in numerous disease states, including gastrointestinal diseases, metabolic syndrome, cardiovascular disease, periodontal disease, and osteoporosis [49]. The hallmark of maintaining a healthy intestinal ecosystem is the integrity of the interstitial barrier [151], and probiotics employ their beneficial effects by modulating immunologic response, strengthening gut barrier function and competing with pathogenic bacteria [152]. Numerous *in vitro* and animal studies have implied the significance of improving the mucosal barrier function by probiotic treatment [153]; however, extrapolating these studies to humans is challenging. For example, some probiotic species, such as *Akkermansia muciniphila*, VSL#3 encompassing *Lactobacillus* and *Bifidobacteria* strains, and *L. plantarum* Dad-13, have proven benefits of protecting against obesity, dyslipidemia, insulin resistance, and fat mass development in mice [46, 48, 52, 154]; however, this has not been significantly reproduced in human studies. While multiple clinical trials have attempted to evaluate the prophylactic and therapeutic effect of probiotics in different disease states, the quality of evidence to support clinical use of probiotics is poor. In addition, it is unclear which species and their respective optimal quantity and duration are beneficial for specific disease states. Hence, there is no consensus recommendation for its use. More research is warranted exploring the overall safety of probiotic supplementation. In addition, given the laxity in oversight by the Food and Drug Administration (FDA), allergic reactions and anaphylaxis should be a focus of safety as some probiotic blends can include allergens such as cow milk and chicken egg protein [146]. Systematic reviews published within the last 5 years have highlighted concern about the broad generalization of conclusions, lack of structural classification, variations in bacterial strains and dosages, and incomplete reporting of probiotic supplementation regimens and subject population identification [53, 144, 155]. Moving forward, more randomized controlled trials with larger sample sizes would help strengthen current data surrounding the utility of probiotics and aid in identifying any serious deleterious effects on patients' health.

8. Conclusion

Over the last 20 years, there has been significant basic science, translational, and clinical research into the use of probiotics in the treatment of disease. There is a widespread belief among patients that probiotics preserve a healthy state and even have curative properties. It is widely believed that the beneficial aspects of probiotics involve antagonism against pathogenic molecules, infections, and augmentation of the gut microbiota, thereby maintaining the host's immune homeostasis. Clinical applications of probiotics are diverse, branching well beyond the gastrointestinal system. While often used as a panacea of sorts by the public, there remains limited evidence of specific species and dosage of efficacy for specific diseases. There is a growing body of research supporting the clinical use of probiotics for applications well beyond gastrointestinal ailments. More research and collaboration among basic science researchers and clinicians to specifically define appropriate usage of probiotics based on the disease targets, dosage, and specific strain deployed.

Conflict of interest

The authors declare no conflict of interest.

Author details

John Ryan[1,2], Shruthi Narasimha[1,2], Robert Pattison[1,2], Rasiq Zackria[1,2], Youssef Ghobrial[1,2], Syed Abdul Basit[1,2], Tarek Ammar[1,2], Vijay Jayaraman[1,2], Christian Stone[1,2] and David Shih[1,2]*

1 Sunrise Health GME Gastroenterology Fellowship, Las Vegas, Nevada

2 Comprehensive Digestive Institute of Nevada, Las Vegas, Nevada

*Address all correspondence to: dshih@nevadagastro.com

References

[1] McFarland LV. From yaks to yogurt: The history, development, and current use of probiotics. Clinical Infectious Diseases. 2015;**60**(Suppl. 2):S85-S90

[2] Gasbarrini G, Bonvicini F, Gramenzi A. Probiotics history. Journal of Clinical Gastroenterology. 2016;**50**(Suppl 2, Proceedings from the 8th Probiotics, Prebiotics & New Foods for Microbiota and Human Health meeting held in Rome, Italy on September 13-15, 2015):S116-S1S9

[3] Hill C, Guarner F, Reid G, Gibson GR, Merenstein DJ, Pot B, et al. Expert consensus document. The international scientific Association for Probiotics and Prebiotics consensus statement on the scope and appropriate use of the term probiotic. Nature Reviews. Gastroenterology & Hepatology. 2014;**11**(8):506-514

[4] Dharmani P, Srivastava V, Kissoon-Singh V, Chadee K. Role of intestinal mucins in innate host defense mechanisms against pathogens. Journal of Innate Immunity. 2009;**1**(2):123-135

[5] Caballero-Franco C, Keller K, De Simone C, Chadee K. The VSL#3 probiotic formula induces mucin gene expression and secretion in colonic epithelial cells. American Journal of Physiology. Gastrointestinal and Liver Physiology. 2007;**292**(1):G315-G322

[6] Kulkarni N, Reddy BS. Inhibitory effect of Bifidobacterium longum cultures on the azoxymethane-induced aberrant crypt foci formation and fecal bacterial beta-glucuronidase. Proceedings of the Society for Experimental Biology and Medicine. 1994;**207**(3):278-283

[7] Karczewski J, Troost FJ, Konings I, Dekker J, Kleerebezem M, Brummer RJ, et al. Regulation of human epithelial tight junction proteins by lactobacillus plantarum in vivo and protective effects on the epithelial barrier. American Journal of Physiology. Gastrointestinal and Liver Physiology. 2010;**298**(6):G851-G859

[8] Zhang W, Zhu YH, Yang JC, Yang GY, Zhou D, Wang JF. A selected lactobacillus rhamnosus strain promotes EGFR-independent Akt activation in an Enterotoxigenic Escherichia coli K88-infected IPEC-J2 cell model. PLoS One. 2015;**10**(4):e0125717

[9] Plaza-Diaz J, Ruiz-Ojeda FJ, Gil-Campos M, Gil A. Mechanisms of action of probiotics. Advances in Nutrition. 2019;**10**(suppl_1):S49-S66

[10] Corthésy B. Multi-faceted functions of secretory IgA at mucosal surfaces. Frontiers in Immunology. 2013;**4**:185

[11] Chaplin DD. Overview of the immune response. The Journal of Allergy and Clinical Immunology. 2010;**125** (2 Suppl. 2):S3-S23

[12] Sierra S, Lara-Villoslada F, Sempere L, Olivares M, Boza J, Xaus J. Intestinal and immunological effects of daily oral administration of lactobacillus salivarius CECT5713 to healthy adults. Anaerobe. 2010;**16**(3):195-200

[13] Zhou H, Coveney AP, Wu M, Huang J, Blankson S, Zhao H, et al. Activation of both TLR and NOD signaling confers host innate immunity-mediated protection against microbial infection. Frontiers in Immunology. 2018;**9**:3082

[14] Asgari F, Falak R, Teimourian S, Pourakbari B, Ebrahimnezhad S, Shekarabi M. Effects of oral probiotic feeding on toll-like receptor gene expression of the chicken's cecal tonsil. Reports of Biochemistry and Molecular Biology. 2018;**6**(2):151-157

[15] Jin B, Sun T, Yu XH, Yang YX, Yeo AE. The effects of TLR activation on T-cell development and differentiation. Clinical & Developmental Immunology. 2012;**2012**:836485

[16] Azad MAK, Sarker M, Wan D. Immunomodulatory effects of probiotics on cytokine profiles. BioMed Research International. 2018;**2018**:8063647

[17] Molero-Abraham M, Glutting JP, Flower DR, Lafuente EM, Reche PA. EPIPOX: Immunoinformatic characterization of the shared T-cell epitome between Variola virus and related pathogenic orthopoxviruses. Journal of Immunology Research. 2015;**2015**:738020

[18] Zhu X, Zhu J. CD4 T helper cell subsets and related human immunological disorders. International Journal of Molecular Sciences. 2020;**21**(21):8011

[19] Chassaing B, Kumar M, Baker MT, Singh V, Vijay-Kumar M. Mammalian gut immunity. Biomedical Journal. 2014;**37**(5):246-258

[20] Jung C, Hugot JP, Barreau F. Peyer's patches: The immune sensors of the intestine. International Journal of Inflammation. 2010;**2010**:823710

[21] Lycke NY, Bemark M. The role of Peyer's patches in synchronizing gut IgA responses. Frontiers in Immunology. 2012;**3**:329

[22] Bakema JE, van Egmond M. The human immunoglobulin a fc receptor FcαRI: A multifaceted regulator of mucosal immunity. Mucosal Immunology. 2011;**4**(6):612-624

[23] Galdeano CM, Perdigón G. Role of viability of probiotic strains in their persistence in the gut and in mucosal immune stimulation. Journal of Applied Microbiology. 2004;**97**(4):673-681

[24] Delcenserie V, Martel D, Lamoureux M, Amiot J, Boutin Y, Roy D. Immunomodulatory effects of probiotics in the intestinal tract. Current Issues in Molecular Biology. 2008;**10**(1-2):37-54

[25] Takahashi T, Nakagawa E, Nara T, Yajima T, Kuwata T. Effects of orally ingested *Bifidobacterium longum* on the mucosal IgA response of mice to dietary antigens. Bioscience, Biotechnology, and Biochemistry. 1998;**62**(1):10-15

[26] Lai HH, Chiu CH, Kong MS, Chang CJ, Chen CC. Probiotic. Nutrients. 2019;**11**:5

[27] Pozo-Rubio T, Olivares M, Nova E, De Palma G, Mujico JR, Ferrer MD, et al. Immune development and intestinal microbiota in celiac disease. Clinical & Developmental Immunology. 2012;**2012**:654143

[28] Sánchez E, Donat E, Ribes-Koninckx C, Fernández-Murga ML, Sanz Y. Duodenal-mucosal bacteria associated with celiac disease in children. Applied and Environmental Microbiology. 2013;**79**(18):5472-5479

[29] Collado MC, Donat E, Ribes-Koninckx C, Calabuig M, Sanz Y. Specific duodenal and faecal bacterial groups associated with paediatric coeliac disease. Journal of Clinical Pathology. 2009;**62**(3):264-269

[30] Laparra JM, Sanz Y. Bifidobacteria inhibit the inflammatory response induced by gliadins in intestinal epithelial cells via modifications of toxic peptide generation during digestion. Journal of Cellular Biochemistry. 2010;**109**(4):801-807

[31] Borruel N, Carol M, Casellas F, Antolín M, de Lara F, Espín E, et al. Increased mucosal tumour necrosis factor alpha production in Crohn's disease can be downregulated ex vivo by probiotic bacteria. Gut. 2002;**51**(5):659-664

[32] Livingston M, Loach D, Wilson M, Tannock GW, Baird M. Gut commensal Lactobacillus reuteri 100-23 stimulates an immunoregulatory response. Immunology and Cell Biology. 2010;**88**(1):99-102

[33] Reséndiz-Albor AA, Reina-Garfias H, Rojas-Hernández S, Jarillo-Luna A, Rivera-Aguilar V, Miliar-García A, et al. Regionalization of pIgR expression in the mucosa of mouse small intestine. Immunology Letters. 2010;**128**(1):59-67

[34] Spinler JK, Taweechotipatr M, Rognerud CL, Ou CN, Tumwasorn S, Versalovic J. Human-derived probiotic lactobacillus reuteri demonstrate antimicrobial activities targeting diverse enteric bacterial pathogens. Anaerobe. 2008;**14**(3):166-171

[35] O'Shea EF, Cotter PD, Stanton C, Ross RP, Hill C. Production of bioactive substances by intestinal bacteria as a basis for explaining probiotic mechanisms: Bacteriocins and conjugated linoleic acid. International Journal of Food Microbiology. 2012;**152**(3):189-205

[36] Collado MC, Meriluoto J, Salminen S. Role of commercial probiotic strains against human pathogen adhesion to intestinal mucus. Letters in Applied Microbiology. 2007;**45**(4):454-460

[37] Belenguer A, Duncan SH, Calder AG, Holtrop G, Louis P, Lobley GE, et al. Two routes of metabolic cross-feeding between Bifidobacterium adolescentis and butyrate-producing anaerobes from the human gut. Applied and Environmental Microbiology. 2006;**72**(5):3593-3599

[38] Turroni F, Özcan E, Milani C, Mancabelli L, Viappiani A, van Sinderen D, et al. Glycan cross-feeding activities between bifidobacteria under in vitro conditions. Frontiers in Microbiology. 2015;**6**:1030

[39] McNulty NP, Yatsunenko T, Hsiao A, Faith JJ, Muegge BD, Goodman AL, et al. The impact of a consortium of fermented milk strains on the gut microbiome of gnotobiotic mice and monozygotic twins. Science Translational Medicine. 2011;**3**(106):106ra

[40] Cox MJ, Huang YJ, Fujimura KE, Liu JT, McKean M, Boushey HA, et al. Lactobacillus casei abundance is associated with profound shifts in the infant gut microbiome. PLoS One. 2010;**5**(1):e8745

[41] Preidis GA, Saulnier DM, Blutt SE, Mistretta TA, Riehle KP, Major AM, et al. Probiotics stimulate enterocyte migration and microbial diversity in the neonatal mouse intestine. The FASEB Journal. 2012;**26**(5):1960-1969

[42] Eisenhauer N, Scheu S, Jousset A. Bacterial diversity stabilizes community productivity. PLoS One. 2012;**7**(3):e34517

[43] Manichanh C, Rigottier-Gois L, Bonnaud E, Gloux K, Pelletier E, Frangeul L, et al. Reduced diversity of faecal microbiota in Crohn's disease

revealed by a metagenomic approach. Gut. 2006;**55**(2):205-211

[44] Forno E, Onderdonk AB, McCracken J, Litonjua AA, Laskey D, Delaney ML, et al. Diversity of the gut microbiota and eczema in early life. Clinical and Molecular Allergy. 2008;**6**:11

[45] Pawar R, Dhawal P, Nabar B, Barve S, Zambare V. Mechanism and applications of probiotics in healthcare industry. In: Barh D, editor. Biotechnology in Healthcare: Applications and Initiative. Vol. 2. London, UK: Elsevier; 2022. pp. 225-245. DOI: 10.1016/B978-0-323-90042-3.00002-5. ISBN: 978-0-323-90042-3

[46] Rajkumar H, Mahmood N, Kumar M, Varikuti SR, Challa HR, Myakala SP. Effect of probiotic (VSL#3) and omega-3 on lipid profile, insulin sensitivity, inflammatory markers, and gut colonization in overweight adults: A randomized, controlled trial. Mediators of Inflammation. 2014;**2014**:348959

[47] McFarland LV, Surawicz CM, Stamm WE. Risk factors for *Clostridium difficile* carriage and *C. difficile*-associated diarrhea in a cohort of hospitalized patients. The Journal of Infectious Diseases. 1990;**162**(3):678-684

[48] Rahayu ES, Mariyatun M, Putri Manurung NE, Hasan PN, Therdtatha P, Mishima R, et al. Effect of probiotic. World Journal of Gastroenterology. 2021;**27**(1):107-128

[49] Stavropoulou E, Bezirtzoglou E. Probiotics in medicine: A long debate. Frontiers in Immunology. 2020;**11**:2192

[50] Rodriguez H, Miller JE. Do prophylactic probiotics prevent the incidence of *Clostridium difficile* colitis infection in hospitalized patients? The Journal of the Oklahoma State Medical Association. 2019;**112**(1):18-19

[51] Negroni A, Costanzo M, Vitali R, Superti F, Bertuccini L, Tinari A, et al. Characterization of adherent-invasive *Escherichia coli* isolated from pediatric patients with inflammatory bowel disease. Inflammatory Bowel Diseases. 2012;**18**(5):913-924

[52] Martín-Muñoz MF, Fortuni M, Caminoa M, Belver T, Quirce S, Caballero T. Anaphylactic reaction to probiotics. Cow's milk and hen's egg allergens in probiotic compounds. Pediatric Allergy and Immunology. 2012;**23**(8):778-784

[53] van den Nieuwboer M, Brummer RJ, Guarner F, Morelli L, Cabana M, Claassen E. Safety of probiotics and synbiotics in children under 18 years of age. Benef Microbes. 2015;**6**(5):615-630

[54] de Souza M, Barbalho S, Goulart R, de Carvalho A. The current and future role of drugs and probiotics in the management of inflammatory bowel disease. Journal of Biosciences and Medicines. 2015;**3**(8):76-85

[55] Warner BB, Deych E, Zhou Y, Hall-Moore C, Weinstock GM, Sodergren E, et al. Gut bacteria dysbiosis and necrotising enterocolitis in very low birthweight infants: A prospective case-control study. Lancet. 2016;**387**(10031):1928-1936

[56] Pammi M, Cope J, Tarr PI, Warner BB, Morrow AL, Mai V, et al. Intestinal dysbiosis in preterm infants preceding necrotizing enterocolitis: A systematic review and meta-analysis. Microbiome. 2017;**5**(1):31

[57] Walker WA. Mechanisms of action of probiotics. Clinical Infectious Diseases.

2008;**46**(Suppl. 2):S87-S91; discussion S144-51

[58] McFarland LV. Diarrhoea associated with antibiotic use. BMJ. 2007;**335**(7610):54-55

[59] Kopacz K, Phadtare S. Probiotics for the prevention of antibiotic-associated diarrhea. Healthcare (Basel). 2022;**10**(8):1450

[60] Lherm T, Monet C, Nougière B, Soulier M, Larbi D, Le Gall C, et al. Seven cases of fungemia with *Saccharomyces boulardii* in critically ill patients. Intensive Care Medicine. 2002;**28**(6):797-801

[61] Knezević M, Cvetinović M, Jović N, Stosić S. Benign symmetric lipomatosis of the neck. Vojnosanitetski Pregled. 1992;**49**(6):588-590

[62] Chu W, Lu F, Zhu W, Kang C. Isolation and characterization of new potential probiotic bacteria based on quorum-sensing system. Journal of Applied Microbiology. 2011;**110**(1):202-208

[63] Cotter PD, Hill C, Ross RP. Bacteriocins: Developing innate immunity for food. Nature Reviews. Microbiology. 2005;**3**(10):777-788

[64] Servin AL. Antagonistic activities of lactobacilli and bifidobacteria against microbial pathogens. FEMS Microbiology Reviews. 2004;**28**(4):405-440

[65] Ashraf R, Shah NP. Immune system stimulation by probiotic microorganisms. Critical Reviews in Food Science and Nutrition. 2014;**54**(7):938-956

[66] Kato K, Mizuno S, Umesaki Y, Ishii Y, Sugitani M, Imaoka A, et al. Randomized placebo-controlled trial assessing the effect of bifidobacteria-fermented milk on active ulcerative colitis. Alimentary Pharmacology & Therapeutics. 2004;**20**(10):1133-1141

[67] Goldenberg JZ, Lytvyn L, Steurich J, Parkin P, Mahant S, Johnston BC. Probiotics for the prevention of pediatric antibiotic-associated diarrhea. Cochrane Database of Systematic Reviews. 2015;(12):CD004827

[68] Blaabjerg S, Artzi DM, Aabenhus R. Probiotics for the prevention of antibiotic-associated diarrhea in outpatients-a systematic review and meta-analysis. Antibiotics (Basel). 2017;**6**(4):21

[69] Szajewska H, Canani RB, Guarino A, Hojsak I, Indrio F, Kolacek S, et al. Probiotics for the prevention of antibiotic-associated diarrhea in children. Journal of Pediatric Gastroenterology and Nutrition. 2016;**62**(3):495-506

[70] Sun X, Hirota SA. The roles of host and pathogen factors and the innate immune response in the pathogenesis of *Clostridium difficile* infection. Molecular Immunology. 2015;**63**(2):193-202

[71] Barbut F, Petit JC. Epidemiology of *Clostridium difficile*-associated infections. Clinical Microbiology and Infection. 2001;**7**(8):405-410

[72] Carroll KC, Bartlett JG. Biology of *Clostridium difficile*: Implications for epidemiology and diagnosis. Annual Review of Microbiology. 2011;**65**:501-521

[73] Mayfield JL, Leet T, Miller J, Mundy LM. Environmental control to reduce transmission of *Clostridium difficile*. Clinical Infectious Diseases. 2000;**31**(4):995-1000

[74] Pakyz AL, Jawahar R, Wang Q, Harpe SE. Medication risk factors

associated with healthcare-associated *Clostridium difficile* infection: A multilevel model case-control study among 64 US academic medical centres. The Journal of Antimicrobial Chemotherapy. 2014;**69**(4):1127-1131

[75] Brown KA, Khanafer N, Daneman N, Fisman DN. Meta-analysis of antibiotics and the risk of community-associated *Clostridium difficile* infection. Antimicrobial Agents and Chemotherapy. 2013;**57**(5):2326-2332

[76] Castagliuolo I, LaMont JT, Nikulasson ST, Pothoulakis C. Saccharomyces boulardii protease inhibits *Clostridium difficile* toxin a effects in the rat ileum. Infection and Immunity. 1996;**64**(12):5225-5232

[77] Castagliuolo I, Riegler MF, Valenick L, LaMont JT, Pothoulakis C. Saccharomyces boulardii protease inhibits the effects of *Clostridium difficile* toxins a and B in human colonic mucosa. Infection and Immunity. 1999;**67**(1):302-307

[78] Su GL, Ko CW, Bercik P, Falck-Ytter Y, Sultan S, Weizman AV, et al. AGA clinical practice guidelines on the role of probiotics in the management of gastrointestinal disorders. Gastroenterology. 2020;**159**(2):697-705

[79] Martini E, Krug SM, Siegmund B, Neurath MF, Becker C. Mend your fences: The epithelial barrier and its relationship with mucosal immunity in inflammatory bowel disease. Cellular and Molecular Gastroenterology and Hepatology. 2017;**4**(1):33-46

[80] Takiishi T, Fenero CIM, Câmara NOS. Intestinal barrier and gut microbiota: Shaping our immune responses throughout life. Tissue Barriers. 2017;**5**(4):e1373208

[81] Shih DQ, Targan SR. Insights into IBD pathogenesis. Current Gastroenterology Reports. 2009;**11**(6):473-480

[82] Frank DN, Robertson CE, Hamm CM, Kpadeh Z, Zhang T, Chen H, et al. Disease phenotype and genotype are associated with shifts in intestinal-associated microbiota in inflammatory bowel diseases. Inflammatory Bowel Diseases. 2011;**17**(1):179-184

[83] Khan I, Ullah N, Zha L, Bai Y, Khan A, Zhao T, et al. Alteration of gut microbiota in inflammatory bowel disease (IBD): Cause or consequence? IBD treatment targeting the gut microbiome. Pathogens. 2019;**8**(3):126

[84] Zuo W, Wang B, Bai X, Luan Y, Fan Y, Michail S, et al. 16S rRNA and metagenomic shotgun sequencing data revealed consistent patterns of gut microbiome signature in pediatric ulcerative colitis. Scientific Reports. 2022;**12**(1):6421

[85] Carvalho FA, Barnich N, Sivignon A, Darcha C, Chan CH, Stanners CP, et al. Crohn's disease adherent-invasive *Escherichia coli* colonize and induce strong gut inflammation in transgenic mice expressing human CEACAM. The Journal of Experimental Medicine. 2009;**206**(10):2179-2189

[86] Barnich N, Carvalho FA, Glasser AL, Darcha C, Jantscheff P, Allez M, et al. CEACAM6 acts as a receptor for adherent-invasive *E. coli*, supporting ileal mucosa colonization in Crohn disease. The Journal of Clinical Investigation. 2007;**117**(6):1566-1574

[87] Vazeille E, Buisson A, Bringer MA, Goutte M, Ouchchane L, Hugot JP, et al. Monocyte-derived macrophages from Crohn's disease patients are impaired in the ability to control intracellular

adherent-invasive *Escherichia coli* and exhibit disordered cytokine secretion profile. Journal of Crohn's & Colitis. 2015;**9**(5):410-420

[88] Darfeuille-Michaud A, Boudeau J, Bulois P, Neut C, Glasser AL, Barnich N, et al. High prevalence of adherent-invasive *Escherichia coli* associated with ileal mucosa in Crohn's disease. Gastroenterology. 2004;**127**(2):412-421

[89] Raso T, Crivellaro S, Chirillo MG, Pais P, Gaia E, Savoia D. Analysis of *Escherichia coli* isolated from patients affected by Crohn's disease. Current Microbiology. 2011;**63**(2):131-137

[90] Martinez-Medina M, Aldeguer X, Lopez-Siles M, González-Huix F, López-Oliu C, Dahbi G, et al. Molecular diversity of *Escherichia coli* in the human gut: New ecological evidence supporting the role of adherent-invasive E. coli (AIEC) in Crohn's disease. Inflammatory Bowel Diseases. 2009;**15**(6):872-882

[91] Matsuoka K, Kanai T. The gut microbiota and inflammatory bowel disease. Seminars in Immunopathology. 2015;**37**(1):47-55

[92] Dalile B, Van Oudenhove L, Vervliet B, Verbeke K. The role of short-chain fatty acids in microbiota-gut-brain communication. Nature Reviews. Gastroenterology & Hepatology. 2019;**16**(8):461-478

[93] Kruis W, Fric P, Pokrotnieks J, Lukás M, Fixa B, Kascák M, et al. Maintaining remission of ulcerative colitis with the probiotic *Escherichia coli* Nissle 1917 is as effective as with standard mesalazine. Gut. 2004;**53**(11):1617-1623

[94] Fedorak RN, Feagan BG, Hotte N, Leddin D, Dieleman LA, Petrunia DM, et al. The probiotic VSL#3 has anti-inflammatory effects and could reduce endoscopic recurrence after surgery for Crohn's disease. Clinical Gastroenterology and Hepatology. 2015;**13**(5):928-35.e2

[95] Štofilová J, Kvaková M, Kamlárová A, Hijová E, Bertková I, Guľašová Z. Probiotic-based intervention in the treatment of ulcerative colitis: Conventional and new approaches. Biomedicine. 2022;**10**(9):2236

[96] Kühbacher T, Ott SJ, Helwig U, Mimura T, Rizzello F, Kleessen B, et al. Bacterial and fungal microbiota in relation to probiotic therapy (VSL#3) in pouchitis. Gut. 2006;**55**(6):833-841

[97] Zocco MA, dal Verme LZ, Cremonini F, Piscaglia AC, Nista EC, Candelli M, et al. Efficacy of lactobacillus GG in maintaining remission of ulcerative colitis. Alimentary Pharmacology & Therapeutics. 2006;**23**(11):1567-1574

[98] Mimura T, Rizzello F, Helwig U, Poggioli G, Schreiber S, Talbot IC, et al. Once daily high dose probiotic therapy (VSL#3) for maintaining remission in recurrent or refractory pouchitis. Gut. 2004;**53**(1):108-114

[99] Gionchetti P, Rizzello F, Venturi A, Brigidi P, Matteuzzi D, Bazzocchi G, et al. Oral bacteriotherapy as maintenance treatment in patients with chronic pouchitis: A double-blind, placebo-controlled trial. Gastroenterology. 2000;**119**(2):305-309

[100] Gionchetti P, Rizzello F, Helwig U, Venturi A, Lammers KM, Brigidi P, et al. Prophylaxis of pouchitis onset with probiotic therapy: A double-blind, placebo-controlled trial. Gastroenterology. 2003;**124**(5):1202-1209

[101] Shen B, Brzezinski A, Fazio VW, Remzi FH, Achkar JP, Bennett AE, et al.

Maintenance therapy with a probiotic in antibiotic-dependent pouchitis: Experience in clinical practice. Alimentary Pharmacology & Therapeutics. 2005;**22**(8):721-728

[102] Pesce M, Seguella L, Del Re A, Lu J, Palenca I, Corpetti C, et al. Next-generation probiotics for inflammatory bowel disease. International Journal of Molecular Sciences. 2022;**23**(10):5466

[103] Denning TL, Bhatia AM, Kane AF, Patel RM, Denning PW. Pathogenesis of NEC: Role of the innate and adaptive immune response. Seminars in Perinatology. 2017;**41**(1):15-28

[104] Gómez-Llorente C, Muñoz S, Gil A. Role of toll-like receptors in the development of immunotolerance mediated by probiotics. The Proceedings of the Nutrition Society. 2010;**69**(3):381-389

[105] Zbinden A, Zbinden R, Berger C, Arlettaz R. Case series of *Bifidobacterium longum* bacteremia in three preterm infants on probiotic therapy. Neonatology. 2015;**107**(1):56-59

[106] Underwood MA, German JB, Lebrilla CB, Mills DA. Bifidobacterium longum subspecies infantis: Champion colonizer of the infant gut. Pediatric Research. 2015;**77**(1-2):229-235

[107] AlFaleh K, Anabrees J. Probiotics for prevention of necrotizing enterocolitis in preterm infants. Cochrane Database of Systematic Reviews. 2014;(4):CD005496

[108] Costeloe K, Hardy P, Juszczak E, Wilks M, Millar MR, Group PiPISC. *Bifidobacterium breve* BBG-001 in very preterm infants: A randomised controlled phase 3 trial. Lancet. 2016;**387**(10019):649-660

[109] Hunter C, Dimaguila MA, Gal P, Wimmer JE, Ransom JL, Carlos RQ, et al. Effect of routine probiotic, lactobacillus reuteri DSM 17938, use on rates of necrotizing enterocolitis in neonates with birthweight < 1000 grams: A sequential analysis. BMC Pediatrics. 2012;**12**:142

[110] Kumar A, Wu H, Collier-Hyams LS, Kwon YM, Hanson JM, Neish AS. The bacterial fermentation product butyrate influences epithelial signaling via reactive oxygen species-mediated changes in cullin-1 neddylation. Journal of Immunology. 2009;**182**(1):538-546

[111] Rivera-Chávez F, Lopez CA, Bäumler AJ. Oxygen as a driver of gut dysbiosis. Free Radical Biology & Medicine. 2017;**105**:93-101

[112] Niño DF, Sodhi CP, Hackam DJ. Necrotizing enterocolitis: New insights into pathogenesis and mechanisms. Nature Reviews. Gastroenterology & Hepatology. 2016;**13**(10):590-600

[113] Lovell RM, Ford AC. Global prevalence of and risk factors for irritable bowel syndrome: A meta-analysis. Clinical Gastroenterology and Hepatology. 2012;**10**(7):712-21.e4

[114] Agarwal N, Spiegel BM. The effect of irritable bowel syndrome on health-related quality of life and health care expenditures. Gastroenterology Clinics of North America. 2011;**40**(1):11-19

[115] Zhang Y, Li L, Guo C, Mu D, Feng B, Zuo X, et al. Effects of probiotic type, dose and treatment duration on irritable bowel syndrome diagnosed by Rome III criteria: A meta-analysis. BMC Gastroenterology. 2016;**16**(1):62

[116] Korterink JJ, Ockeloen L, Benninga MA, Tabbers MM, Hilbink M, Deckers-Kocken JM. Probiotics for childhood functional gastrointestinal

disorders: A systematic review and meta-analysis. Acta Paediatrica. 2014;**103**(4):365-372

[117] Guglielmetti S, Mora D, Gschwender M, Popp K. Randomised clinical trial: *Bifidobacterium bifidum* MIMBb75 significantly alleviates irritable bowel syndrome and improves quality of life—A double-blind, placebo-controlled study. Alimentary Pharmacology & Therapeutics. 2011;**33**(10):1123-1132

[118] Andresen V, Gschossmann J, Layer P. Heat-inactivated *Bifidobacterium bifidum* MIMBb75 (SYN-HI-001) in the treatment of irritable bowel syndrome: A multicentre, randomised, double-blind, placebo-controlled clinical trial. The Lancet Gastroenterology & Hepatology. 2020;**5**(7):658-666

[119] Simon E, Călinoiu LF, Mitrea L, Vodnar DC. Probiotics, prebiotics, and synbiotics: Implications and beneficial effects against irritable bowel syndrome. Nutrients. 2021;**13**(6):2112

[120] Min YW, Rezaie A, Pimentel M. Bile acid and gut microbiota in irritable bowel syndrome. Journal of Neurogastroenterology and Motility. 2022;**28**(4):549-561

[121] Arthur LE, Kizor RS, Selim AG, van Driel ML, Seoane L. Antibiotics for ventilator-associated pneumonia. Cochrane Database of Systematic Reviews. 2016;**10**(10):CD004267

[122] Branch-Elliman W, Wright SB, Howell MD. Determining the ideal strategy for ventilator-associated pneumonia prevention. Cost-benefit analysis. American Journal of Respiratory and Critical Care Medicine. 2015;**192**(1):57-63

[123] Moggia E, Koti R, Belgaumkar AP, Fazio F, Pereira SP, Davidson BR, et al. Pharmacological interventions for acute pancreatitis. Cochrane Database of Systematic Reviews. 2017;**4**(4):CD011384

[124] Hempel S, Newberry S, Ruelaz A, Wang Z, Miles JN, Suttorp MJ, et al. Safety of probiotics used to reduce risk and prevent or treat disease. Evidence Report/Technology Assessment. 2011;**200**:1-645

[125] Doron SI, Hibberd PL, Gorbach SL. Probiotics for prevention of antibiotic-associated diarrhea. Journal of Clinical Gastroenterology. 2008;**42**(Suppl. 2): S58-S63

[126] Ochman H, Lawrence JG, Groisman EA. Lateral gene transfer and the nature of bacterial innovation. Nature. 2000;**405**(6784):299-304

[127] Lerner A, Matthias T, Aminov R. Potential effects of horizontal gene exchange in the human gut. Frontiers in Immunology. 2017;**8**:1630

[128] Egervärn M, Lindmark H, Olsson J, Roos S. Transferability of a tetracycline resistance gene from probiotic lactobacillus reuteri to bacteria in the gastrointestinal tract of humans. Antonie Van Leeuwenhoek. 2010;**97**(2):189-200

[129] Lerner A, Matthias T. Changes in intestinal tight junction permeability associated with industrial food additives explain the rising incidence of autoimmune disease. Autoimmunity Reviews. 2015;**14**(6):479-489

[130] Matthias T, Jeremias P, Neidhöfer S, Lerner A. The industrial food additive, microbial transglutaminase, mimics tissue transglutaminase and is immunogenic in celiac disease patients. Autoimmunity Reviews. 2016;**15**(12):1111-1119

[131] Bassetti S, Frei R, Zimmerli W. Fungemia with Saccharomyces cerevisiae

after treatment with *Saccharomyces boulardii*. The American Journal of Medicine. 1998;**105**(1):71-72

[132] Burkhardt O, Köhnlein T, Pletz M, Welte T. *Saccharomyces boulardii* induced sepsis: Successful therapy with voriconazole after treatment failure with fluconazole. Scandinavian Journal of Infectious Diseases. 2005;**37**(1):69-72

[133] Zein EF, Karaa S, Chemaly A, Saidi I, Daou-Chahine W, Rohban R. Lactobacillus rhamnosus septicemia in a diabetic patient associated with probiotic use: A case report. Annales de Biologie Clinique. 2008;**66**(2):195-198

[134] Kunz AN, Noel JM, Fairchok MP. Two cases of *Lactobacillus bacteremia* during probiotic treatment of short gut syndrome. Journal of Pediatric Gastroenterology and Nutrition. 2004;**38**(4):457-458

[135] Land MH, Rouster-Stevens K, Woods CR, Cannon ML, Cnota J, Shetty AK. Lactobacillus sepsis associated with probiotic therapy. Pediatrics. 2005;**115**(1):178-181

[136] Mackay AD, Taylor MB, Kibbler CC, Hamilton-Miller JM. *Lactobacillus endocarditis* caused by a probiotic organism. Clinical Microbiology and Infection. 1999;**5**(5):290-292

[137] Presterl E, Kneifel W, Mayer HK, Zehetgruber M, Makristathis A, Graninger W. Endocarditis by *Lactobacillus rhamnosus* due to yogurt ingestion? Scandinavian Journal of Infectious Diseases. 2001;**33**(9):710-714

[138] Besselink MG, van Santvoort HC, Buskens E, Boermeester MA, van Goor H, Timmerman HM, et al. Probiotic prophylaxis in predicted severe acute pancreatitis: A randomised, double-blind, placebo-controlled trial. Lancet. 2008;**371**(9613):651-659

[139] Vitetta L, Coulson S, Thomsen M, Nguyen T, Hall S. Probiotics, D-lactic acidosis, oxidative stress and strain specificity. Gut Microbes. 2017;**8**(4):311-322

[140] Rao SSC, Yu S, Tetangco EP, Yan Y. Probiotics can Cause D-Lactic Acidosis and Brain Fogginess: Reply to Quigley et al. Clinical and Translational Gastroenterology. 2018;**9**(11):207

[141] Papagaroufalis K, Fotiou A, Egli D, Tran LA, Steenhout P. A randomized double blind controlled safety trial evaluating d-lactic acid production in healthy infants fed a lactobacillus reuteri-containing formula. Nutrition and Metabolic Insights. 2014;**7**:19-27

[142] Ewaschuk JB, Naylor JM, Zello GA. D-lactate in human and ruminant metabolism. The Journal of Nutrition. 2005;**135**(7):1619-1625

[143] Rao SSC, Rehman A, Yu S, Andino NM. Brain fogginess, gas and bloating: A link between SIBO, probiotics and metabolic acidosis. Clinical and Translational Gastroenterology. 2018;**9**(6):162

[144] Doron S, Snydman DR. Risk and safety of probiotics. Clinical Infectious Diseases. 2015;**60**(Suppl. 2):S129-S134

[145] Van den Nieuwboer M, Brummer RJ, Guarner F, Morelli L, Cabana M, Claasen E. The administration of probiotics and synbiotics in immune compromised adults: Is it safe? Beneficial Microbes. 2015;**6**(1):3-17

[146] Sanders ME, Akkermans LM, Haller D, Hammerman C, Heimbach J, Hörmannsperger G, et al. Safety assessment of probiotics for human use. Gut Microbes. 2010;**1**(3):164-185

[147] Johnston BC, Supina AL, Ospina M, Vohra S. Probiotics for the prevention of pediatric antibiotic-associated diarrhea. Cochrane Database of Systematic Reviews. 2007;(2):CD004827

[148] Katz JA. Probiotics for the prevention of antibiotic-associated diarrhea and Clostridium difficile diarrhea. Journal of Clinical Gastroenterology. 2006;**40**(3):249-255

[149] McFarland LV. Meta-analysis of probiotics for the prevention of antibiotic associated diarrhea and the treatment of *Clostridium difficile* disease. The American Journal of Gastroenterology. 2006;**101**(4):812-822

[150] Rocha-Ramírez LM, Pérez-Solano RA, Castañón-Alonso SL, Moreno Guerrero SS, Ramírez Pacheco A, García Garibay M, et al. Probiotic. J. Immunologic Research. 2017;**2017**:4607491

[151] Bron PA, Kleerebezem M, Brummer RJ, Cani PD, Mercenier A, MacDonald TT, et al. Can probiotics modulate human disease by impacting intestinal barrier function? The British Journal of Nutrition. 2017;**117**(1):93-107

[152] Mathipa MG, Thantsha MS. Probiotic engineering: Towards development of robust probiotic strains with enhanced functional properties and for targeted control of enteric pathogens. Gut Pathogens. 2017;**9**:28

[153] Plovier H, Everard A, Druart C, Depommier C, Van Hul M, Geurts L, et al. A purified membrane protein from Akkermansia muciniphila or the pasteurized bacterium improves metabolism in obese and diabetic mice. Nature Medicine. 2017;**23**(1):107-113

[154] Yadav H, Lee JH, Lloyd J, Walter P, Rane SG. Beneficial metabolic effects of a probiotic via butyrate-induced GLP-1 hormone secretion. The Journal of Biological Chemistry. 2013;**288**(35):25088-25097

[155] Lawley TD, Clare S, Walker AW, Stares MD, Connor TR, Raisen C, et al. Targeted restoration of the intestinal microbiota with a simple, defined bacteriotherapy resolves relapsing *Clostridium difficile* disease in mice. PLoS Pathogens. 2012;**8**(10):e1002995

Chapter 2

Nonalcoholic Fatty Liver Disease, Procalcitonin, and Gut Microbiota: Players in the Same Team

Doina Georgescu, Ana Lascu, Ioana Ionita, Oana-Elena Ancusa, Mihai Ionita, Ciprian Rosca, Despina Calamar-Popovici and Daniel Lighezan

Abstract

The study aimed to assess the link between procalcitonin (PCT) and gut dysbiosis in patients with nonalcoholic fatty liver disease (NAFLD). A total of 125 research participants, 100 patients with NAFLD (59% women and 41% men) age between 43 and 84 years and 25 healthy controls, joined this observational study. Patients were consecutively enrolled into two groups: 50 with gut dysbiosis and 50 without gut dysbiosis, after several conditions have been ruled out. Patients from dysbiotic group displayed significantly lesser use of biguanides and statins and elevation of fatty liver index (FLI), PCT, C-reactive protein (CRP), and alanine aminotransferase (ALT). Their gut microbiome was characterized by *Bacteroides* and *Prevotella* sp. dominant enterotype (74%) and by *Ruminococcus* sp. in only 26% of cases. The decrease of H index of biodiversity was observed in 64% of patients as well as of *Firmicutes/Bacteroidetes* (F/B) ratio and *Akkermansia muciniphila* in 60%. The increase of lipopolysaccharide positive bacteria was noted in 62% of patients. PCT strongly correlated with the level of CRP and ALT as well as to stool's H index of biodiversity and F/B ratio. Dysbiotic patients with NAFLD exhibited significant elevation of PCT that correlated well with the H index of stool's microbiota biodiversity, F/B ratio, CRP level, and severity of cytolytic syndrome.

Keywords: nonalcoholic fatty liver disease, procalcitonin, gut dysbiosis, gut microbiota, C-reactive protein

1. Introduction

Nonalcoholic fatty liver disease (NAFLD) represents the accumulation of fat of more than 5% of liver cells, not related to alcohol abuse. It can manifest as simple steatosis, inflammation with hepatocytes necrosis, known as nonalcoholic steatohepatitis (NASH), or in serious situations as end-stage chronic liver disease (NASH-related cirrhosis) with severe fibrosis and architectural damages [1, 2]. Over the past few decades, given the increased incidence of metabolic syndrome, NAFLD became a leading actor in liver diseases, with an exponentially upward trend, especially in developed countries [3]. As result, NAFLD features as a problem of public health due to its evolutionary potential with propensity of development fibrosis, cirrhosis, hepatocellular carcinoma, and liver-related morbidity and mortality, not to mention the increase risk for cardiovascular diseases in conjunction to associated metabolic issues [4, 5].

The development of NAFLD/NASH could be triggered by multiple conditions such as genetic disorders, particularities of life style and diet with high intake of carbohydrates and fats, hormones imbalance and insulin resistance, host-derived features like age, ethnicity, gender, antibiotic use, and inflammatory state, as well as imbalance of gut microbiota [6].

Procalcitonin (PCT), a peptide 13-kD glycoprotein, which is a precursor of calcitonin, without hormonal activity, rises in serum as a response to proinflammatory conditions, especially related to those of bacterial origin. In this context, PCT along with C-reactive protein (CRP), interleukins (ILs), and various cytokines could be considered as an acute phase reactant [7, 8].

Interestingly, while PCT levels should decline in patients with liver diseases and hepatocytes insufficiency, however, it was observed an increase of those levels, even without a bacterial infection. Those observations shed a new light upon the relation PCT and liver conditions. In patients with acute liver failure, it seems that procalcitonin elevation is not related to bacterial infection but more to cellular injury [9, 10].

The relation between NAFLD and gut microbiota dysbiosis was observed three decades ago in rats with blind intestinal loop and small intestinal bacterial overgrowth [11]. Gut microbiota dysbiosis could intervene in NAFLD pathogenesis by modulating the energy metabolism and insulin resistance, increasing free fatty acids (FFA), decreasing choline production, increasing gut permeability, upregulating hepatic de novo lipogenesis and triglyceride synthesis, releasing hepatotoxic compounds, eliciting endogenous alcohol production, and eventually producing hepatocyte's fat accumulation as droplets of triglycerides [12].

Some studies have demonstrated that gut microbiota dysbiosis may be involved in the perturbation of the hepatic metabolism of carbohydrates and lipids that consecutively could disturb the balance between pro- and anti-inflammatory local liver cytokines, giving the possibility of development NAFLD or NASH [13].

The so-called gut-liver axis represents not only a proximity anatomical relationship but also a perfect functional link between liver and the gastrointestinal tract. Through this axis, a direct connection is made, so that many metabolites related to the gut microbiota could rapidly reach receptors located at the liver surface and consecutively trigger the activation of numerous pathogenic pathways, resulting in serious events such as insulin resistance, liver inflammation, hepatocyte destruction, and fibrosis [14, 15].

The increase of gut permeability seems to play an important role in NAFLD by releasing into the portal vein stream of several substances resulted from bacterial metabolism, such as lipopolysaccharides (LPS), bacterial components, short-chain fatty acids (SCFAs), bile acids (BAs), choline metabolites, and endogenous ethanol that reach the liver and seem to contribute to the pathogenesis of NAFLD [16].

A human study based on histology-proven fatty liver (FL) disease has demonstrated that the severity of NAFLD is related not only to gut microbiota dysbiosis per se but also to important metabolic functional modifications of the gut microbiome. It was observed that *Bacteroides* sp. were significantly increased in patients with NASH and *Ruminococcus* sp. were associated to higher stages of fibrosis: $F \geq 2$. The authors attempted to make a stratification of NAFLD related to enterotypes of gut microbiota and hypothesized that the imbalance of microbiota could be used as a possible predictor of NAFLD [17].

2. Aim of the study

The aim of the study was to assess whether there is a link between PCT and gut dysbiosis in noncirrhotic patients with nonalcoholic fatty liver disease (NAFLD). The study was approved by the Ethics Committee of Scientific Research of the University of Medicine and Pharmacy "Victor Babes" from Timisoara, Romania, Nr. 15/10.05.2021 and was conducted in accordance with the Declaration of Helsinki. All the participants provided written informed consent before the beginning of the study.

3. Patients and methods

3.1 Inclusion criteria

A total of 125 research participants, 100 patients with NAFLD (59% women and 41% men) having a mean age of 48.67 ± 8.66 years and 25 healthy controls, joined this observational study. Patients were consecutively enrolled, being assigned into two groups, based on the presence or absence of the gut dysbiosis (DB): 50 with DB, the study group and 50 without DB, the comparison group, after several diseases and conditions have been ruled out.

3.2 Exclusion criteria

Exclusion criteria include exposure to toxics such as alcohol abuse with heavy drinking more than 40 g/day in men and 30 g/day in women, over the past 10 years, or exposure to industrial toxic substances, as well as to several groups of drugs with liver toxicity, and other liver conditions either inherited or acquired like hemochromatosis, $alpha_1$ antitrypsin deficiency, Wilson disease, autoimmune hepatitis, primary biliary cirrhosis, infection with viral B, D, or C hepatitis. Many other conditions such as organ insufficiency (heart, lungs, liver, or kidney), cancer, recent trauma and surgery, burning, myocadial infarction and cardiogenic shock, stroke, bacterial infectious diseases and sepsis, pancreatic diseases, thyroid diseases, long-standing parenteral nutrition, inflammatory bowel disease, and other entities resulting in malnutrition syndromes, as well as recent treatment with antibiotics or probiotics have been ruled out.

3.3 Examination approach and laboratory work-up

Patients underwent measurements of waist circumference and blood pressure (BP), body mass index (BMI) assessment, as well as thoroughly clinical examination. *Laboratory work-up:* complete blood count (CBC), routine liver tests including hepatitis B surface (HBs) antigen, Delta antigen, anti-HCV antibodies, plasma iron and copper, alpha 1 antitrypsin, antinuclear antibodies (ANA), antimitochondrial antibodies (AMA), lipase, thyroid stimulating hormone, as well as C-reactive protein (CRP), procalcitonin (PCT), fasting plasma glucose (FPG), HbA_1c, total cholesterol, low-density lipoprotein (LDL) and high-density lipoprotein (HDL), triglycerides, creatinine and uric acid, microproteinuria, urine and stool microbiology were run, using standardized, accredited methods.

Stool's microbiological assessment: Sterile containers with collected stool samples were frozen at −20°C and initially processed in order to determine possible aerobe, anaerobe, or microaerophiles species [18]. After identifying different types of stool species by the matrix-assisted laser desorption ionization time-of-flight mass spectrometry (MALDI-TOF-MS) method, they were expressed as colony formatting units (CFU)/gram stool and the severity of gut microbiota DB was semiquantitative scored as follows: 0 = absent, 1 = mild, 2 = medium, 3 = severe [19]. In the case of dysbiosis, frozen stools were further processed by the 16S rRNA next-generation sequencing (NGS) method in order to assess the enterotype, H index of alpha-biodiversity, and several bioindicators of the gut microbiome [20].

3.4 Noninvasive assessment of NAFLD

3.4.1 Imaging assessment

Every study participant was performed high-resolution real-time duplex ultrasonography with semiquantitative assessment of steatosis as follows: mild, moderate, and severe [21]. Point shear wave elastography was performed in order to rule out severe fibrosis (F4) [22]. Each patient also underwent abdominal helical computed tomography (CT) with evidence of the decrease of liver density consecutive to lipid accumulation [23].

3.4.2 Fatty liver index (FLI)

The FLI was calculated based on a mathematical formula that included measurements of waist circumference (cm), BMI (kg/m^2), gamma-glutamyl-transpeptidase (GGT) (U/l), and triglycerides (mg/dl), as follows: FLI = (e 0.953*log e (triglycerides) + 0.139*BMI + 0.718*log e (GGT) + 0.053*waist circumference − 15.745)/(1 + e 0.953*log e (triglycerides) + 0.139*BMI + 0.718*log e (GGT) + 0.053*waist circumference − 15.745) × 100. The values could range between 0 and 100. If the FLI is under 30, there is a very low probability of fatty liver (FL), but an FLI over 60 substantially magnifies the risk for FL, prompting complementary examinations [24].

3.4.3 Fibromax (BioPredictive®)

Fibromax (BioPredictive®) with the calculation of SteatoTest® and NashTest® based on some biochemical blood variables, such as alpha-2 macroglobulin, haptoglobin, apolipoprotein A1, total bilirubin, gamma-glutamyl-transpeptidase (GGT), alanine—aminotransferase (ALT), aspartate—aminotransferase (AST), fasting plasma glucose (FPG), cholesterol, and triglycerides, as well as on some clinical parameters such as age, gender, weight, and height was used in this study, in order to assess NAFLD in enrolled patients [25].

3.5 Body mass index

BMI was calculated based on patients' height and weight, using the formula: BMI = weight(kg)/height(m)^2 and interpreted as underweight (≤18.5 kg/m^2), normal

(18.5–24.9 kg/m^2), overweight (25.0–29.9 kg/m^2), obese (30.0–39.9 kg/m^2), and morbidly obese (≥40 kg/m^2).

3.6 Blood pressure measurements

At least two measurements of blood pressure (BP) were taken in the morning, with patients at rest, in a sitting position, using the same standardized device (OMRON M2 HEM-7121E). The final value of BP represented the mean of these primary two measurements. The diagnostic of hypertension was made according to European guidelines [26].

3.7 Assessment of diabetes mellitus (DM)

According to American Diabetes Association (ADA) criteria, a fasting plasma glucose (FPG) of 126 mg% or higher, or a 2-hour plasma glucose level of 200 mg% during 75-g oral glucose tolerance test, is consistent with the diagnosis of DM [27].

3.8 Assessment of dyslipidemia

The assessment of dyslipidemia was based on the presence of abnormal concentrations of lipids or lipoproteins in the blood, resulting in low level of high-density lipoprotein (HDL), high blood levels of low-density lipoprotein (LDL), or high blood levels of triglycerides. In this study, the cutoffs were considered as follows: total cholesterol <200 mg%, LDL < 100 mg%, HDL > 50 mg%, and triglycerides <150 mg% [28].

3.9 Assessment of chronic kidney disease (CKD)

CKD diagnosis was performed using creatinine serum level and estimated glomerular filtration rate (GFR), presence of microproteinuria (30–300 mg/24 hours) and imagistic characterization of kidney [29].

4. Statistical analysis

Graph Pad Prism 9.4.1 software (Graph Pad Software, Inc., La Jolla, CA, USA) was used for statistical analysis. Given exploratory, pilot study, no sample size calculation was needed. Quantitative variables were expressed as mean values (MV) ± standard deviation (SD). Chi-squared test was used to compare the two of groups, in cases of qualitative variables expressed as percentages. The unpaired t test was calculated and $p \leq 0.05$ was considered statistically significant, with confidence interval CI = 95%. Nonparametric Pearson's correlation test was also performed in order to establish the "r" coefficient, drawing the direction and magnitude of possible links between variables.

5. Results

This is an observational, cross-sectional study concerning 125 research participants: 100 patients with NAFLD, 50 with gut dysbiosis and 50 patients without gut dysbiosis, and 25 healthy controls.

Variables	**DB (+)**	**DB (−)**	**CON**	**P_1 DB (+) vs. CON**	**P_2 DB (−) vs. CON**	**P_3DB(+)vs. DB(−)**
Age (years)	50.31 ± 8.34	49.45 ± 8.55	50.52 ± 4.03	0.87	0.42	0.61
Gender W/ M	62%/38%	58%/42%	56%/44%	0.77	1	0.77
U/R residence	70%/30%	66%/34%	80%/20%	0.2785	0.2785	1
Hb (g/dl)	13.51 ± 1.22	13.21 ± 1.33	13.77 ± 0.91	0.34	0.06	0.25
L/mm^3	$7.55x10^3 \pm 2.45x10^3$	$7.12x10^3 \pm 2.14x10^3$	$7.11x10^3 \pm 0.8\ x10^3$	0.38	0.98	0.45
Plt/mm^3	$310.11x10^3 \pm 112.22x10^3$	$290.15x10^3 \pm 115.16\ x10^3$	$278.1x10^3 \pm 51.40\ x10^3$	0.18	0.62	0.38
ALT (IU)	57.43 ± 9.32	43.81 ± 6.32	19.92 ± 4.16	**<0.0001**	**<0.0001**	**0.02**
Creat (mg/dl)	1.05 ± 0.66	1.01 ± 0.55	0.64 ± 0.1	**0.0029**	**0.0014**	0.74
FPG (mg/dl)	105.34 ± 19.97	100.54 ± 6.75	80.56 ± 7.28	**<0.0001**	**<0.0001**	0.10
HbA$_1$c	5731 ± 0,288	5255 ± 0,215	5.122 ± 0.311	**<0.0001**	**<0.0001**	**<0.0001**
LDL-C(mg/dl)	137.25 ± 25.72	124.22 ± 31.43	101 ± 21.01	**<0.0001**	**<0.0001**	**0.02**
HDL-C (mg/dl)	40.78 ± 18.45	44.77 ± 7.89	54.28 ± 13.54	**0.0018**	**0.0003**	0.1629
Tgl (mg/dl)	177.85 ± 43.12	127.89 ± 51.11	87.99 ± 11.56	**<0.0001**	**<0.0001**	**<0.0001**
PCT (ng/ml)	1.520 ± 0.045	0.512 ± 0.198	0.1364 ± 0.0418	**<0.0001**	**<0.0001**	**<0.0001**
CRP(g/dl)	2.32 ± 0.86	0.85 ± 0.52	0.2 ± 0.05	**<0.0001**	**<0.0001**	**<0.0001**
Microproteinuria	36%	32%	4%	**0.0028**	**0.0067**	0.6744
Variables	DB (+)	DB (−)	CON	P_1 DB (+) vs. CON	P_2 DB (−) vs. CON	P_3DB(+)vs. DB(−)
Age (years)	50.31 ± 8.34	49.45 ± 8.55	50.52 ± 4.03	0.87	0.42	0.61
Gender W/ M	62%/38%	58%/42%	56%/44%	0.77	1	0.77
U/R residence	70%/30%	66%/34%	80%/20%	0.2785	0.2785	1
Hb (g/dl)	13.51 ± 1.22	13.21 ± 1.33	13.77 ± 0.91	0.34	0.06	0.25
L/mm^3	$7.55x10^3 \pm 2.45x10^3$	$7.12x10^3 \pm 2.14x10^3$	$7.11x10^3 \pm 0.8\ x10^3$	0.38	0.98	0.45
Plt/mm^3	$310.11x10^3 \pm 112.22x10^3$	$290.15x10^3 \pm 115.16\ x10^3$	$278.1x10^3 \pm 51.40\ x10^3$	0.18	0.62	0.38

DOI: http://dx.doi.org/10.5772/intechopen.110134

Variables	DB (+)	DB (−)	CON	P_1 DB (+) vs. CON	P_2 DB (−) vs. CON	P_3DB(+)vs. DB(−)
ALT (IU)	57.43 ± 9.32	43.81 ± 6.32	19.92 ± 4.16	**<0.0001**	**<0.0001**	**0.02**
Creat (mg/dl)	1.05 ± 0.66	1.01 ± 0.55	0.64 ± 0.1	**0.0029**	**0.0014**	0.74
FPG (mg/dl)	105.34 ± 19.97	100.54 ± 6.75	80.56 ± 7.28	**<0.0001**	**<0.0001**	0.10
HbA_1c	5731 ± 0,288	5255 ± 0,215	5.122 ± 0.311	**<0.0001**	**<0.0001**	**<0.0001**
LDL-C(mg/dl)	137.25 ± 25.72	124.22 ± 31.43	101 ± 21.01	**<0.0001**	**<0.0001**	**0.02**
HDL-C (mg/dl)	40.78 ± 18.45	44.77 ± 7.89	54.28 ± 13.54	**0.0018**	**0.0003**	0.1629
Tgl (mg/dl)	177.85 ± 43.12	127.89 ± 51.11	87.99 ± 11.56	**<0.0001**	**<0.0001**	**<0.0001**
PCT (ng/ml)	1.520 ± 0.045	0.512 ± 0.198	0.1364 ± 0.0418	**<0.0001**	**<0.0001**	**<0.0001**
CRP(g/dl)	2.32 ± 0.86	0.85 ± 0.52	0.2 ± 0.05	**<0.0001**	**<0.0001**	**<0.0001**
Microproteinuria	36%	32%	4%	**0.0028**	**0.0067**	0.6744

DB = dysbiosis, CON = controls, W/M = women/men, Hb = hemoglobin, L = leukocytes, Plt = platelets, ALT = alanine-aminotransferase, creat = creatinine, FPG = fasting plasma glucose, HbA1c = glycosylated hemoglobin, LDL = low-density lipoprotein, HDL = high-density lipoprotein, Tgl = triglycerides, PCT = procalcitonin, CRP = C-reactive protein, p bold = significant difference.

Table 1.
Baseline demographic and biological data in research participants.

As seen in **Table 1**, that illustrates demographic and biological baseline aspects in all research participants, patients either dysbiotic or not displayed significant differences when compared with controls, related to several variables, such as ALT, FPG, HbA1C, LDL, and HDL-cholesterol, triglycerides, creatinine, microproteinuria, CRP, and PCT. However, no significant differences were noted when compared patients' age, gender, location, and complete blood count (CBC), to those of control's group. Dysbiotic patients from the study group displayed significant elevation of PCT, C-reactive protein (CRP), and cytolytic enzymes: alanine aminotransferase (ALT), LDL-cholesterol, triglycerides, and HbA1c when compared to patients with NAFLD and no dysbiosis. No significant statistical differences were recorded between dysbiotic and normobiotic patients related to age, gender, location, CBC, creatinine, and HDL-cholesterol.

As seen in **Table 2**, that depicts the comparison of several clinical studied in patients included in this study, patients from dysbiotic group exhibited significant differences related to higher FLI, severity of fatty liver either simple steatosis or NASH, as well as less frequent treatment with biguanides and statins. The other variables, such as smoking history, sedentary life style, obesity, dyslipidemia, hypertension, G-I associated conditions, GSD, T2DM, IGT, CKD, and cardiovascular conditions, showed comparable results when compared dysbiotic patients with those with normobiosis.

As presented in **Table 3**, that displays stool's microbiota main alterations in patients with NAFLD and associated gut dysbiosis, the gut microbiome of the study

Variables	DB (+)	DB (−)	p
Smoking history	54%	38%	0.1102
Sedentary lifestyle	62%	50%	0.2291
BMI > 30 kg/m^2	58%	42	0.1114
HT	36%	28%	0.3936
FLI (units)	77.42 ± 8.44	69.23 ± 7.82	**<0.0001**
Simple steatosis	36%	58%	**0.00283**
NASH	64%	42%	**0.00283**
G-I associated conditions	56%	46%	0.3196
GSD	38%	34%	0.1567
T2DM/IGT	58%	46%	0.4005
Oral antidiabetics other than biguanides	4%	0%	0.3191
Insulin therapy	8%	0%	0.1538
Biguanides	24%	44%	**0.0357**
Statins	36%	58%	**0,0283**
Fibrates	42%	44%	0.8407
Dyslipidemia	40%	36%	0.2183
CKD	36%	32%	0.6641
C-V conditions	56%	44%	0.6897

DB = dysbiosis, BMI = body mass index, HT = hypertension, NASH = nonalcoholic steatohepatitis, G-I = gastrointestinal, GSD = gallstone disease, T2DM/IGT = type 2 diabetes mellitus/Impaired glucose tolerance, CKD = chronic kidney disease, C-V = cardiovascular, p bold = significant difference.

Table 2.
Clinical baseline aspects in patients with NAFLD.

Variables	DB +
Overall DB score	1.62 ± 0.69
Decreased F/B	64%
F/B	2.77 ± 0.68
Biodiversity Shannon-Wiener H index	2.68 ± 0.51
Decreased Shannon- Wiener H index	76%
Increased LPS (+) bacteria	60%
Decreased *Akkermansia muciniphila*	62%

DB = dysbiosis, F/B = Firmicutes/Bacteroidetes, LPS = lipopolysaccharide.

Table 3.
Stool's microbiota bioindicator alterations in dysbiotic patients.

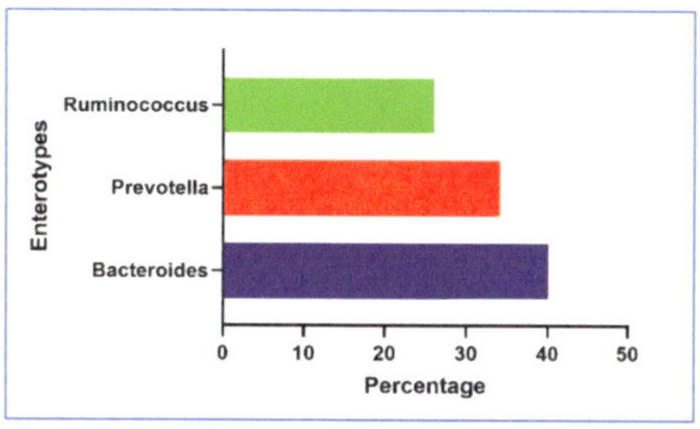

Figure 1.
Distribution of enterotypes in dysbiotic patients with NAFLD.

group was characterized by several alterations, expressed either by the decrease of various bioindicators, such as H index of biodiversity, observed in 76% of patients, *Akkermansia muciniphila* sp. in 62% of patients, and F/B ratio in 64%, or by the increase of LPS (+) bacteria in 60% of patients.

The study of the stool's microbiota enterotypes based on the mathematical analysis of the proportional relationship between *Bacteroides* sp., *Prevotella* sp., and *Ruminococcus* sp. in dysbiotic patients with NAFLD was expressed in percentages and is depicted in **Figure 1**.

As seen in **Figure 1**, patients with NAFLD and gut microbiota dysbiosis were characterized by a microbiological picture in which predominated *Bacteroides* sp. and *Prevotella* spp. dominant enterotype, observed in 74% of cases. *Ruminococcus spp.* dominant enterotype was noted in only 26% of cases.

Correlations of PCT to several blood biological variables such as CRP and ALT, as well as to stool's microbiota variables like F/B ratio, and H index of alpha biodiversity were analyzed in dysbiotic patients with NAFLD and are displayed in **Figure 2**.

As illustrated in **Figure 2**, PCT positively strong correlated ($p < 0.0001$) to the serum levels of ALT and to the F/B ratio of the gut microbiome ($p < 0.0001$). PCT also positively strong correlated with the stool's microbiota dysbiosis bioindicator, represented by the H index of alpha biodiversity ($p = 0.005$) and to the serum levels of CRP ($p = 0.0031$).

Figure 3 depicts the correlations of the gut microbiota dysbiosis intensity to Fibromax analyzed scores, such as SteatoTest, that expressed the severity of simple

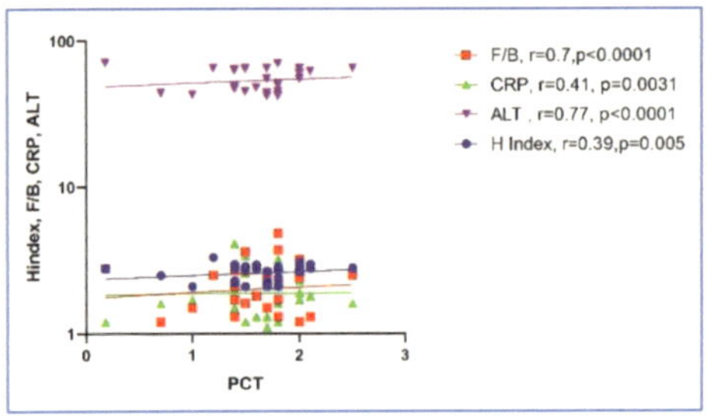

Figure 2.
Correlations of PCT in patients with NAFLD and gut dysbiosis.

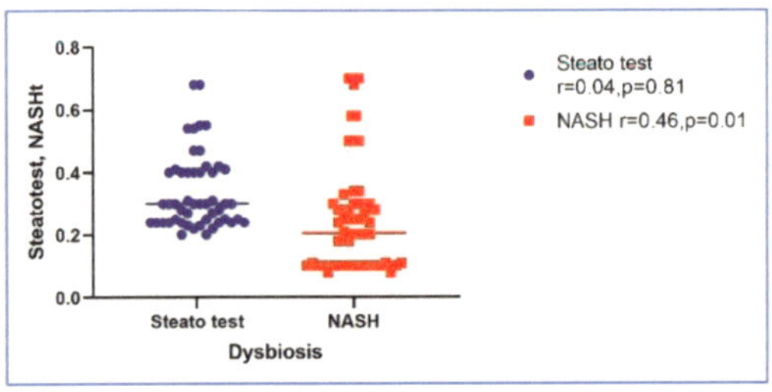

Figure 3.
Correlations of severity to steatosis and NASH scores.

steatosis, and NashTest, that expressed the level of necro-inflammatory activity caused by the metabolic condition.

As illustrated in **Figure 3**, significantly positive correlations were noted between the severity of gut microbiota dysbiosis and the NASH scores according to Fibromax test, but no significant correlations were observed between the gut microbiota dysbiosis range and the severity of simple steatosis, represented by SteatoTest scores.

6. Discussions

In the present study, as we observed strong correlations between the levels of inflammation expressed by PCT, CRP, and the severity of cytolytic syndrome, comparable results were also reported by other researches, related to various causes of liver pathologies. Thus, the correlation of PCT and transaminases levels were noted in patients suffering from various forms of acute liver failure, where authors observed that PCT identified not the potential bacterial infections but the severity of the liver cell injury [30]. Another study published in 2019 reported that the levels of serum CRP and serum PCT were positively correlated with transaminases levels and alkaline phosphatase as well, in patients with acute pancreatitis and associated liver injury [31].

As far as we know, at the moment, there are not so many studies addressing the relationship between NAFLD/NASH, procalcitonin, and gut dysbiosis. One case control study that included 50 patients with NAFLD proven by histology did not reveal significant increase of PCT when compared with healthy controls. However, CRP was considered useful in the diagnosis of NAFLD being significant augmented in patients by comparing to controls, but was not capable to discriminate between NASH and simple steatosis [32]. An important relationship between inflammation and NAFLD was observed by others, as we also noted in the present study. One cross-sectional study that included 55 patients over 30 years old, diagnosed with NAFLD, demonstrated a relationship between fatty liver and CRP levels, bringing additional proof regarding the role of inflammation in NAFLD. Of the proinflammatory cytokines, it seems that tumor necrosis factor-alpha (TNF-alpha) may play a pivotal role in liver inflammation. Also, proinflammatory cytokines and several interleukins (ILs) as well as LPS could trigger reactive oxygen species (ROS). As a consequence, the augmentation of the hepatocyte damage will develop, accompanied by activation of Kupffer cells and further increase of expression of TNF-α and IL-6 that will increase the levels of local and systemic proinflammatory cytokines [33]. A recent review starting from the known phenomenon of persistent inflammation in NAFLD discussed the relationship between continuing subclinical inflammation in NAFLD and the risk for developing hepatocellular carcinoma [34].

According to the Pearson's parametric correlation analysis, the present paper revealed that the levels of PCT correlated strong with certain characteristics of the bioindicators of the intestinal microbiota, namely, the Shannon-Wiener index of alpha biodiversity and the F/B ratio. We have not found in the literature similar studies that analyze this relationship, PCT-gut DB in patients with NAFLD. Regarding this particular relationship between PCT and DB, recently, literature studies have been especially focused on the DB-PCT relationship mostly in COVID-19-infected patients. Thus, in patients suffering from COVID-19 infection and associated hyperinflammatory reaction with augmentation of CRP $\geq$ 10 mg/dl, PCT $\geq$ 5 ng/ml, and WBC $\geq$ 15 G/l, alterations of the gut microbiota finger print were reported, with modification characterized by increase of *Parabacteroides* sp. and *Lachnoclostridium* sp., and reduction of *Blautia* sp., *Faecalibacterium* sp., and *Ruminococcus* sp. [35]. Other studies reported that the so-called triad in patients infected by COVID-19, expressed by the dysbiosis of the gut microbiota, augmented immune response, and high inflammatory state could make the difference between patients, regarding the way they can cope, either being resilient or being fragile and developing the "cytokine storm" with its consecutive severe outcome [36]. Understanding the changes in the intestinal microbiome in COVID-infected patients that could associate a particular host response could explain the unfavorable evolution of those with severe inflammation and increase of CRP and PCT, as well as the persistence of some symptoms as a consequence of remnant dysbiosis [37]. If situations that result in more or less expressed inflammatory syndrome, in which it was demonstrated the increase of the level of CRP and PCT, that were associated with some specific changes in the intestinal microbiota, we could hypothesize that the dysbiosis associated with NAFLD would generate an inflammation and would result in the growth of inflammatory proteins of the acute phase, such as CRP and PCT.

As others and we previously reported, several alterations of the gut microbiome were observed in the present study regarding dysbiotic patients with NAFLD [38, 39]. These modifications were characterized by the decrease of biodiversity of the F/B ratio and of *Akkermansia muciniphila* sp. and by the increase of the LPS (+) bacteria. Modifications of the enterotypes of the microbiota in patients with NAFLD and associated dysbiosis were also seen; thus, *Bacteroides* sp. and *Prevotella* sp. were the dominant enterotypes (enterotypes I and II) in three-fourth of patients, only one-fourth expressing *Ruminococcus* sp. (enterotype III) [40, 41].

Many studies advocated the anti-inflammatory role of statins, but only recently researchers have reported a relationship between statins and gut microbiome. We also observed that patients with NAFLD, obesity, and associated metabolic issues exhibited alterations of gut microbiota and were less treated with statins for their dyslipidemia. Recent studies reported that patients with obesity presented gut dysbiosis that was negatively associated with statin treatment. Thus, patients displayed alterations of gut microbiota with modifications of the enterotypes of study participants [42]. Others also hypothesize the possibility of statins to even modulate the gut microbiome [43, 44].

Results of the present study showed that patients with NAFLD and dysbiosis with increase of LPS positive bacteria and decrease of *Akkermansia* sp. were less treated with biguanides, by comparing with those without dysbiosis. Alteration of gut microbiota and antidiabetic drugs especially biguanides is a subject to recent debates. Researchers reported that metformin could associate an increase of small chain fatty acid (SCFA)-producing bacteria and may favor some species such as *Proteobacteria phylum*, *Allobaculum Lactobacillus* genera, and *Verrucomicrobia phylum*. The mucin-degrading bacteria are also abundant, such as *Akkermansia* sp. It was also observed that metformin increases *Escherichia* sp. and decreases *Intestinibacter* sp. in human gut microbiota and some species such as *Bifidobacterium adolescentis* were negatively correlated with HbA1c. From this point of view, the lowering effect of the glucose level can also be mediated by the microbiome modifications induced by metformin [45].

7. Conclusion

Dysbiotic patients having NAFLD displayed significant elevation of inflammatory acute phase reactant proteins such as PCT and CRP. Significant increase of the cytolytic enzymes like alanine aminotransferase (ALT) and other biological variables like LDL-cholesterol, triglycerides, and HbA1c was also noted. Patients with NAFLD from the dysbiotic group exhibited significant differences related to higher FLI and severity of fatty liver either simple steatosis or NASH. Less often treatment with biguanides and statins was recorded in patients with fatty liver and gut dysbiosis. The gut microbiome of the patients with NAFLD was characterized by various alterations. The decrease of some bioindicators, such as H index of biodiversity, *A. muciniphila* sp., and F/B ratio, was frequently observed. However, other species, namely, LPS (+), were often found abundant. The enterotypes of patients with NAFLD and dysbiosis were characterized mostly by *Bacteroides* sp. and *Prevotella* spp. and rarely by *Ruminococcus spp.* Strong positive correlations were observed between PCT and some blood biological variables, such as ALT and CRP, as well as between PCT and some stool's microbiota bioindicators, such as F/B ratio and stool's H index of alpha biodiversity. Gut dysbiosis of patients with NAFLD was significantly positively correlated with the severity of NASH scores. All these correlations between PCT and various bioindicators of the gut microbiome and also between dysbiosis and NASH severity suggest that these three entities, namely, PCT, dysbiosis, and NAFLD, are closely related.

Conflict of interest

The authors declare no conflict of interest.

Author details

Doina Georgescu[1*], Ana Lascu[2], Ioana Ionita[1], Oana-Elena Ancusa[1], Mihai Ionita[1], Ciprian Rosca[1], Despina Calamar-Popovici[1] and Daniel Lighezan[1]

1 Department of Internal Medicine I, "V Babes" University of Medicine and Pharmacy, Timisoara, Romania

2 Department of Functional Sciences, "V Babes" University of Medicine and Pharmacy, Timisoara, Romania

*Address all correspondence to: doina.georgescu@umft.ro

References

[1] Williams CD, Stengel J, Asike MI, et al. Prevalence of NAFLD and NASH among a largely middle –aged population utilizing ultrasound and liver biopsy: A prospective study. Gastroenterology. 2011;**140**:124

[2] Chasalani N, Younossi Z, Lanvine JE, et al. The diagnostic and management of NAFLD: Practice guidance from AASLD. Hepatology. 2018;**67**:328

[3] Perumpail BJ, Khan MA, Yoo ER, et al. Clinical epidemiology and disease burden of NAFLD. World Journal of Gastroenterology. 2017;**23**(47):8263

[4] Marjot T, Moolla A, Cobbold JF, Hodson L, Tomlinson JW. Nonalcoholic fatty liver disease in adults: Current concepts inetiology, outcomes, and management. Endocrine Reviews. 2020;**41**(1):66-117. DOI: 10.1210/endrev/bnz009

[5] Younossi ZM, Paik JM, Al Shabeeb R, Golabi P, Younossi I, Henry L. Are there outcome differences between NAFLD and metabolic-associated fatty liver disease? Hepatology. 2022;**76**(5):1423-1437. DOI: 10.1002/hep.32499

[6] Ancusa OE, Georgescu D, Iurciuc S, et al. Acute phase inflammatory proteins, uut microbiota dysbiosis and severity of nonalcoholic fatty liver disease in patients with type 2 diabetes mellitus. Review Chimica. 2020;**71**(5):290-298. DOI: 10.37358/Rev

[7] Gomez-Cerquera JM, Daroca-Perez R, Baeza-Trinida R, et al. Validity of procalcitonin on the diagnosis of bacterial infection in elderly patients. Enfermedades Infecciosas y Microbiología Clínica. 2015;**33**:52

[8] Lu J, Cl C, Jin JD, et al. Continuous elevation of procalcitonin in cirrhosis combined with hepatic carcinoma: A case report. BMC Infectious Diseases. 2021;**21**:29. DOI: 10.1186/s12879-020-05684- 2

[9] Dong R, Wan B, Lin S, et al. Procalcitonin and liver disease; a literature review. Journal of Clinical and Translational Hepatology. 2019;**7**(1):51

[10] Rule JA, Hynan LS, Attar N, Sanders C, Korzun WJ, Lee WM, et al. Procalcitonin identifies cell injury, not bacterial infection, in acute liver failure. PLoS One. 2015;**10**(9):e0138566. DOI: 10.1371/journal.pone.0138566

[11] Lichtman SN, Keku J, Schwab JH, Sartor RB. Hepatic injury associated with small bowel bacterial overgrowth in rats is prevented by metronidazole and tetracycline. Gastroenterology. 1991;**100**:513-519

[12] Auguet T, Bertran L, Binetti J. Intestinal dysbiosis and non-alcoholic fatty liver disease. In: Beloborodova NV, Grechko AV, editors. Human Microbiome. London: IntechOpen; 2020. DOI: 10.5772/intechopen.92972

[13] Kolodziejczyk AA, Zheng D, Shibolet O, Elinav E. The role of the microbiome in NAFLD and NASH. EMBO Molecular Medicine. 2019;**11**:e9302

[14] Brandl K, Kumar V, Eckmann L. Gut-liver axis at the frontier of host-microbial interactions. American Journal of Physiology-Gastrointestinal and Liver Physiology. 2017;**312**:G413-G419

[15] Khan A, Ding Z, Ishaq M, et al. Understanding the effects of gut microbiota dysbiosis on nonalcoholic

fatty liver disease and the possible probiotics role: Recent updates. International Journal of Biological Science. 2021;**17**(3):818-833. DOI: 10.7150/ijbs.56214

[16] Janssen S, Depoortere I. Nutrient sensing in the gut: New roads to therapeutics? Trends in Endocrinology and Metabolism. 2013;**24**(2):92-100. DOI: 10.1016/j.tem.2012.11.006

[17] Boursier J, Mueller O, Barret M, et al. The severity of nonalcoholic fatty liver disease is associated with gut dysbiosis and shift in the metabolic function of the gut microbiota. Hepatology. 2016;**63**(3):764-775

[18] Brown R, Poxton IR, Wilkinson JF. Centrifuges, colorimeters and bacterial counts. In: Collee JG, Duguid JP, Fraser AG, Marmion BP, editors. Mackie and McCartney Practical Medical Microbiology. 14th ed. Edinburgh, Churchill Livingstone; 1999. pp. 200-247

[19] Sandrin TR, Goldstein JE, Shoemaker S. MALDI TOF MS profiling of bacteria at the strain level: A review. Mass Spectrometry Reviews. 2013;**32**(3):188

[20] Ji B, Nielsen J. From next generation sequencing to systemic modeling of the gut microbiome. Frontiers in Genetics. 2015;**6**:219

[21] Li Q, Dhyani M, Grajo JR, et al. Current status of imaging in NAFLD. World Journal of Hepatology. 2018;**10**(8):530

[22] Sirli R, Sporea I, Popescu A, Danila M. Ultrasound-based elastography for the diagnosis of portal hypertension in cirrhotics. World Journal of Gastroenterology. 2015;**21**(41):11542-11551

[23] Zhang YN, Fowler KJ, Hamilton G. Liver fat imaging—A clinical overview of ultrasound, CT, and MR imaging. The British Journal of Radiology. 2018;**91**(1089):20170959

[24] Begogni G, Bellentani S, Miglioli L, et al. The fatty liver index: A simple and accurate prediction of hepatic steatosis in general population. BMJ Gastroenterology. 2006;**6**(1):33

[25] Morra R, Munteanu M, Imbert-Bismut F, et al. Fibromax: Towards a new universal biomarker of liver disease? Expert Review of Molecular Diagnostics. 2007;7:5

[26] Mancia G, Fagard R, Narkiewicz K, et al. ESH/ESC Guidelines for the management of arterial hypertension. In: 23rd European Meeting on Hypertension & Cardiovascular Protection. 2013. http://www.esh2013.org/wordpress/wp-content/uploads/2013/06/ESC-ESH-Guidelines-2013

[27] American Diabetes Association. Diagnostic and classification of diabetes mellitus. Diabetes Care. 2014;**37**(suppl1):S81-S90

[28] Grundy SM, Cleeman JL, Merz CN, et al. Implications of recent clinical trials for the National Cholesterol Education Program Adult Treatment Panel III guidelines. Circulation. 2004;**110**:227

[29] Johnson CA, Levey AS, Coresh J, et al. Clinical practice guidelines for chronic kidney disease in adults: Part I. definition, disease stages, evaluation, treatment, and risk factors. American Family Physician. 2004;**70**(5):869

[30] Sugihara T, Koda M, Okamoto T, et al. Serum procalcitonin in patients with acute liver failure. Yonago Acta

Medica. 2017;**60**(1):40-46. PMID: 28331420; PMCID: PMC5355843

[31] Li XC, Y, Liu Z, Chen, H Mao H. The relationship between liver injury and serum levels of C-reactive protein and procalcitonin in patients with acute pancreatitis. Journal of the College of Physicians and Surgeons Pakistan. 2019;**29**(3):287-289

[32] Oruc N, Ozutemiz O, Yuce G, et al. Serum procalcitonin and CRP levels in non-alcoholic fatty liver disease: A case control study. BMC Gastroenterology. 2009;**9**:16. DOI: 10.1186/1471-230X-9-16

[33] Foroughi M, Maghsoudi Z, Khayyatzadeh S, Ghiasvand R, Askari G, Iraj B. Relationship between non-alcoholic fatty liver disease and inflammation in patients with non-alcoholic fatty liver. Advanced Biomedical Research. 2016;**5**:28

[34] Peiseler M, Tacke F. Inflammatory mechanisms underlying nonalcoholic teatohepatitis and the transition to hepatocellular carcinoma. Cancers (Basel). 2021;**13**(4):730. DOI: 10.3390/cancers13040730

[35] Schult D, Reitmeier S, Koyumdzhieva P, et al. Gut bacterial dysbiosis and instability is associated with the onset of complications and mortality in COVID-19. Gut Microbes. 2022;**14**(1):2031840. DOI: 10.1080/19490976.2022.2031840

[36] Ferreira C, Viana SD, Reis F. Is gut microbiota dysbiosis a predictor of increased susceptibility to poor outcome of COVID-19 patients? An update. Microorganisms. 2020;**9**(1):53. DOI: 10.3390/microorganisms9010053

[37] Yeoh YK, Zuo T, Lui GC, et al. Gut microbiota composition reflects disease severity and dysfunctional immune responses in patients with COVID-19. Gut. 2021;**70**:698-706

[38] Georgescu D, Iurciuc M, Ionita I, et al. Portal vein thrombosis and gut microbiota: understanding the burden. Revista de Chimie. 2019;**70**(6):2181-2185. DOI: 10.37358/RC.70.19

[39] Georgescu D, Ionita I, Lascu A, et al. Gallstone disease and bacterial performance of gut microbiota in middle aged and older people. International Journal of General Medicine. 2022;**15**:5513. DOI: 10.2147/IJGM.S350104

[40] Salzman ET, Palacios T, Thomsen M, Vitetta L. Intestinal microbiome shifts, dysbiosis, inflammation and nonalcoholic fatty liver disease. Frontiers in Microbiology. 2018;**9**:61

[41] Grabherr F, Grander C, Effenberger M, Adolph TE, Tilg H. Gut dysfunction and non-alcoholic fatty liver disease. Frontiers in Endocrinology. 2019;**10**:611

[42] Vieira- Silva S, Falony G, Belda E, et al. Statin therapy is associated with lower prevalence of gut microbiota dysbiosis. Nature. 2020;**581**:310-315. DOI: 10.1038/s41586-020-2269-x

[43] Dias AM, Cordeiro G, Estevinho MM, et al. Gut bacterial microbiome composition and statin intake - a systematic review. Pharmacology Research & Perspectives. 2020;**8**:e00601. DOI: 10.1002/prp2.601

[44] Lim GB. Improved gut microbiota profile in individuals with obesity taking statins. Nature Reviews. Cardiology. 2020;**17**:385. DOI: 10.1038/s41569-020-0396-6

[45] Montandon SA, Jornayvaz FR. Effects of antidiabetic drugs on gut microbiota composition. Genes. 2017;**8**:250. DOI: 10.3390/genes810025

Chapter 3

Personalized and Targeted Gut Microbiome Modulation in the Prevention and Treatment of Chronic Diseases

Alojz Bomba and Martin Haranta

Abstract

The gut microbiota is being recognized as a factor with a significant influence on host physiology, health maintenance, and disease prevention. Distinct alterations of the gut microbiota are correlated with several chronic diseases. Currently, gut microbiota can be modulated by diet, probiotics, prebiotics, postbiotics, pharmabiotics, and fecal microbiota transplantation. An effective strategy in gut microbiota modulation is needed for the prevention and supportive treatment of chronic diseases. New and more effective approaches toward gut microbiota modulation are emerging, namely personalization and targeted modulation. The composition of novel products and treatments based on the individual gut microbiome, metabolome, strain specificity, and clinical data analysis can reveal and address specific changes to the diversity, composition, and function of gut microbiota. These analyses enable the development of personalized and targeted gut microbiota modulation, by the application of beneficial microorganisms, their consortia, their metabolites, and their effective combination.

Keywords: gut microbiota, microbiome, dysbiosis, chronic diseases, personalized medicine, probiotics

1. Introduction

The gastrointestinal tract is a major immunological organ that evolved to tolerate commensal and dietary antigens, yet retains the ability to mount a protective immune response to pathogens. The complex co-evolved community of the gut microbiota impacts the development of immunity and health of an individual. Although much of the gut microbiota is deemed non-culturable.,the advent of high-throughput sequencing techniques has greatly improved the ability to clarify gut microbiota composition and function. New technologies enable to include estimation of the gut microbiome diversity as well as species and novel gene identification. Average human gut microbiota is now better defined and has been estimated to exceed 1000 bacterial species [1, 2]. Bacteroidetes and Firmicutes represent predominantly in the gut microbiota. Other phyla such as Proteobacteria, Actinobacteria, Cyanobacteria, and Verrucomicrobia, as well as methanogenic Archaea, mainly *Methanobrevibacter smithii*, are present in the gut microbiota only in a minority [3, 4]. The distribution of these phyla in the gut depends on a wide range of host factors including genetics, epigenetics, local immune response, oxygen gradient, dietary intake, and interactions among microbes.

Gastrointestinal microorganisms can influence host processes to impact host physiology, immunology, and metabolism. The composition, diversity, and functionality of the gut microbiota can alter signaling events between the microbiome and the host to influence gut homeostasis and host health [5]. Analysis of the microbiota can be performed in different states of diseases, and its results together with the application to animal experimental models can provide a simpler system in which the disease pathogenesis can be examined [5].

Reduction of the bacterial diversity and overall disbalance of the gut microbiota also known as dysbiosis is associated with many chronic diseases [6]. In some instances, gut microbiota alterations can affect intestinal permeability, allowing the transfer of lipopolysaccharide originating from the walls of gram-negative bacteria into the circulation, leading to endotoxemia and low-grade inflammation in different parenchymatous organs, resulting in metabolic disorders and chronic diseases [7].

The etiology of chronic diseases is often multifactorial, and gut microbiota is also one of the key factors. Current therapy for chronic diseases mostly does not reflect this fact, which limits its overall effectiveness. A better understanding of gut microbiota cross-talk mechanisms and their subsequent effects could provide new insights into the role of gut microbiota and dysbiosis in disease pathogenesis. This knowledge and technology can allow the development of potentially effective alternative approaches for preventive and therapeutic measures based on gut microbiota modulation [5, 8, 9]. More effective methods and biotherapeutics are needed for personalized and targeted gut microbiota modulation as supportive therapy for chronic diseases.

Targeted modulation of the gut microbiota represents an approach when specific bacterial strains have clinically proven effects of changes in the microbiota and human health. These bacteria are used in products to deliver specific predetermined effects for the host based on his disease and microbiota composition.

2. The gut microbiota in chronic diseases

The gut microbiota alterations are observed in almost all chronic diseases, including inflammatory bowel diseases (IBD), irritable bowel syndrome, metabolic syndrome, obesity, diabetes, cardiovascular diseases, cancer, neurodegenerative diseases, and mental disorders. Microbiota alterations appear characteristic for each disease state. To date, it is unclear if dysbiosis is a cause or a consequence of the disease [6].

Inflammatory bowel disease is an umbrella term for ulcerative colitis (UC) and Crohn's disease (CD). Changes in the composition of the gut microbiota are reported in patients with IBD, namely a decrease in populations of Firmicutes and Bacteroidetes and an increased Enterobacteriaceae. Other significant differences in gut microbial composition for CD include increased representation by *Ruminococcus gnavus* and decreased beneficial bacteria *Faecalibacterium prausnitzii*, *Bifidobacterium adolescentis*, *Dialister invisus*, as well as an uncharacterized cluster of Clostridium XIVa. IBD patients have a reduced number of butyrate-producing bacteria and an increased number of sulfate-reducing bacteria, which promote further inflammatory processes [10]. The loss of obligate anaerobes with an increase of facultative anaerobes was also observed in patients with IBD [11]. It has been found that patients with IBD have altered metabolism including defective microbial and intestinal bile acid metabolism [6, 12, 13]. A higher level of fecal trypsin was detected in patients with CD suggesting altered protein degradation [14].

Decreased gut microbial diversity is associated with metabolic syndrome and obesity. The gut microbiota changes in these diseases are characterized by an increased ratio of Firmicutes to Bacteroidetes [15]. It seems that gut microbiota is in close correlation with obesity and can affect the transfer of the number of calories from the diet to the host and the host metabolism of absorbed calories [16].

Type 1 diabetes mellitus (T1D) and type 2 diabetes mellitus (T2D) differ in the mechanisms of pathogenesis. Both types of diabetes are associated with dysbiosis, but with different characteristic patterns. T1D is associated with a decrease in mucin degrading bacteria, *Bifidobacteria*, *Lactobacillus*, and *Prevotella* and an increase in *Bacteroidetes* and *Clostridium.* T2D is characterized by a decrease in *Clostridium* and an increase in *Lactobacillus* and *Bacteroidetes*. In both types of diabetes mellitus, changes of the microbiota were observed such as a decrease in the gut microbiota diversity, a decrease in butyrate-producing bacteria and Firmicutes, disrupted epithelial barrier integrity, and increased gut permeability [12].

Autism spectrum disorders (ASD) are characterized by social and communication deficits and repetitive behaviors. A significant increase in the Firmicutes/Bacteroidetes ratio was found in autistic individuals due to a decrease in the relative abundance of Bacteroidetes. At the genus level, a decrease in the relative abundance of *Alistipes*, *Bilophila,* and *Parabacteroides* was detected, while *Corynebacterium* and *Lactobacillus* were significantly increased. The increase in Clostridiales bacteria in constipated autistic individuals can be important in the pathogenesis of autism by the production of propionic acid, which can permeate into the brain and cause cognitive impairments [17]. It was also observed that the relative proportion of the fungal genus *Candida* was more than double in autistic than neurotypical subjects, but this difference was only partially significant due to a larger dispersion of values [18].

Dysbiosis in patients with colorectal cancer (CRC) is characterized by a decrease of butyrate-producing bacteria and an increase in the proportion of several potentially pathogenic bacteria. It has been suspected that bacterial species, such as *Bacteroides fragilis*, *Clostridium septicum*, *Fusobacterium spp*., and *Escherichia coli,* are involved in colorectal carcinogenesis. A decrease in Firmicutes and an increase in Proteobacteria, Bacteroidetes, and Fusobacteria were observed in CRC. In colorectal cancer tissue, an increase in the population of *Akkermansia muciniphila* and *Fusobacterium nucleatum* has been detected. It was found that the composition and numbers of dominant microbial species in CRC-associated dysbiosis in the gut lumen differ depending on disease severity and tumor stage [19, 20].

3. Current possibilities of the gut microbiota modulation in chronic diseases and future development

Current knowledge suggests that gut microbiota and gut dysbiosis could play an important role in the etiology and pathogenesis of chronic diseases and gut microbiota modulation could be an effective tool for their supportive treatment.

Nutrition significantly affects the diversity, composition, and function of the gut microbiota and human health at an early age, in adulthood, and also in old age. Diet high in fiber, fermented foods, and a diet containing omega- 3 fatty acids have a very positive effect on the composition and metabolic activity of beneficial microorganisms of the gastrointestinal tract. Diet represents a safe, readily modifiable, and cheap method of early intervention in chronic diseases, which may have significant health benefits by regulating the gut microbiota and mucous barrier [21].

New knowledge about the mutual communication between gut microorganisms and the whole organism makes it possible to develop new and effective methods of modulating the gut microbiota using beneficial microorganisms or their metabolites [22].

Probiotics are proposed as alternatives to antimicrobial drugs, and they can be an adjuvant therapy in the treatment of diseases associated with gut dysbiosis. Prebiotics modulate gut microbiota by stimulating the growth and metabolic activity of gut-beneficial microorganisms [23]. It has been shown that the positive effect of probiotic bacteria, prebiotics, or natural bioactive substances in functional foods can effectively reduce the incidence of chronic diseases [24]. The beneficial effects of probiotics on the host can be significantly improved by potentiated probiotics [25], which contain a suitable combination of probiotic bacteria with natural bioactive substances such as oligosaccharides, polyunsaturated fatty acids, and plant extracts [26–29]. Experiments in gnotobiotic piglets have shown that polyunsaturated fatty acids increased the adherence ability of lactobacilli and their inhibitory effect on the adhesion of *Escherichia coli* O8: K88ab: H9 in the gut [26, 27]. Effects of probiotic (PRO) *Lactobacillus plantarum* and combination of PRO and prebiotic (PRE) inulin enriched with oligofructose (2%) and PRO with Linioleum virginale (O) on gut bacteria in 1,2-dimethylhydrazine exposed rats were studied. It was shown that combinations of PRO-O and PRO-PRE had a synergistic effect which was higher than the effect of administering only PRO [28]. Preventive application of *L. plantarum* LS/07 alone or in combination with inulin to rats with chronic inflammation reduced the inflammatory process in the gut mucosa by down-regulating of pro-inflammatory cytokine synthesis and suppression of NF-κB activity in mucosal cells [29].

The next-generation probiotics hold promise to treat diverse medical conditions, and they can be more effective than single or multi-strains commercial probiotics. Moreover, several different strains with proven health benefits such as *Akkermansia muciniphila*, *Faecalibacterium prausnitzii*, *Bacteroides fragilis, Bacteroides uniformis*, *Eubacterium hallii,* and members of the Clostridia clusters IV, XIVa, and XVIII. can be considered candidates for the next generation of probiotics and other microbiota-based drugs. The development of the next generation probiotics holds promise for innovation in both the food/feed sector and the pharmaceutical industry [30].

New knowledge of the role of microbiota in health and diseases allows to expand the possibilities of administration of probiotics, in relation to their application form, depending on the intended use. Increasing interest in the application of probiotics in clinical practice will likely require specific regulatory approaches, if they are administered in a diseased population. More recently, the European Food Safety Authority has defined a new “live biotherapeutic products” (LBP) category, clarifying pharmaceutical expectations. Similar to all products intended to prevent or treat diseases, LBPs will have to be registered as medicinal products to reach the market in the USA and Europe [31].

Fecal microbiota transplantation (FMT) is the administration of fecal microbiota from a healthy person (donor) to a patient with a disease associated with dysbiosis. FMT is an effective therapeutic alternative for *Clostridium difficile* infection (CDI) but could be a promising therapeutic approach in patients with other diseases such as inflammatory bowel diseases (IBD), irritable bowel syndrome, metabolic syndrome, and obesity [32, 33]. It is hypothesized that FMT improves colonization resistance of recipient gut microbiota, but the mechanisms are not well understood. Fecal microbiota can be transplanted also in lyophilized encapsulated form. Another possibility of FMT is to use human gut microbiota cultured anaerobically in vitro. In choosing the route of FMT administration, the indication should be taken into account [12, 34–36].

Next-generation-based therapies, including synthetic stool products or bacterial consortia, currently have been coming to the fore, as an alternative to FMT, as they have much fewer side effects. It was shown that gut microbiota could be effectively modulated by the administration of defined microbiota. Application of 33 bacterial strains, isolated from human stool or a stool substitute mixture comprising a multi-species community of bacteria, may be protective against *C. difficile* or S. *typhimurium* enteral infection. The defined consortium of 8 bacterial strains (altered Schaedler flora) could be effective to diminish fecal urease activity and ammonia production [12, 37, 38].

Autoprobiotic technology can be applied to modulate gut microbiota using selected indigenous probiotic bacteria isolated from a healthy donor. The isolated bacteria are stored in cryobanks and returned to the host if dysbiotic conditions occur [39].

One of the new therapeutic approaches targeting the gut microbiota is based on metabolites of microorganisms—"postbiotics". They are produced, modulated, or degraded by the microbiota and act directly on the host with their metabolic and signaling function. These metabolites, such as short-chain fatty acids, flavonoids, or organic acid taurine, serve as a means of communication in interactions between hosts and microorganisms. Postbiotics target microbial signaling pathways by mitigating the negative effects of deficiency or excess of metabolites involved in signaling pathways. Postbiotics do not affect the gut dysbiosis, but have the potential to correct its negative effects. In contrast to the application of living microorganisms, their dosage and methods of application follow the principles of pharmacokinetics [40]. The term "pharmabiotics" refers not only to living microorganisms but also to dead or altered microorganisms, such as bacteria, but also their metabolites [41].

4. Personalized and targeted microbiota modulation and its potential for more efficient prevention and treatment of chronic diseases

Current knowledge suggests that the gut microbiome plays an extraordinary role in the development of chronic diseases. A better understanding of the mechanisms of its involvement in the pathogenesis of diseases is crucial for successful and effective microbiota modulation. The composition and functional characteristics of a healthy microbiome remain to be defined. Certain parameters such as the diversity of the microbiota, an abundance of certain genera (i.e., *Bifidobacteria*, *Lactobacillus*, etc.), or specific ratios between main bacterial phyla are considered markers of a healthy microbiota. The characterization of a healthy microbiota would make it possible to optimize nutrition and modify the microbiota to prevent diseases and to improve the effectiveness of therapy in people with gut dysbiosis and associated diseases [42].

Although some diseases have been correlated with dysbiosis, it is not clear if dysbiosis is a cause or consequence. Several trials have shown that therapies correcting dysbiosis, including fecal microbiota transplantation and probiotics, are promising in inflammatory bowel disease [10]. However, current knowledge shows that fecal microbiota transplantation does not have the same high effectiveness in inflammatory bowel disease as it does in *Clostridium difficile* infection. Dysbiosis occurs in both diseases, but the etiology and pathogenesis of inflammatory bowel disease are more complex in comparison with *Clostridium difficile* infection [43] and the same problem of complexity applies to many other diseases. Various strategies have emerged in the modulation of the gut microbiota in the prevention or treatment of diseases. Progress in this area is hampered due to ambiguities in the exact role of the microbiota in a given disorder, variations in the phenotype of the human disease, and variability in the formulation and delivery of the intended therapies. The use of gut microbiota modulation in medical practice requires a significant shift on all these fronts [41]. It is known that pathogenic microorganisms can cause various diseases, including cancer, and gut dysbiosis plays a very negative role in the pathogenesis of diseases. It is, therefore, reasonable to assume that modulation of gut microbiota may be a very effective means of prevention, but also supportive therapy for many chronic diseases shortly.

We have effective means to fight against chronic diseases through gut microbiota modulation. The suitable diet, probiotics, prebiotics, postbiotics, and gut microbiota transplantation represent them. However, what we need the most is a strategy for their effective use to the patient in individual's illness. Personalized and targeted modulation of gut microbiota has all the prerequisites to become a key strategy for the prevention and supportive therapy of chronic diseases [44, 45]. Personalized and precision medicine creates prerequisites for the application of new methods of treatment for many chronic diseases aimed at modifying the gut microbiome, including cancer therapy. Taking into account the role of gut microorganisms in disease pathogenesis could significantly contribute to increasing the effectiveness of their treatment [46].

Patient-tailored manipulation of the human microbiome may enable the development of precision microbiome-targeting treatment for a variety of multi-factorial disorders. More effective methods of adjusting the gut microbiome can be personalized probiotics and prebiotics, personalized nutrition taking into account the composition and functionality of the gut microbiota, postbiotics containing metabolites of microorganisms affecting the communication of microorganisms with the host, and phage therapy. However, their use in clinical practice requires the establishment of standard sampling procedures, their analysis, and interpretation of the obtained results. The use of personalized and precision medicine procedures will thus make it possible to streamline the diagnosis and therapy of diseases in which the gut microbiome plays an important role [47].

The development of precision probiotics, next-generation prebiotics resulting from a better understanding of metabolic interactions among members of the microbial ecosystem, and personalized dietary therapies tailored to an individual's microbiota will form the new frontier in the field of personalized medicine [48].

It can be assumed that new knowledge will make it possible to increasingly use the modulation of the gut microbiota to improve the effectiveness of disease prevention and their supportive therapy. It is highly likely that a suitable solution will be the application of a personalized approach using various possibilities of gut microbiota modulation through beneficial microorganisms or diet. However, it will be necessary to gain new knowledge about the composition and functionality of the optimal gut microbiota and the role of gut dysbiosis in the pathogenesis of diseases [49].

Effective modulation of the gut microbiome will require research and development of more effective methods and products for personalized and targeted modulation of the gut microbiome [24, 45]. Personalized medicine uses and combines genomic and clinical data to more accurately predict an individual's susceptibility towards development of the disease and his response to treatment. Personalized approach thus allows optimization of patient care. Personalized medicine approach and targeted approach in gut microbiota modulation should be based on analyses of the patient's clinical data and an analysis of the patient's gut microbiome and metabolome that reveals the specific changes in his gut microbiota diversity, composition, and function. These analyses allow using personalized and targeted gut microbiota modulation, by the application of beneficial microorganisms, their consortia, and their metabolites. It can be assumed that this method of modulation will in many cases require a combination of personalized probiotics, probiotic strains with specific effects, and metabolites of microorganisms—postbiotics.

The study of the application of personalized probiotics was conducted on 48 patients. The aim of this study was to determine changes in selected markers within the microbiota after 3 months of treatment by the personalized probiotic supplement. The probiotic composition (species, number of species, and number of CFU) of the probiotic mixture was designed based on gut microbiome analysis and prepared for each patient separately. After 3 months of probiotic supplementation, control samples were analyzed. Data confirmed a statistically significant increase of specific beneficial bacterial groups (lactobacilli, bifidobacteria, and actinobacteria) as well as the total number of species, thus increasing the overall diversity of the microbiota, which is considered a marker of a healthy gut microbiome. Results showed that the probiotic supplementation improved stool frequency in both cases—constipation and also diarrhea. The study confirmed the significance of a personalized approach in probiotic supplementation [50]. Of course, further data and studies are needed to demonstrate the effectiveness of a personalized approach in the clinical field.

It can be expected that also a new method of personalized and targeted modulation of gut microbiome combined with the auto-transplantation of *ex vivo* modulated patient's gut microbiota will be developed in near future for clinical practice [45, 51]. Innovative animal experimental models and clinical studies will greatly aid the shift in gut microbiome research and modulation that will enable the production of high-quality products for the patients [52].

5. Conclusions

Gut microbiota has an important role in the health and etiology and pathogenesis of chronic diseases. Future research on gut microbiome in chronic disease should be aimed to clarify the association between gut microbiota dysbiosis and disease pathogenesis. Diet, probiotics, prebiotics, postbiotics, and fecal microbiota transplantation can be used for gut microbiota modulation. Research on gut microbiota and its role in health and disease constantly brings new knowledge, which in the foreseeable future will significantly streamline not only prevention but also supportive therapy of many chronic diseases. New strategies such as personalized and targeted modulation of gut microbiota are emerging based on analysis of the patient's microbiome, metabolome, and clinical data. They will result in the application of beneficial microorganisms, their consortia, and metabolites to address the specific problem for specific people. The analysis of the patient's gut microbiota could also serve for early diagnosis in people at risk of chronic disease, and intervention can be made that will prevent chronic disease from occurring.

Conflict of interest

The authors declare no conflict of interest.

Author details

Alojz Bomba[1,2*] and Martin Haranta[1,2]

1 Perbiotix Ltd., Kysucké Nové Mesto, Slovak Republic

2 ARCOBIOME Advanced Research Center of Microbiome, Joint Research Center, Pavol Jozef Šafárik University in Košice, Faculty of Medicine, Slovak Republic and Perbiotix Ltd, Slovak Republic

*Address all correspondence to: alojz.bomba@iprobio.sk

References

[1] Wang WL, Xu SY, Ren ZG, Tao L, Jiang JW, Zheng SS. Application of metagenomics in the human gut microbiome. World Journal of Gastroenterology. 2015;**21**:803-814. DOI: 10.3748/wjg.v21.i3.803

[2] Karlsson F, Tremaroli V, Nielsen J, Bäckhed F. Assessing the human gut microbiota in metabolic diseases. Diabetes. 2013;**62**:3341-3349. DOI: 10.2337/db13-0844

[3] Eckburg PB, Bik EM, Bernstein CN, Purdom E, Dethlefsen L, Sargent M, et al. Diversity of the human intestinal microbial flora. Science. 2005;**308**:1635-1638. DOI: 10.1126/science.1110591

[4] Qin J, Li Y, Cai Z, Li S, Zhu J, Zhang F, et al. A metagenome-wide association study of gut microbiota in type 2 diabetes. Nature. 2012;**490**:55-60. DOI: 10.1038/nature11450

[5] Tlaskalová-Hogenová H, Štepanková R, Kozáková H, Hudcovic T, Vannucci L, Tučkova L, et al. The role of gut microbiota (commensal bacteria) and the mucosal barrier in the pathogenesis of inflammatory and autoimmune diseases and cancer: Contribution of germ-free and gnotobiotic animal models of human diseases. Cellular & Molecular Immunology. 2011;**8**:110-120. DOI: 10.1038/cmi.2010.67

[6] Carding S, Verbeke K, Vipond DT, Corfe BM, Owen LJ. Dysbiosis of the gut microbiota in disease. Microbiol Ecology and Health Disease. 2015;**26**:26191. DOI: 10.3402/mehd.v26.26191

[7] Cani PD, Bibiloni R, Knauf C, Waget A, Neyrinck AM, Delzenne MN, et al. Changes in gut microbiota control metabolic endotoxemia-induced inflammation in high-fat diet-induced obesity and diabetes in mice. Diabetes. 2008;**57**:1470-1481. DOI: 10.2337/db07-1403

[8] Laparra JM, Sanz Y. Interactions of gut microbiota with functional food components and nutraceuticals. Pharmacological Research. 2010;**61**:219-225. DOI: 10.1016/j.phrs.2009.11.001

[9] Sekirov I, Russell SL, Antunes LCM, Finlay BB. Gut microbiota in health and disease. Physiological Reviews. 2010;**90**:859-904. DOI: 10.1152/physrev.00045.2009

[10] Matsuoka K, Kanai T. The gut microbiota and inflammatory bowel disease. Seminars in Immunopathology. 2015;**37**:47-55. DOI: 10.1007/s00281-014-0454-4

[11] Nagao-Kitamoto H, Shreiner AB, Gillilland MG 3rd, Kitamoto S, Ishii C, Hirayama A, et al. Functional characterization of inflammatory bowel disease–associated gut dysbiosis in gnotobiotic mice. Cellular and Molecular Gastroenteroly and Hepatology. 2016;**2**:468-481. DOI: 10.1016/j.jcmgh.2016.02.003

[12] DeGruttola AK, Low D, Mizoguchi A, Mizoguchi E. Current understanding of dysbiosis in disease in human and animal models. Inflammatory Bowel Diseases. 2016;**22**:1137-1150. DOI: 10.1097/MIB.0000000000000750

[13] Duboc H, Rajca S, Rainteau D, Benarous D, Maubert MA, Quervain E, et al. Connecting dysbiosis, bile-acid dysmetabolism and gut inflammation in inflammatory bowel diseases. Gut. 2013;**62**:531-539. DOI: 10.1136/gutjnl-2012-302578

[14] Scott KP, Antoine JM, Midtvedt T, van Hemert S. Manipulating the gut microbiota to maintain health and treat disease. Microbial Ecology in Health and Disease. 2015;**26**:25877. DOI: 10.3402/mehd.v26.25877

[15] Ley RE, Bäckhed F, Turnbaugh P, Lozupone CA, Knight RD, Gordon JI. Obesity alters gut microbial ecology. Proceedings of the National Academy of Sciences of the United States of America. 2005;**102**:11070-11075. DOI: 10.1073/pnas.0504978102

[16] Turnbaugh PJ, Bäckhed F, Fulton L, Gordon JL. Diet-induced obesity is linked to marked but reversible alterations in the mouse distal gut microbiome. Cell Host & Microbe. 2008;**3**:213-223. DOI: 10.1016/j.chom.2008.02.015

[17] Li Q, Han Y, Dy ABC, Hagerman RJ. The gut microbiota and autism spectrum disorders. Frontiers in Cellular Neuroscience. 2017;**11**:120. DOI: 10.3389/fncel.2017.00120

[18] Strati F, Cavalieri D, Albanese D, De Felice C, Donati C, Hayek J, et al. New evidences on the altered gut microbiota in autism spectrum disorders. Microbiome. 2017;**5**:24. DOI: 10.1186/s40168-017-0242-1

[19] Gagnière J, Raisch J, Veziant J, Barnich N, Bonnet R, Buc E, et al. Gut microbiota imbalance and colorectal cancer. World Journal of Gastroenterology. 2016;**22**:501-518. DOI: 10.3748/wjg.v22.i2.501

[20] Castellarin M, Warren R, Freeman J, Dreolini L, Krzywinski M, Strauss J, et al. Fusobacterium nucleatum infection is prevalent in human colorectal carcinoma. Genome Research. 2012;**22**:299-306. DOI: 10.1101/gr.126516.111

[21] Alemao CA, Budden KF, Gomez HM, Rehman SF, Marshall JE, Shukla SD, et al. Impact of diet and the bacterial microbiome on the mucous barrier and immune disorders. Allergy. 2021;**76**:714-734. DOI: 10.1111/all.14548

[22] Hrncir T. Gut microbiota dysbiosis: Triggers, consequences, diagnostic and therapeutic options. Microorganism. 2022;**10**:578. DOI: 10.3390/microorganisms10030578

[23] Kvakova M, Bertkova I, Stofilova J, Savidge TC. Co-encapsulated synbiotics and immobilized probiotics in human health and gut microbiota modulation. Food. 2021;**10**:1297. DOI: 10.3390/foods10061297

[24] Bubnov RV, Spivak MY, Lazarenko LM, Bomba A, Boyko NV. Probiotics and immunity: Provisional role for personalized diets and disease prevention. EPMA Journal. 2015;**6**:14. DOI: 10.1186/s13167-015-0036-0

[25] Bomba A, Nemcová R, Mudroňová D, Guba P. The possibilities of potentiating the efficacy of probiotics. Trends in Food Science & Technology. 2002;**13**:121-126. DOI: 10.1016/S0924-2244(02)00129-2

[26] Bomba A, Nemcová R, Gancarčíková S, Herich R, Guba P, Mudroňová D. Improvement of the probiotic effect of micro-organisms by their combination with maltodextrins, fructo-oligosaccharides and polyunsaturated fatty acids. British Journal of Nutrition. 2002;**88** (Suppl.1):S95-S99. DOI: 10.1079/BJN2002634

[27] Nemcová R, Borovská D, Koščová J, Gancarčíková S, Mudroňová D, Buleca V, et al. The effect of supplementation of flax-seed oil on interaction of Lactobacillus plantarum-Biocenol™ LP96 and Escherichia coli O8:K88ab:H9 in the gut of germ-free piglets. Research

in Veterinary Science. 2012;**93**:39-41. DOI: 10.1016/j.rvsc.2011.07.031

[28] Strojný L, Bomba A, Hijová E, Chmelárová A, Mojžišová G, Bertková I, et al. Effects of a probiotic in combination with prebiotics on intestinal lactobacilli and coliforms and activities of bacterial enzymes in 1,2-dimethylhydrazine exposed rats. Czech Journal of Animal Science. 2011;**56**:99-106. DOI: 10.17221/56/2010-CJAS

[29] Štofilová J, Szabadosová V, Hrčková G, Salaj R, Bertková I, Hijová E, et al. Bomba A. Co-administration of a probiotic strain Lactobacillus plantarum LS/07 CCM7766 with prebiotic inulin alleviates the intestinal inflammation in rats exposed to N,N-dimethylhydrazine. International Immunopharmacology. 2015;**24**:361-368. DOI: 10.1016/j.intimp.2014.12.022

[30] El Hage R, Hernandez-Sanabria E, Van de Wieofle T. Emerging trends in "smart probiotics": Functional consideration for the development of novel health and industrial applications. Frontiers in Microbiology. 2017;**8**:1889. DOI: 10.3389/fmicb.2017.01889

[31] Cordaillat-Simmons M, Rouanet A, Pot B. Live biotherapeutic products: The importance of a defined regulatory framework. Experimental & Molecular Medicine. 2020;**52**:1397-1406. DOI: 10.1038/s12276-020-0437-6

[32] Konturek PC, Haziri D, Brzozowski T, Hess T, Heyman S, Kwiecien S, et al. Emerging role of fecal microbiota therapy in the treatment of gastrointestinal and extra-gastrointestinal diseases. Journal of Physiology and Pharmacology. 2015;**66**:483-491. PMID: 26348073

[33] Paramsothy S, Kamm MA, Kaakoush NO, Walsh AJ, van den Bogaerde J, Samuel D, et al. Multidonor intensive faecal microbiota transplantation for active ulcerative colitis: A randomised placebo-controlled trial. Lancet. 2017;**389**:1218-1128. DOI: 10.1016/S0140-6736(17)30182-4

[34] Norin E. Anaerobicaly cultivated human intestinal microbiota. How to overcome intestinal problems in patients with a diverse intestinal microbiota. In: Proceedings of The Joint Congress of The 19th International Symposium on Gnotobiology, The 50th Congress of Japanese Association of Germfree Life and Gnotobiology and the 39th Congress of the Society for Microbial Ecology and Disease. Tokyo; 2017. p. 47

[35] Seekatz AM, Aas J, Gesser CE, Rubin TA, Saman DM, Bakken JS, et al. Recovery of the gut microbiome following fecal microbiota transplantation. MBio. 2014;**5**:e00893-e00814. DOI: 10.1128/mBio.00893-14

[36] Vrieze A, de Groot PF, Kootte RS, Knaapen M, van Nood E, Nieuwdorp M. Fecal transplant: A safe and sustainable clinical therapy for restoring intestinal microbial balance in human disease? Best Practice & Research Clinical Gastroenterology. 2013;**27**:127-137. DOI: 10.1016/j.bpg.2013.03.003

[37] Petrof EO, Gloor GB, Vanner SJ, Weese SJ, Carter D, Daigneault MC, et al. Stool substitute transplant therapy for the eradication of Clostridium difficile infection: 'RePOOPulating' the gut. Microbiome. 2013;**1**:3. DOI: 10.1186/2049-2618-1-3

[38] Shen TC, Albenberg L, Bittinger K, Chehoud C, Chen YY, Judge CA, et al. Engineering the gut microbiota to treat hyperammonemia. European Journal of Clinical Investigation. 2015;**125**:2841-2850. DOI: 10.1172/JCI79214

[39] Suvorov A. Gut microbiota, probiotics, and human health. Bioscience of Microbiota, Food and Health. 2013;**32**:81-91. DOI: 10.12938/bmfh.32.81

[40] Wong AC, Levy M. New approaches to microbiome-based therapies. mSystems. 2019;**4**:e00122-e00119. DOI: 10.1128/mSystems.00122-19

[41] Quigley EMM, Gajula P. Recent advances in modulating the microbiome. F1000Research. 2020;**9**:F100. DOI: 10.12688/f1000research.20204.1

[42] Bäckhed F, Fraser CM, Ringel Y, Sanders ME, Sartor RB, Sherman PM, et al. Defining a healthy human gut microbiome: Current concepts, future directions, and clinical applications. Cell Host & Microbe. 2012;**12**:611-622. DOI: 10.1016/j.chom.2012.10.012

[43] Lopez J, Grinspan A. Fecal microbiota transplantation for inflammatory bowel disease. Gastroenterology & Hepatology (N Y). 2016;**12**:374-379

[44] Takáčová M, Bomba A, Tóthová C, Micháľová A, Turňa H. Any future for faecal microbiota transplantation as a novel strategy for gut microbiota modulation in human and veterinary medicine? Life. 2022;**12**:723. DOI: 10.3390/life12050723

[45] Bomba A, Strojný L, Ambro L, Link R. Gut microbiome and its targeted modulation: Where it is heading? In: Proceedings of the international scientific conference on probiotics, prebiotics, gut microbiota and health. Prague; 2019

[46] Behrouzi A, Nafari AH, Siadat SD. The significance of microbiome in personalized medicine. Clinical and Translational Medicine. 2019;**8**:16. DOI: 10.1186/s40169-019-0232-y

[47] Zmora N, Zeevi D, Korem T, Segal E, Elinav E. Taking it personally: Personalized utilization of the human microbiome in health and disease. Cell Host & Microbe. 2016;**19**:12-20. DOI: 10.1016/j.chom.2015.12.016

[48] Kashyap PC, Chia N, Nelson H, Segal E, Elinav E. Microbiome at the frontier of personalized medicine. Mayo Clinic Proceedings. 2017;**92**(12):1855-1864. DOI: 10.1016/j.mayocp.2017.10.004

[49] Wargo JA. Modulating gut microbes. Science. 2020;**369**(6509):1302-1303. DOI: 10.1126/science.abc3965

[50] Ryšávka P, Kohutková-Lánová M, Netušil R, Pospíšilová E, Hanáčková E, Čmielová J, et al. Targeted modulation of gut microbiota by personalized probiotics. Internatiomal Journal of Probiotics α Prebiotics. 2022;**17**:33-41

[51] Kort R. Personalized therapy with probiotics from the host by TripleA. Trends in Biotechnology. 2014;**32**:291-293. DOI: 10.1016/j.tibtech.2014.04.002

[52] Gancarcikova S, Lauko S, Hrckova G, Andrejcakova Z, Hajduckova V, Madar M, et al. Innovative animal model of DSS-induced ulcerative colitis in pseudo germ-free mice. Cell. 2020;**9**:2571. DOI: 10.3390/cells9122571

Chapter 4

Probiotic Effects on Disease Prevention and Treatment

Kajal Farahmandi and Sadegh Sulaimany

Abstract

Research on the probiotic effect in preventing or treating diseases has attracted scientists' attention for many decades. Findings of probiotics effects on human health indicate that they are not only no detrimental but also may have a beneficial effect on the host. Indeed, the effectiveness of probiotics depends on the type of utilized strain, duration, dose administration, and single or combined strains used that can be different in a specific disease. Therefore, probiotics can play a significant role in the treatment and prevention of different diseases through several mechanisms; for instance, stimulating respiratory immunity in the airway and enhancing resistance to respiratory tract infections, can prevent or reduce the duration of respiratory system diseases. By ameliorating glucose metabolism, reducing inflammation and oxidative stress in pancreatic cells, and preventing the destruction of β-pancreatic cells, may prevent the onset of diabetes and the pathogenesis of diabetic retinopathy as well. Moreover, using their metabolites, especially short-chain fatty acids production, probiotics may have an important effect on weight modifications. Finally, from the regulation of important neurotransmitters and regulation of inflammatory markers, it may be effective in mental disorders improvement.

Keywords: probiotics, microbiota, diarrhea, irritable bowel syndrome, inflammatory bowel disease, Crohn's disease, ulcerative colitis, respiratory diseases, metabolic disorders, mental disorders, diabetes, obesity

1. Introduction

Research on the probiotic effect in preventing or treating diseases has attracted researchers' attention for many decades. The importance of probiotics in such areas can be indicated by close to 300 meta-analyses published from 2000 to 2020 investigating the efficacy of probiotics in preventing and treating diseases. Probiotics are defined as live non-pathogenic microorganisms that confer beneficial health to the host when administered in a sufficient number [1] (1×10^9 colony forming units (CFU) per serving [2]). However, a concern has increased that probiotics may not survive in sufficient numbers when they are added to dairy products or pass through the gastrointestinal tract and may not be helpful as would be expected [3, 4]. Therefore, improving the shelf-life of probiotic strains is important. According to research, microencapsulation of probiotic strain by spray drying through adding additives like tragacanth to skim milk could remarkably enhance the survival of the cells during drying [5]. Amara and Shibl showed that probiotics are not only helpful in supporting health or managing pathogenic infections, but also effective for the treatment and controlling of diseases [6]. In addition, the utilization of fermented foods which are the usual source of lactic acid bacteria can confer remarkable health benefits, such as decreasing the incidence rate of type 2 diabetes and cardiovascular illnesses [7], and also helpful metabolic effects [8].

Categorizing 294 meta-analysis articles have been done from the year of 2000 until 2020, on the effects of probiotics in the prevention and treatment of diseases, demonstrated that only 21% of these studies reported the ineffectiveness of probiotics in the prevention or treatment of various diseases but 79% showed a positive effect. It is worth saying that no analysis was found to report a negative effect of probiotics. This shows the importance of probiotics on human health that they are not only not detrimental but also may have a beneficial effect on the host. Besides, the statistics of the efficacy percentage of probiotics on diseases indicate that probiotic supplements may be more effective in preventing or treating some diseases (80.95–100%), including; diabetes, infections, irritable bowel syndrome, enterocolitis, and diarrhea. It is worth mentioning that these results have been conducted with more than 14 meta-analysis articles from 2000 to 2020 on each of these diseases (**Figure 1**).

Probiotics have been used to modulate the microbial community in a beneficial way and as a result, immunity improves against many infections that threaten human and animal lives [9]. Probiotics exert their beneficial effects on the host through different mechanisms different mechanisms including straightly eliminating or inhibiting the growth of pathogens by producing antimicrobial substances, destroying toxins, regulating the immune system, reintroducing the microbiota balance, competing with pathogenic microbes for adhesion sites and nutrients, enhancing intestinal barrier function, and immunomodulation [10–13].

Using antibiotics in a large amount unselectively annihilates normal intestine and genital tract flora, and damages the host's mechanisms of immunity [14]. Nowadays, spreading antibiotic resistance among human pathogens is a major public health concern in the world. It can affect people at any stage of life, as well as the healthcare, veterinary, and agriculture industries. As it is clear

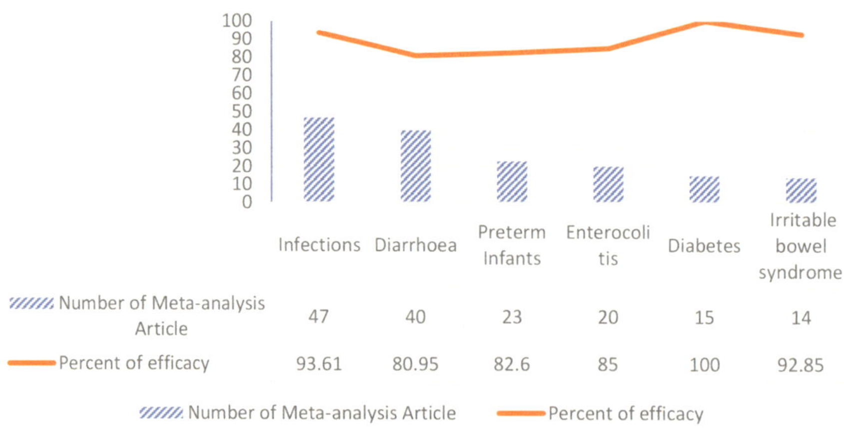

Figure 1.
The effectiveness percent of probiotics on diseases with the highest number of studies (from 2000 to 2020).

antimicrobial resistance is increasing nowadays due to the overuse or misuse of antibiotics against infections; however, probiotics can be used as a great alternative to them [15, 16]. As probiotics help to balance the intestinal microbiota composition, they can protect the host against diseases [17]. However, it should be noted that to produce probiotic supplements for humans or animals, strains containing antibiotic resistance genes must be distinguished from other strains, as there is a possible risk of spreading resistance genes to other pathogenic or non-pathogenic strains [18].

It is the purpose of this chapter to provide a comprehensive review of the research that has been conducted on the importance of probiotics in the prevention/treatment of several common human diseases.

2. Distribution of probiotic articles by type disease

Figure 2 shows the distribution of meta-analysis probiotic articles published from 2000 to 2020 by anatomical of physiological target. The greatest number of studies were associated with digestive system diseases (139 out of 283 or 49.11% of the total) and the least of them were related to disorders of the nervous system, eye, and adnexa. **Figure 2** illustrates the proportion of probiotics in the treatment of different diseases as well.

3. Efficacy of probiotics on gastrointestinal diseases

Probiotics have a positive effect on intestinal function. They enhance the structure of mucus barrier and make intestinal connections closer by boosting the amount of mucus produced. They decrease inflammation and restore normal bowel movements as well [19, 20]. So, these mechanisms of action lead to probiotics having a major role in the management of gastrointestinal disorders.

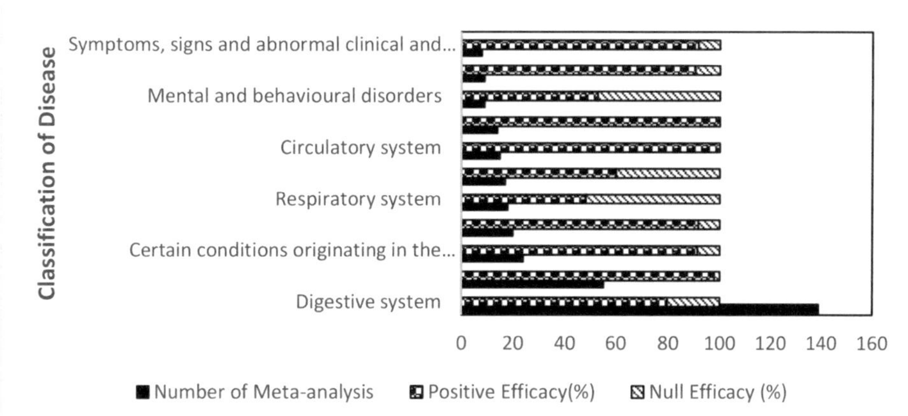

Figure 2.
Distribution of probiotics-disease-related meta-analysis articles based on the category of diseases (2000–2020). The effectiveness of probiotics was defined as the percentage of completed curing or just improvement of some parameters in patients based on the result of each meta-analysis study.

3.1 Diarrhea

Among the probiotic studies conducted on digestive system diseases, diarrhea is approximately the most studied case. Evidence demonstrates that epidemiological relevance of acute diarrhea, whether caused by virus or associated by using antibiotic, is very high in the world, particularly, in developing countries [21]. Evidence show *Limosilactobacillus reuteri* ATCC 55730 [22, 23] and *Saccharomyces boulardii* [24, 25] play an important role in treating acute diarrhea in children. Research shows that two probiotic strains including *Lactobacillus GG* and *Saccharomyces boulardii* play important role in preventing antibiotic-associated diarrhea in both adult patients and children as well [21, 26]. Research reported that treatment by probiotics could reduce acute diarrheal illness by approximately 1 day [27–32].

Probiotics' preventive or therapeutic effect in almost all types of diarrheas is related to some parameters including strain type, the antimicrobial and anti-inflammatory properties of the probiotic strain, and utilized dosage [11–13]. The effectiveness of probiotics on diarrhea has been imputed to their immunostimulatory effect and also restoring gut microflora to the balance situation [33, 34].

3.2 Irritable bowel syndrome (IBS)

In rodents with intestinal inflammation, it has been proven that probiotics can reduce intestinal cytokine secretion and improve epithelial barrier function [35]. And a reduction of IBS symptoms happened in IBS patients due to enhanced cytokine profile [36] after probiotic supplementation was used [19, 37–39]. A meta-analysis of 15 human studies including 1793 IBS patients also indicated that probiotic therapy reduced pain and symptom severity scores in these people [40]. Furthermore, studies both in humans and animals show that different probiotic strains can be effective in alleviating abdominal pain and decreasing visceral hypersensitivity by changing the expression of neurotransmitters and receptors which are associated with the pain pathways such as the opioid or the cannabinoid receptors [41, 42]. However, taking into account the effectiveness of probiotics based on the type of strain used, duration, dose of administration, and single or combined strains used, can be different in a specific disease. Although many research showed the efficacy of probiotics on IBS patients, however, Connell et al. reported that VSL#3 probiotic supplement which is the combination of eight bacterial strains, not had any positive effect on abdominal pain, stool consistency, abdominal bloating, or quality of life in patients with IBS [43].

3.3 Inflammatory bowel disease (IBD)

IBD is a collective term used to describe Crohn's disease (CD), ulcerative colitis (UC), and nonspecific colitis [44]. The inflammation of the gastrointestinal tract is in common characteristic of these diseases although each of them has distinct features, the inflammation may lead to pain, diarrhea, and bleeding [44]. The precise cause of IBS is unknown; however, it is thought that a multifactor is involved, the complex interplay of genetics and epigenome, environmental factors, and microbiome [45].

It is shown that probiotic administration alleviated the severity of the colitis by decreasing the NF-κB DNA binding activity, and also reducing the accumulation of leukocytes, and downregulating IL-6 and TNF-α production. Probiotics also might be useful in preserving remission and preventing relapse of UC [46, 47]. Other researchers demonstrated the efficacy of probiotics on this disease as well [48, 49]. It should be noted that based on investigating all meta-analysis studies of probiotics on UC published from 2000 to 2020, probiotics supplementations was 100% effective for remission induction and preventing relapse of UC. Therefore, probiotic therapy seems to be a safe and effective method for patient with UC, however, evidence has not proven efficacy of this supplement on CD patients so far [49–52]. A clinical trial confirmed this statement. In a randomized, double-blind, placebo-controlled trial of adult patients with UC and CD, treatment with a multi-strain probiotic supplement or placebo for 4 weeks. The result showed that utilizing probiotics could reduce intestinal inflammation in patients with UC, but not in CD [53].

4. Efficacy of probiotics on respiratory diseases

Studies report that probiotics can play a significant role in treatment and preventing or reducing the duration of respiratory system diseases [54–56] and it might be a practical alternative to promote recovery from these diseases [57, 58]. Besides, some evidence showed that probiotics may stimulate respiratory immunity by improving T regulatory response in the airway and enhance resistance to respiratory tract infections caused by bacteria and viruses [59–61]. Probiotics impact lung microbiota [62] and then exert anti-inflammatory activity in the lungs [63]. For instance, orally administered of *Lactobacillus helveticus* can modulated the immune response in a positive way [64–67]. And this probiotic strain by increasing the number of cells secreting IgA in the intestine and bronchial-associated lymphoid tissue has an immunoprotective impact on mucosal immunity [68]. Evidence indicates that lactic acid bacteria and their metabolites move from gut to lung and exert various immunomodulatory actions [69]. Different probiotic strains including *Bifidobacterium* and *Lactobacillus* were reported to be a great option in treating rotavirus infection in both animals and humans [70–72]. Besides, among chronic respiratory diseases, some probiotic strains have improved at least one symptom of allergic rhinitis (AR). In particular, *Lactobacillus paracasei* LP-33 can enhance the quality of life of patients with AR, according to a meta-analysis study carried out recently [73].

4.1 Influenza

An animal study was done by Lu et al. [69] evaluated the effect of *Lactobacillus mucosae* 1025, *Bifidobacterium breve* CCFM1026, and their mixture on mice infected with the influenza virus for 19 days. The result shows that the clinical symptoms were improved by probiotic treatments. *L. mucosae* 1025 could directly decrease viral loading in the lung, and *B. breve* CCFM1026 might alter the immune responses. However, the mixture reduced viral loading and increased the antiviral protein MxA expression, which none of the single strains alone were not able to increase MxA expression. It is reported this is because of increasing the amount of butyrate production resulting from changing the gut microbiota composition [69]. In addition, other probiotic strains which are tested in mice with influenza infection and their effectiveness were determined are *Bacillus subtilis* 3 [74], *Lactobacillus rhamnosus* M21 [75], *Bacillus subtilis* PY79 [76]. Studies indicate *Bacillus subtilis* 3 is not only effective for the prevention and treatment of influenza but also helpful in the prevention and treatment of bacterial infections in both animal models [77, 78] and humans [78, 79]. The antibacterial property of this strain is due to its ability to produce an antibiotic named aminocoumarin which can suppress a wide range of pathogens and also strengthen host resistance [80]. Furthermore, a double-blinded, placebo-controlled trial of the combination of different probiotic strains containing *Lacticaseibacillus paracasei* subsp. *paracasei, Lactobacillus casei* 431 and *Lactobacillus fermentum* PCC on patients with a common cold and influenza-like infections was conducted by Zhang et al. [81]. In this trial, probiotic mixture 50–60% compared to the placebo group decreased the outbreak of common cold and influenza-like symptoms [81].

4.2 Covid-19

The evidence indicates that gut microbiota dysbiosis happened in COVID-19 patients even 6 months after recovery [82]. Restoring gut microbiota balance has been demonstrated to promote host resistance to viruses or invading pathogens at the respiratory mucosa level [83, 84]. Therefore, administration of prebiotics and probiotics are suggested to COVID-19 patients, to modulate the balance of gut microbiota and decrease the risk of secondary infection due to bacterial translocation [85].

In Covid-19 infected patients, reducing probiotic strains, especially *Lactobacillus* and *Bifidobacterium* may postpone recovery. Consequently, it is suggested that host-microbiota balance should be preserved in the gut and lung which can be beneficial in fighting against COVID-19 [86]. Besides, Mahooti et al. [87] recommend that because probiotics have antiviral properties against other viruses, so they can be a complementary treatment against SARS CoV-2.

In numerous human studies, it has been shown that probiotics, especially, *Lactobacillus rhamnosus* GG, has the ability to improve the barrier of intestinal and lung and homeostasis, by increasing regulatory T cells, enhancing anti-viral defense, and reduce pro-inflammatory cytokines in systemic and respiratory infections. These immunomodulatory agents may be helpful in individuals who have been infected or are at risk of developing, COVID-19 [88].

4.3 Pneumonia

It seems probiotic therapy is a fascinating option as a nonantibiotic method for protection of the host microbiota balance and VAP prevention. Probiotics may probably decrease the incidence of VAP through diverse local and systemic effects that limit the colonization of pathogen species or improve host immune defenses [89]. Numerous studies confirmed the promising efficacy of probiotics on the prevention of VAP [90–95].

A RCT shows that the combination of four probiotic strains including *Lactobacillus acidophilus LA-5*, *Lactobacillus plantarum*, *Bifidobacterium lactis* BB-12, and *Saccharomyces boulardii* could reduce the incidence of VAP by 11.9%, the time of stay in the intensive care unit (ICU) and the length of hospital stay [96]. In addition, a clinical trial shows that using a mixture of probiotic supplements containing *Lactobacillus*, *Bifidobacterium*, and Streptococcus spp. for 14 days, can significantly reduce the length of ICU and hospital stays in VAP patients [97].

Despite a meta-analysis of including 15 randomized controlled trials involving 2039 patients which reported that probiotic therapy could prevent ventilator-associated pneumonia (VAP), and decrease the duration of antibiotic treatment of VAP, however, they had not shown any significant impact on the duration of mechanical ventilation, ICU length of stay and mortality [98]. Another meta-analysis also confirmed that there was no remarkable difference in ICU length of stay between probiotics and placebo groups [92].

Among the investigation we have done on reviewing probiotic meta-analysis studies until 2020, out of 6 studies on pneumonia, 5 of them related to VAP, and one study was on nosocomial pneumonia. The statistics show that probiotic supplementation could be 66.66% effective to prevent ventilator-associated pneumonia.

5. Efficacy of probiotics on metabolic diseases

Many hypotheses surround the feasible involvement of the intestinal microbiota in metabolic disorders such as diabetes and obesity.

5.1 Diabetes

Some evidence suggests that in diabetic patients, disruption in antioxidant defenses happens and free radicals are produced in large amounts [99, 100]. Oxidative stress is considered as one of the major factors in insulin resistance [101], the onset of diabetes and the pathogenesis of diabetic retinopathy as well [102, 103]. Evidence recommends that some probiotic strains are effective in reducing inflammation and oxidative stress in pancreatic cells [104, 105], and they play an important role in preventing the destruction of β-pancreatic cells [106, 107]. A preclinical study of the effect of probiotics on diabetic rats showed that the combination of two probiotic strains including *Lactobacillus acidophilus* and *Lactobacillus casei* could significantly suppress oxidative damage by repressing the lipid peroxidation and protecting the antioxidant content of glutathione, superoxide dismutase, catalase and glutathione peroxidase in their pancreases [108]. It has also been demonstrated that *Bifidobacterium adolescentis* enhances insulin sensitivity [109] by increasing the amount of production of glucagon-like peptide 1 (GLP-1) [110]. GLP-1, a growth factor for pancreatic cells, through complicated mechanisms like modulation of insulin secretion, pancreatic cell mass and food consumption improve glucose tolerance [111]. Furthermore, probiotics have also been found to be effective in reducing blood glucose levels [112–114]. This may be because of properties of probiotics that can ameliorate glucose metabolism via increasing the bioavailability of gliclazide, suppressing or postponing the intestinal absorption of glucose and changing the autonomic nervous activity [115–117]. The result of a clinical trial on 79 diabetic people who had used metformin as a daily treatment, and received multi-probiotic strains or placebo two times a day for 12 weeks, indicates glycated hemoglobin (HbA1c), and weight significantly decreased in the probiotic-utilizing group compared to placebo [118].

5.2 Obesity

Many recent meta-analysis studies proved that probiotics significantly had a promising effect on weight loss and body mass index (BMI) improvement [119–122]. Besides, in one study, it was shown that when the combination of different probiotic strains was used for more than 8 weeks, reducing the body weight and BMI happened [123]. However, some other meta-analysis studies did not approve this statement [124, 125]. Furthermore, in another research was done by million and colleagues reported different species of *Lactobacillus* have different effects on weight in both humans and animals [126]. According to this research probiotic strains associated with weight gain in animals were *Lactobacillus fermentum* and *Lactobacillus ingluviei*.

And a probiotic strain with anti-obesity effect was *Lactobacillus plantarum*, in addition, *Lactobacillus gasseri* was an effective strain for weight loss in both humans and animals [126]. Contradictory results on the effect of probiotics in weight modifications may be due to differences in the probiotic strains and host.

The gut microbiota effects on energy regulation can be a prime factor in the development of obesity [127, 128]. Human intestinal microbiota is a complicated ecosystem that includes numerous kinds of microorganisms like bacteria, viruses, archaea, fungi, protists, nematodes, and phages, involved in various functions of host metabolism [129]. A higher proportion in the strains of *Bacteroides fragilis*, *Clostridium leptum*, and *Bifidobacterium catenulatum* and a lower percentage of *Clostridium coccoides*, *Lactobacillus sensu lato*, and *Bifidobacterium* display considerable weight loss [130, 131], therefore, probiotics may be a powerful tool in modulating obesity by changing the gut microbiota composition [132, 133].

The gut microbiota remarkedly can ferment the indigestible carbohydrates into short-chain fatty acids (SCFAs). SCFAs are the main metabolites of intestinal microbiota which have an important role in energy, glucose, lipid homeostasis and intestinal health [134, 135]. The most plentiful SCFAs are acetate, butyrate, and propionate (encompass 95% of all SCFAs), which are the main substrates for glucose metabolism [129]. Multiple animal studies have shown that the gut microbiota and their metabolites, especially SCFAs, have a significant role in obesity [136–138] and also in the prevention and treatment of obesity-associated insulin resistance [139–142]. Therefore, it is recommended that SCFAs have the ability to control host energy metabolism in the advancement of diet-induced weight and also can be applied for de-novo synthesis of lipid and glucose [143]. However, in human studies, there is contradiction in the association between SCFAs and obesity. For instance, some studies have demonstrated a positive interaction between fecal SCFAs levels [144–146] and obesity while others reported an unfavorable result [147]. Evidence shows that acetate plays an important role in the hypothalamic control of appetite [139] and also increase anorexigenic neuropeptide expression [139] so it is suggested that acetate may be a functional treatment for obesity. Among acetate-producing probiotic strains we can suggest *Methanobrevibacter smithii* and *Blautia hydrogenotrophica* [148]. Chambers et al. have demonstrated that colonic propionate can acutely lessen energy intake and prevent long-term weight gain in people [149]. Considering probiotics, the species of genera *Lactobacillus* and *Bifidobacterium* basically create butyrate and propionate [150]. Butyrate has the ability to alleviate obesity and other metabolic complications which are very usual in western nations [151]. For presentation, a decrease in the number of microbes that produce butyrate in humans is connected with an elevated threat of metabolic disease [152]. *Clostridium butyricum, Faecalibacterium prausnitzii*, *Eubacterium rectale*, *Roseburia* are some of probiotic strains found in the intestines of healthy animals and humans which produce butyrate [153, 154].

5.3 Other metabolic disorders

Meta-analysis studies reporting the effectiveness of probiotic supplementation on lipid and glucose metabolism on pregnant women [155] and patients with diabetes [156]. And also, the result of another meta-analysis study suggests that probiotics should be used as a new way to control and management of lipid profile and blood pressure in type 2 diabetic patients [157]. Probiotics play their role in reducing serum cholesterol (hypocholesterolemia) through some mechanisms including binding cholesterol and fatty acids to the probiotic bacteria's cellular membrane [147], deconjugation of bile acids by the presence of bile salts hydrolase enzymes in lactic acid bacteria [139, 148–150], the transformation of cholesterol to coprostanol and excreted into feces [147]. A clinical trial of 84 pregnant women with gestational diabetes mellitus (GDM) receiving 300 mg/day of yogurt contained two probiotic strains including *Lactobacillus acidophilus* and *Bifidobacterium lactis* or placebo (ordinary yogurt) for 2 months reported that consumption of yogurt probiotics can manage blood glucose better and also the rate of macrosomia might be reduced in pregnant women by GDM through this regimen [158].

6. Effect of probiotics on mental illnesses

6.1 Depression and anxiety

Depression and anxiety are common psychological disorders that they are highly comorbid with each other, and are important public health problems. The efficacy of probiotics on depression and anxiety through meta-analysis studies over the course of 20 years (from 2000 to 2020) was reviewed comprehensively. Half of these studies showed that probiotics could improve the symptoms of these patients [159–162] while the other half reported, probiotic therapy for these mental disorders is not proven [163–166]. In a randomized, double-blind, placebo-controlled trial treatment of 65 multiple sclerosis patients with multi-strain probiotics, promoted mental health parameters [167]. Recent research found that two hypotheses may explain the potential positive effect of probiotics on mood and cognition; one theory is controlling important neurotransmitters and the other is regulating inflammatory markers by these probiotics [168]. Studies exhibit that cytokines increase by inflammatory factors, and subsequently, cytokines effect on synthesis, release, and absorption of neurotransmitters [169–171]. Ultimately, the increased levels of proinflammatory cytokines are associated with neurological disorders such as depression and anxiety. Probiotics improve mood and insomnia in depressed patients [172–174] by reducing inflammatory cytokines Interleukin-1 beta (IL-1β), [175, 176], Interleukin-6 (IL-6), tumor necrosis factor-alpha (TNF-α) [172–174, 176].

7. Conclusion

The effects of probiotics have been widely investigated in a broad spectrum of diseases and are currently suggested as a possible treatment or prevention for several diseases. Different mechanisms are known for the beneficial effects of probiotics, including directly eliminating or preventing pathogens growth by producing antimicrobial substances, eliminating toxins, competing for binding to receptors of epithelial cells, regulating the immune response, reintroducing the microbiota balance, enhancing tight intestinal connections, and also increasing mucus production. Probiotic therapy seems to be a safe and effective method especially, for patients with UC for remission induction and preventing relapse of UC, but, evidence has not proven the efficacy of this supplement on CD patients so far. However, it is needed to taking into account that the biological effects of probiotics on a special disease can be distinctly strain-specific. Therefore, more randomized clinical trials of various probiotic strains in both form of single and mixture on those patients are needed to definitively prove the effectiveness of probiotic microorganisms on these diseases.

Conflict of interest

The authors declare no conflict of interest.

Author details

Kajal Farahmandi[1] and Sadegh Sulaimany[2]*

1 Department of Industrial and Environmental Biotechnology, National Institute of Genetic Engineering and Biotechnology (NIGEB), Tehran, Iran

2 Social and Biological Network Analysis Laboratory (SBNA), Department of Computer Engineering, University of Kurdistan, Sanandaj, Iran

*Address all correspondence to: s.sulaimany@uok.ac.ir

References

[1] Reid G. Probiotics: Definition, scope and mechanisms of action. Best Practice & Research. Clinical Gastroenterology 2016;**30**(1):17-25

[2] Accepted Claims about the Nature of Probiotic Microorganisms in Food—Canada.ca [Internet]. 2022. Available from: https://www.canada.ca/en/health-canada/services/food-nutrition/food-labelling/health-claims/accepted-claims-about-nature-probiotic-microorganisms-food.html

[3] Yao M, Xie J, Du H, McClements DJ, Xiao H, Li L. Progress in microencapsulation of probiotics: A review. Comprehensive Reviews in Food Science and Food Safety. 2020;**19**(2):857-874

[4] Scourboutakos MJ, Franco-Arellano B, Murphy SA, Norsen S, Comelli EM, L'Abbé MR. Mismatch between probiotic benefits in trials versus food products. Nutrients. 2017;**9**(4):400

[5] Farahmandi K, Rajab S, Tabandeh F, Shahraky MK, Maghsoudi A, Ashengroph M. Efficient spray-drying of Lactobacillus rhamnosus PTCC 1637 using total CFU yield as the decision factor. Food Bioscience. 2021;**40**:100816

[6] Amara AA, Shibl A. Role of probiotics in health improvement, infection control and disease treatment and management. Saudi Pharmaceutical Journal. 2015;**23**(2):107-114

[7] Marco ML, Heeney D, Binda S, Cifelli CJ, Cotter PD, Foligné B, et al. Health benefits of fermented foods: Microbiota and beyond. Current Opinion in Biotechnology. 2017;**44**:94-102

[8] Taylor BC, Lejzerowicz F, Poirel M, Shaffer JP, Jiang L, Aksenov A, et al. Consumption of fermented foods is associated with systematic differences in the gut microbiome and metabolome. mSystems [Internet]. 2020;**5**(2). Available from: https://journals.asm.org/doi/10.1128/mSystems.00901-19

[9] Fuller R. Probiotics in man and animals. The Journal of Applied Bacteriology. 1989;**66**(5):365-378

[10] Wan MLY, Forsythe SJ, El-Nezami H. Probiotics interaction with foodborne pathogens: A potential alternative to antibiotics and future challenges. Critical Reviews in Food Science and Nutrition. 2019;**59**(20):3320-3333

[11] Roussel C, Sivignon A, de Vallée A, Garrait G, Denis S, Tsilia V, et al. Anti-infectious properties of the probiotic Saccharomyces cerevisiae CNCM I-3856 on enterotoxigenic E. coli (ETEC) strain H10407. Applied Microbiology and Biotechnology. 2018;**102**(14):6175-6189

[12] De Vrese M, Offick B. Probiotics and prebiotics: Effects on diarrhea. Bioactive Foods in Promoting Health. 2010. pp. 205-227

[13] Patel R, DuPont HL. New approaches for bacteriotherapy: Prebiotics, new-generation probiotics, and synbiotics. Clinical Infectious Diseases. 2015;**60**(suppl_2):108-121

[14] Tegegne BA, Kebede B. Probiotics, their prophylactic and therapeutic applications in human health development: A review of the literature. Heliyon. 2022;**8**(6):e09725

[15] Stavropoulou E, Tsigalou C, Bezirtzoglou E. Spreading of

antimicrobial resistance (AMR) across clinical borders. Erciyes Medical Journal. 2019;**41**:238-243

[16] Bezirtzoglou E, Alexopoulos A, Voidarou C. Apparent antibiotic misuse in environmental ecosystems and food. Microbial Ecology in Health and Disease. 2008;**20**(4):197-198

[17] Choudhari G, Zambare V, Pawar R. Screening, isolation and characterization of probiotically safe lactic acid bacteria from human faeces for biofilm formation. International Journal of Research in BioSciences. 2018;**7**(2):10-18

[18] Pawar R, Zambare V, Nabar B. Comparative assessment of antibiotic resistance in lactic acid bacteria isolated from healthy human adult and infant feces. Nepal Journal of Biotechnology. 2020;**8**(2):69-75

[19] McFarland LV, Dublin S. Meta-analysis of probiotics for the treatment of irritable bowel syndrome. World Journal of Gastroenterology. 2008;**14**(17):2650-2661

[20] Whelan K, Quigley EMM. Probiotics in the management of irritable bowel syndrome and inflammatory bowel disease. Current Opinion in Gastroenterology. 2013;**29**(2):184-189

[21] Cremonini F, Di Caro S, Nista EC, Bartolozzi F, Capelli G, Gasbarrini G, et al. Meta-analysis: The effect of probiotic administration on antibiotic-associated diarrhoea. Alimentary Pharmacology & Therapeutics. 2002;**16**(8):1461-1467

[22] Chmielewska A, Ruszczyński M, Szajewska H. Lactobacillus reuteri strain ATCC 55730 for the treatment of acute infectious diarrhoea in children: A meta-analysis of randomized controlled trials. Pediatria Wspolczesna. 2008;**10**(1):32-36

[23] Szajewska H, Urbańska M, Chmielewska A, Weizman Z, Shamir R. Meta-analysis: *Lactobacillus reuteri* strain DSM 17938 (and the original strain ATCC 55730) for treating acute gastroenteritis in children. Beneficial Microbes. 2014;**5**(3):285-293

[24] Jun P, Jiang H, Xusheng Q, Ziliang T. A meta analysis of the efficacy of *Saccharomyces boulardii* in children with acute diarrhea. African Journal of Pharmacy and Pharmacology. 2012;**6**(21):1508-1514

[25] Dinleyici EC, Eren M, Yargic ZA, Vandenplas Y. Costeffectiveness of add-on probiotics (*Saccharomyces boulardii*) in children with acute rotavirus diarrhea in Turkey (SB-cosTR). In: Proceedings of the 44th Annual Meeting of the European Society for Paediatric Gastroenterology, Hepatology, and Nutrition. 2011. pp. 25-28

[26] Hawrelak JA, Whitten DL, Myers SP. Is *Lactobacillus rhamnosus* GG effective in preventing the onset of antibiotic-associated diarrhoea: A systematic review. Digestion. 2005;**72**(1):51-56

[27] Bhat S, Shreekrishna GN, Savio CD. Efficacy of probiotics in acute diarrhoea in children. International Journal of Contemporary Pediatrics. 2018;**5**(4):1646-1650

[28] Alien SJ, Okoko B, Martínez E, Gregorio G, Dans LF. Probiotics for treating infectious diarrhoea. Cochrane Database of Systematic Reviews. 2003;(4):CD003048. DOI: 10.1002/14651858

[29] Huang JS, Bousvaros A, Lee JW, Diaz A, Davidson EJ. Efficacy of probiotic use in acute diarrhea in children: A meta-analysis. Digestive Diseases and Sciences. 2002;**47**(11):2625-2634

[30] Van Niel CW, Feudtner C, Garrison MM, Christakis DA. Lactobacillus therapy for acute infectious diarrhea in children: A meta-analysis. Pediatrics. 2002;**109**(4):678-684

[31] Szajewska H, Mrukowicz JZ. Probiotics in the treatment and prevention of acute infectious diarrhea in infants and children: A systematic review of published randomized, double-blind, placebo-controlled trials. Journal of Pediatric Gastroenterology and Nutrition. 2001;**33**:S17-S25

[32] Chen K, Xin J, Zhang G, Xie H, Luo L, Yuan S, et al. A combination of three probiotic strains for treatment of acute diarrhoea in hospitalised children: An open label, randomised controlled trial. Beneficial Microbes. 2020;**11**(4):339-346

[33] Isolauri E, Sütas Y, Kankaanpää P, Arvilommi H, Salminen S. Probiotics: Effects on immunity. The American Journal of Clinical Nutrition. 2001;**73**(2):444s-450s

[34] Erickson KL, Hubbard NE. Probiotic immunomodulation in health and disease. The Journal of Nutrition. 2000;**130**(2):403S-409S

[35] Madsen K, Cornish A, Soper P, McKaigney C, Jijon H, Yachimec C, et al. Probiotic bacteria enhance murine and human intestinal epithelial barrier function. Gastroenterology. 2001;**121**(3):580-591

[36] O'Mahony L, McCarthy J, Kelly P, Hurley G, Luo F, Chen K, et al. Lactobacillus and bifidobacterium in irritable bowel syndrome: Symptom responses and relationship to cytokine profiles. Gastroenterology. 2005;**128**(3):541-551

[37] Nikfar S, Rahimi R, Rahimi F, Derakhshani S, Abdollahi M. Efficacy of probiotics in irritable bowel syndrome: A meta-analysis of randomized, controlled trials. Diseases of the Colon & Rectum. 2008;**51**(12):1775-1780

[38] Zhang Y, Li L, Guo C, Mu D, Feng B, Zuo X, et al. Effects of probiotic type, dose and treatment duration on irritable bowel syndrome diagnosed by Rome III criteria: A meta-analysis. BMC Gastroenterology. 2016;**16**(1):62

[39] Cayzeele-Decherf A, Pélerin F, Leuillet S, Douillard B, Housez B, Cazaubiel M, et al. *Saccharomyces cerevisiae* CNCM I-3856 in irritable bowel syndrome: An individual subject meta-analysis. World Journal of Gastroenterology. 2017;**23**(2):336-344

[40] Didari T, Mozaffari S, Nikfar S, Abdollahi M. Effectiveness of probiotics in irritable bowel syndrome: Updated systematic review with meta-analysis. World Journal of Gastroenterology. 2015;**21**(10):3072-3084

[41] Rousseaux C, Thuru X, Gelot A, Barnich N, Neut C, Dubuquoy L, et al. *Lactobacillus acidophilus* modulates intestinal pain and induces opioid and cannabinoid receptors. Nature Medicine. 2007;**13**(1):35-37

[42] Verdu EF, Bercik P, Verma-Gandhu M, Huang XX, Blennerhassett P, Jackson W, et al. Specific probiotic therapy attenuates antibiotic induced visceral hypersensitivity in mice. Gut. 2006;**55**(2):182-190

[43] Connell M, Shin A, James-Stevenson T, Xu H, Imperiale TF, Herron J. Systematic review and meta-analysis: Efficacy of patented probiotic, VSL# 3, in irritable bowel syndrome. Neurogastroenterology & Motility. 2018;**30**(12):e13427

[44] Schölmerich J. Treatment of inflammatory bowel disease. Praxis. 2007;**96**(9):337-343

[45] De Souza HSP, Fiocchi C, Iliopoulos D. The IBD interactome: An integrated view of aetiology, pathogenesis and therapy. Nature Reviews. Gastroenterology & Hepatology. 2017;**14**(12):739-749

[46] Hegazy SK, El-Bedewy MM. Effect of probiotics on pro-inflammatory cytokines and NF-κB activation in ulcerative colitis. World Journal of Gastroenterology: WJG. 2010;**16**(33):4145

[47] Sang LX, Chang B, Zhang WL, Wu XM, Li XH, Jiang M. Remission induction and maintenance effect of probiotics on ulcerative colitis: A meta-analysis. World Journal of Gastroenterology. 2010;**16**(15):1908-1915

[48] Elahi B, Nikfar S, Derakhshani S, Vafaie M, Abdollahi M. On the benefit of probiotics in the management of pouchitis in patients underwent Ileal pouch anal anastomosis: A meta-analysis of controlled clinical trials. Digestive Diseases and Sciences. 2008;**53**(5):1278-1284

[49] Rahimi R, Nikfar S, Rahimi F, Elahi B, Derakhshani S, Vafaie M, et al. A meta-analysis on the efficacy of probiotics for maintenance of remission and prevention of clinical and endoscopic relapse in Crohn's disease. Digestive Diseases and Sciences. 2008;**53**(9):2524-2531

[50] Doherty G, Bennett G, Patil S, Cheifetz A, Moss AC. Interventions for prevention of post-operative recurrence of Crohn's disease. Cochrane Database of Systematic Reviews. 2009;(4):Cd006873

[51] Jin X, Chen X, Zhang Z, Hu W, Ou R, Li S, et al. Long noncoding RNA SNHG12 promotes the progression of cervical cancer via modulating miR-125b/STAT3 axis. Journal of Cellular Physiology. 2019;**234**(5):6624-6632

[52] Derwa Y, Gracie DJ, Hamlin PJ, Ford AC. Systematic review with meta-analysis: The efficacy of probiotics in inflammatory bowel disease. Alimentary Pharmacology & Therapeutics. 2017;**46**(4):389-400

[53] Bjarnason I, Sission G, Hayee BH. A randomised, double-blind, placebo-controlled trial of a multi-strain probiotic in patients with asymptomatic ulcerative colitis and Crohn's disease. Inflammopharmacology [Internet]. 2019;**27**(3):465-473. Available from: https://link.springer.com/article/10.1007/s10787-019-00595-4

[54] King S, Glanville J, Sanders ME, Fitzgerald A, Varley D. Effectiveness of probiotics on the duration of illness in healthy children and adults who develop common acute respiratory infectious conditions: A systematic review and meta-analysis. British Journal of Nutrition. 2014;**112**(01):41-54

[55] Liu S, Hu P, Du X, Zhou T, Pei X. *Lactobacillus rhamnosus* GG supplementation for preventing respiratory infections in children: A meta-analysis of randomized, Placebo-controlled Trials. Indian Pediatrics. 2013;**50**(4):377-381

[56] Wang Y, Li X, Ge T, Xiao Y, Liao Y, Cui Y, et al. Probiotics for prevention and treatment of respiratory tract infections in children: A systematic review and meta-analysis of randomized controlled trials. Medicine. 2016;**95**(31):e4509

[57] Darbandi A, Asadi A, Ghanavati R, Afifirad R, Emamie AD, Talebi M. The effect of probiotics on respiratory tract infection with special emphasis on COVID-19: Systemic review 2010-20. International Journal of Infectious Diseases. 2021;**105**:91-104

[58] Hao Q, Dong BR, Wu T. Probiotics for preventing acute upper respiratory

tract infections. Cochrane Database of Systematic Reviews. 2011;**9**:CD006895

[59] Budden KF, Gellatly SL, Wood DLA, Cooper MA, Morrison M, Hugenholtz P, et al. Emerging pathogenic links between microbiota and the gut–lung axis. Nature Reviews. Microbiology. 2017;**15**(1):55-63

[60] Forsythe P. Probiotics and lung immune responses. Annals of the American Thoracic Society. 2014;**11**(Supplement 1):S33-S37

[61] Mortaz E, Adcock IM, Folkerts G, Barnes PJ, Paul Vos A, Garssen J. Probiotics in the management of lung diseases. Mediators of Inflammation. 2013:1-10

[62] Enaud R, Prevel R, Ciarlo E, Beaufils F, Wieërs G, Guery B, et al. The gut-lung axis in health and respiratory diseases: A place for inter-organ and inter-kingdom crosstalks. Frontiers in Cellular and Infection Microbiology. 2020;**10**:9

[63] McAleer JP, Kolls JK. Contributions of the intestinal microbiome in lung immunity. European Journal of Immunology. 2018;**48**(1):39-49

[64] Vinderola G, Matar C, Perdigón G. Milk fermented by *Lactobacillus helveticus* R389 and its non-bacterial fraction confer enhanced protection against Salmonella enteritidis serovar Typhimurium infection in mice. Immunobiology. 2007;**212**(2):107-118

[65] Vinderola G, Matar C, Perdigón G. Milk fermentation products of *L. helveticus* R389 activate calcineurin as a signal to promote gut mucosal immunity. BMC Immunology. 2007;**8**(1):1-10

[66] LeBlanc JG, Matar C, Valdez JC, LeBlanc J, Perdigon G. Immunomodulating effects of peptidic fractions issued from milk fermented with *Lactobacillus helveticus*. Journal of Dairy Science. 2002;**85**(11):2733-2742

[67] LeBlanc J, Fliss I, Matar C. Induction of a humoral immune response following an *Escherichia coli* O157: H7 infection with an immunomodulatory peptidic fraction derived from *Lactobacillus helveticus*-fermented milk. Clinical and Vaccine Immunology. 2004;**11**(6):1171-1181

[68] Matar C, Valdez JC, Medina M, Rachid M, Perdigon G. Immunomodulating effects of milks fermented by *Lactobacillus helveticus* and its non-proteolytic variant. Journal of Dairy Research. 2001;**68**(4):601-609

[69] Lu W, Fang Z, Liu X, Li L, Zhang P, Zhao J, et al. The potential role of probiotics in protection against influenza a virus infection in mice. Food. 2021;**10**(4):902

[70] Kandasamy S, Vlasova AN, Fischer D, Kumar A, Chattha KS, Rauf A, et al. Differential effects of *Escherichia coli* Nissle and *Lactobacillus rhamnosus* strain GG on human rotavirus binding, infection, and B cell immunity. The Journal of Immunology. 2016;**196**(4):1780-1789

[71] Shornikova AV, Casas IA, Mykkänen H, Salo E, Vesikari T. Bacteriotherapy with *Lactobacillus reuteri* in rotavirus gastroenteritis. The Pediatric Infectious Disease Journal. 1997;**16**(12):1103-1107

[72] Lee DK, Park JE, Kim MJ, Seo JG, Lee JH, Ha NJ. Probiotic bacteria, *B. longum* and *L. acidophilus* inhibit infection by rotavirus in vitro and decrease the duration of diarrhea in pediatric patients. Clinics and Research in Hepatology and Gastroenterology. 2015;**39**(2):237-244

[73] Farahmandi K, Mohr AE, McFarland LV. Effects of probiotics on allergic rhinitis: A systematic review and meta-analysis of randomized clinical trials. American Journal of Rhinology & Allergy. 2022;**36**(4):440-450

[74] Starosila D, Rybalko S, Varbanetz L, Ivanskaya N, Sorokulova I. Anti-influenza activity of a *Bacillus subtilis* probiotic strain. Antimicrobial Agents and Chemotherapy. 2017;**61**(7):e00539-e00517

[75] Song JA, Kim HJ, Hong SK, Lee DH, Lee SW, Song CS, et al. Oral intake of *Lactobacillus rhamnosus* M21 enhances the survival rate of mice lethally infected with influenza virus. Journal of Microbiology, Immunology and Infection. 2016;**49**(1):16-23

[76] Song M, Hong HA, Huang JM, Colenutt C, Khang DD, Nguyen TVA, et al. Killed *Bacillus subtilis* spores as a mucosal adjuvant for an H5N1 vaccine. Vaccine. 2012;**30**(22):3266-3277

[77] Sorokulova IB, Kirik DL, Pinchuk IV. Probiotics against *Campylobacter pathogens*. Journal of Travel Medicine. 1997;**4**(4):167-170

[78] Sorokulova I. Preclinical testing in the development of probiotics: A regulatory perspective with Bacillus strains as an example. Clinical Infectious Diseases. 2008;**46**(Supplement_2):S92-S95

[79] Gracheva NM, Gavrilov AF, Solov'eva AI, Smirnov VV, Sorokulova IB, Reznik SR, et al. The efficacy of the new bacterial preparation biosporin in treating acute intestinal infections. Zhurnal Mikrobiologii, Epidemiologii, i Immunobiologii. 1996;(1):75-77

[80] Rybalko SL, Khristova ML, Shapiro AV, Varbanets LD, Zubkova NL, Zadorozhna VI, et al. Usage of new bacterial adjuvants for vaccination by anti-influenza and anti-poliomyelitis vaccines. Biopolymers and Cell. 2003;**19**(3):262-269

[81] Zhang H, Yeh C, Jin Z, Ding L, Liu BY, Zhang L, et al. Prospective study of probiotic supplementation results in immune stimulation and improvement of upper respiratory infection rate. Synthetic and Systems Biotechnology. 2018;**3**(2):113-120

[82] Chen Y, Gu S, Chen Y, Lu H, Shi D, Guo J, et al. Six-month follow-up of gut microbiota richness in patients with COVID-19. Gut. 2022;**71**(1):222-225

[83] Zelaya H, Alvarez S, Kitazawa H, Villena J. Respiratory antiviral immunity and immunobiotics: Beneficial effects on inflammation-coagulation interaction during influenza virus infection. Frontiers in Immunology. 2016;7:633

[84] Racedo S, Villena J, Salva S, Alvarez S. Influence of yogurt consumption on the respiratory immune response. Food and Agricultural Immunology. 2009;**20**(3):231-244

[85] Xu K, Cai H, Shen Y, Ni Q, Chen Y, Hu S, et al. 冠状病毒病 (COVID-19) 诊疗浙江经验 management of COVID-19: The Zhejiang experience. Zhejiang Da Xue Xue Bao. Yi Xue Ban. 2019;**2020**:147-157

[86] Nguyen QV, Chong LC, Hor YY, Lew LC, Rather IA, Choi SB. Role of probiotics in the management of COVID-19: A computational perspective. Nutrients. 2022;**14**(2):274

[87] Mahooti M, Miri SM, Abdolalipour E, Ghaemi A. The immunomodulatory effects of probiotics on respiratory viral infections: A hint for COVID-19 treatment? Microbial Pathogenesis. 2020;**148**:104452

[88] Bottari B, Castellone V, Neviani E. Probiotics and COVID-19. International Journal of Food Sciences and Nutrition. 2021;**72**(3):293-299

[89] Morrow LE, Kollef MH, Casale TB. Probiotic prophylaxis of ventilator-associated pneumonia: A blinded, randomized, controlled trial. American Journal of Respiratory and Critical Care Medicine. 2010;**182**(8):1058-1064

[90] Batra P, Soni KD, Mathur P. Efficacy of probiotics in the prevention of VAP in critically ill ICU patients: An updated systematic review and meta-analysis of randomized control trials. Journal of Intensive Care. 2020;**8**(1):1-14

[91] Su M, Jia Y, Li Y, Zhou D, Jia J. Probiotics for the prevention of ventilator-associated pneumonia: A meta-analysis of randomized controlled trials. Respiratory Care. 2020;**65**(5):673-685

[92] Fan QL, Yu XM, Liu QX, Yang W, Chang Q, Zhang YP. Synbiotics for prevention of ventilator-associated pneumonia: A probiotics strain-specific network meta-analysis. Journal of International Medical Research. 2019;**47**(11):5349-5374

[93] Bo L, Li J, Tao T, Bai Y, Ye X, Hotchkiss RS, et al. Probiotics for preventing ventilator-associated pneumonia. Cochrane Database of Systematic Reviews. 2014;**10**:CD009066

[94] Siempos II, Ntaidou TK, Falagas ME. Impact of the administration of probiotics on the incidence of ventilator-associated pneumonia: A meta-analysis of randomized controlled trials. Critical Care Medicine. 2010;**38**(3):954-962

[95] Shimizu K, Yamada T, Ogura H, Mohri T, Kiguchi T, Fujimi S, et al. Synbiotics modulate gut microbiota and reduce enteritis and ventilator-associated pneumonia in patients with sepsis: A randomized controlled trial. Critical Care. 2018;**22**(1):1-9

[96] Tsilika M, Thoma G, Aidoni Z, Tsaousi G, Fotiadis K, Stavrou G, et al. A four-probiotic preparation for ventilator-associated pneumonia in multi-trauma patients: Results of a randomized clinical trial. International Journal of Antimicrobial Agents. 2022;**59**(1):106471

[97] Mahmoodpoor A, Hamishehkar H, Asghari R, Abri R, Shadvar K, Sanaie S. Effect of a probiotic preparation on ventilator-associated pneumonia in critically ill patients admitted to the intensive care unit: A prospective double-blind randomized controlled trial. Nutrition in Clinical Practice. 2019;**34**(1):156-162

[98] Zhao J, Li L, qing, Chen C yang, Zhang G sheng, Cui W, Tian B ping. Do probiotics help prevent ventilator-associated pneumonia in critically ill patients? A systematic review with meta-analysis. ERJ Open Research. 2021;7(1):00302-2020

[99] Maritim AC, Sanders aRA, Watkins Iii JB. Diabetes, oxidative stress, and antioxidants: A review. Journal of Biochemical and Molecular Toxicology. 2003;**17**(1):24-38

[100] Lipinski B. Pathophysiology of oxidative stress in diabetes mellitus. Journal of Diabetes and its Complications. 2001;**15**(4):203-210

[101] Houstis N, Rosen ED, Lander ES. Reactive oxygen species have a causal role in multiple forms of insulin resistance. Nature. 2006;**440**(7086):944-948

[102] Rösen P, Nawroth PP, King G, Möller W, Tritschler H, Packer L. The

role of oxidative stress in the onset and progression of diabetes and its complications: A summary of a congress series sponsored byUNESCO-MCBN, the American Diabetes Association and the German diabetes society. Diabetes/Metabolism Research and Reviews. 2001;**17**(3):189-212

[103] Behl T, Kaur I, Kotwani A. Implication of oxidative stress in progression of diabetic retinopathy. Survey of Ophthalmology. 2016;**61**(2):187-196

[104] Harisa GI, Taha EI, Khalil AF, Salem MM. Oral administration of Lactobacillus acidophilus restores nitric oxide level in diabetic rats. Australian Journal of Basic and Applied Sciences. 2009;**3**(3):2963-2969

[105] Valladares R, Sankar D, Li N, Williams E, Lai KK, Abdelgeliel AS, et al. Lactobacillus johnsonii N6. 2 mitigates the development of type 1 diabetes in BB-DP rats. PLoS One. 2010;**5**(5):e10507

[106] Lin MY, Yen CL. Antioxidative ability of lactic acid bacteria. Journal of Agricultural and Food Chemistry. 1999;**47**(4):1460-1466

[107] Uskova MA, Kravchenko LV. Antioxidant properties of lactic acid bacteria--probiotic and yogurt strains. Voprosy Pitaniia. 2009;**78**(2):18-23

[108] Yadav H, Jain S, Sinha PR. Oral administration of dahi containing probiotic *Lactobacillus acidophilus* and *Lactobacillus casei* delayed the progression of streptozotocin-induced diabetes in rats. Journal of Dairy Research. 2008;**75**(2):189-195

[109] Chen J, Wang R, Li XF, Wang RL. Bifidobacterium adolescentis supplementation ameliorates visceral fat accumulation and insulin sensitivity in an experimental model of the metabolic syndrome. British Journal of Nutrition. 2012;**107**(10):1429-1434

[110] Cani PD, Daubioul CA, Reusens B, Remacle C, Catillon G, Delzenne NM. Involvement of endogenous glucagon-like peptide-1 (7-36) amide on glycaemia-lowering effect of oligofructose in streptozotocin-treated rats. Journal of Endocrinology. 2005;**185**(3):457-465

[111] Drucker DJ. Glucagon-like peptides: Regulators of cell proliferation, differentiation, and apoptosis. Molecular Endocrinology. 2003;**17**(2):161-171

[112] Pan YQ, Zheng QX, Jiang XM, Chen XQ, Zhang XY, Wu JL. Probiotic supplements improve blood glucose and insulin resistance/sensitivity among healthy and GDM pregnant women: A systematic review and Meta-analysis of randomized controlled trials. Evidence-Based Complementary and Alternative Medicine. 2021;**2021**:1-17

[113] Peng TR, Wu TW, Chao YC. Effect of probiotics on the glucose levels of pregnant women: A meta-analysis of randomized controlled trials. Medicina (B Aires). 2018;**54**(5):77

[114] Nikbakht E, Khalesi S, Singh I, Williams LT, West NP, Colson N. Effect of probiotics and synbiotics on blood glucose: A systematic review and meta-analysis of controlled trials. European Journal of Nutrition. 2018;**57**(1):95-106

[115] Borthakur A, Gill RK, Tyagi S, Koutsouris A, Alrefai WA, Hecht GA, et al. The probiotic Lactobacillus acidophilus stimulates chloride/hydroxyl exchange activity in human intestinal epithelial cells. The Journal of Nutrition. 2008;**138**(7):1355-1359

[116] Al-Salami H, Butt G, Tucker I, Skrbic R, Golocorbin-Kon S,

Mikov M. Probiotic pre-treatment reduces Gliclazide permeation (ex vivo) in healthy rats but increases it in diabetic rats to the level seen in untreated healthy rats. Archives of Drug Information. 2008;**1**(1):35-41

[117] Yamano T, Tanida M, Niijima A, Maeda K, Okumura N, Fukushima Y, et al. Effects of the probiotic strain *Lactobacillus johnsonii* strain La1 on autonomic nerves and blood glucose in rats. Life Sciences. 2006;**79**(20):1963-1967

[118] Madempudi RS, Ahire JJ, Neelamraju J, Tripathi A, Nanal S. Efficacy of UB0316, a multi-strain probiotic formulation in patients with type 2 diabetes mellitus: A double blind, randomized, placebo controlled study. PLoS One. 2019;**14**(11):e0225168. Available from: https://journals.plos.org/plosone/article?id=10.1371/journal.pone.0225168

[119] Koutnikova H, Genser B, Monteiro-Sepulveda M, Faurie JM, Rizkalla S, Schrezenmeir J, et al. Impact of bacterial probiotics on obesity, diabetes and non-alcoholic fatty liver disease related variables: A systematic review and meta-analysis of randomised controlled trials. BMJ Open. 2019;**9**(3):e017995

[120] Wang ZB, Xin SS, Ding LN, Ding WY, Hou YL, Liu CQ, et al. The potential role of probiotics in controlling overweight/obesity and associated metabolic parameters in adults: A systematic review and meta-analysis. Evidence-Based Complementary and Alternative Medicine. 2019;**2019**:1-14

[121] Borgeraas H, Johnson LK, Skattebu J, Hertel JK, Hjelmesaeth J. Effects of probiotics on body weight, body mass index, fat mass and fat percentage in subjects with overweight or obesity: A systematic review and meta-analysis of randomized controlled trials. Obesity Reviews. 2018;**19**(2):219-232

[122] John GK, Wang L, Nanavati J, Singh R, Mullin G. Mo1963—*Lactobacillus probiotics* reduce body mass index, body weight, and fat mass in overweight and obese subjects: A systematic review and meta-analysis of randomized controlled trials. Gastroenterology. 2018;**154**(6):S-865-S-866

[123] Zhang Q, Wu Y, Fei X. Effect of probiotics on body weight and body-mass index: A systematic review and meta-analysis of randomized, controlled trials. International Journal of Food Sciences and Nutrition. 2016;**67**(5):571-580

[124] Suzumura EA, Bersch-Ferreira ÂC, Torreglosa CR, da Silva JT, Coqueiro AY, Kuntz MGF, et al. Effects of oral supplementation with probiotics or synbiotics in overweight and obese adults: A systematic review and meta-analyses of randomized trials. Nutrition Reviews. 2019;**77**(6):430-450

[125] Park S, Bae JH. Probiotics for weight loss: A systematic review and meta-analysis. Nutrition Research. 2015;**35**(7):566-575

[126] Million M, Angelakis E, Paul M, Armougom F, Leibovici L, Raoult D. Comparative meta-analysis of the effect of Lactobacillus species on weight gain in humans and animals. Microbial Pathogenesis. 2012;**53**(2):100-108

[127] Flint HJ, Scott KP, Louis P, Duncan SH. The role of the gut microbiota in nutrition and health. Nature Reviews. Gastroenterology & Hepatology. 2012;**9**(10):577

[128] Moreno-Indias I, Cardona F, Tinahones FJ, Queipo-Ortuño MI. Impact

of the gut microbiota on the development of obesity and type 2 diabetes mellitus. Frontiers in Microbiology. 2014;**5**:190

[129] Cerdó T, García-Santos JA, G. Bermúdez M, Campoy C. The role of probiotics and prebiotics in the prevention and treatment of obesity. Nutrients. 2019;**11**(3):635

[130] Cotillard A, Kennedy SP, Kong LC, Prifti E, Pons N, Le Chatelier E, et al. Dietary intervention impact on gut microbial gene richness. Nature. 2013;**500**(7464):585

[131] Le Chatelier E, Nielsen T, Qin J, Prifti E, Hildebrand F, Falony G, et al. Richness of human gut microbiome correlates with metabolic markers. Nature. 2013;**500**(7464):541

[132] Kadooka Y, Sato M, Ogawa A, Miyoshi M, Uenishi H, Ogawa H, et al. Effect of *Lactobacillus gasseri* SBT2055 in fermented milk on abdominal adiposity in adults in a randomised controlled trial. British Journal of Nutrition. 2013;**110**(9):1696-1703

[133] Zarrati M, Shidfar F, Nourijelyani K, Mofid V, Hossein Zadeh-Attar MJ, Bidad K, et al. *Lactobacillus acidophilus* La5, Bifidobacterium BB12, and *Lactobacillus casei* DN001 modulate gene expression of subset specific transcription factors and cytokines in peripheral blood mononuclear cells of obese and overweight people. BioFactors. 2013;**39**(6):633-643

[134] Murugesan S, Nirmalkar K, Hoyo-Vadillo C, García-Espitia M, Ramírez-Sánchez D, García-Mena J. Gut microbiome production of short-chain fatty acids and obesity in children. European Journal of Clinical Microbiology & Infectious Diseases. 2018;**37**(4):621-625

[135] de Clercq NC, Groen AK, Romijn JA, Nieuwdorp M. Gut microbiota in obesity and undernutrition. Advances in Nutrition. 2016;**7**(6):1080-1089

[136] den Besten G, Lange K, Havinga R, van Dijk TH, Gerding A, van Eunen K, et al. Gut-derived short-chain fatty acids are vividly assimilated into host carbohydrates and lipids. American Journal of Physiology-Gastrointestinal and Liver Physiology. 2013;**305**(12):G900-G910

[137] Liou AP, Paziuk M, Luevano JM Jr, Machineni S, Turnbaugh PJ, Kaplan LM. Conserved shifts in the gut microbiota due to gastric bypass reduce host weight and adiposity. Science Translational Medicine. 2013;**5**(178):178ra41-178ra41

[138] Perry RJ, Peng L, Barry NA, Cline GW, Zhang D, Cardone RL, et al. Acetate mediates a microbiome–brain–β-cell axis to promote metabolic syndrome. Nature. 2016;**534**(7606):213-217

[139] Frost G, Sleeth ML, Sahuri-Arisoylu M, Lizarbe B, Cerdan S, Brody L, et al. The short-chain fatty acid acetate reduces appetite via a central homeostatic mechanism. Nature Communications. 2014;**5**:3611

[140] Li Z, Yi CX, Katiraei S, Kooijman S, Zhou E, Chung CK, et al. Butyrate reduces appetite and activates brown adipose tissue via the gut-brain neural circuit. Gut. 2018;**67**(7):1269-1279

[141] Den Besten G, Bleeker A, Gerding A, van Eunen K, Havinga R, van Dijk TH, et al. Short-chain fatty acids protect against high-fat diet–induced obesity via a PPARγ-dependent switch from lipogenesis to fat oxidation. Diabetes. 2015;**64**(7):2398-2408

[142] Lu Y, Fan C, Li P, Lu Y, Chang X, Qi K. Short chain fatty acids prevent

high-fat-diet-induced obesity in mice by regulating G protein-coupled receptors and gut microbiota. Scientific Reports. 2016;**6**:37589

[143] Kim KN, Yao Y, Ju SY. Short chain fatty acids and fecal microbiota abundance in humans with obesity: A systematic review and meta-analysis. Nutrients. 2019;**11**(10):2512

[144] Rahat-Rozenbloom S, Fernandes J, Gloor GB, Wolever TMS. Evidence for greater production of colonic short-chain fatty acids in overweight than lean humans. International Journal of Obesity. 2014;**38**(12):1525-1531

[145] Fernandes J, Su W, Rahat-Rozenbloom S, Wolever TMS, Comelli EM. Adiposity, gut microbiota and faecal short chain fatty acids are linked in adult humans. Nutrition & Diabetes. 2014;**4**(6):e121-e121

[146] Riva A, Borgo F, Lassandro C, Verduci E, Morace G, Borghi E, et al. Pediatric obesity is associated with an altered gut microbiota and discordant shifts in F irmicutes populations. Environmental Microbiology. 2017;**19**(1):95-105

[147] Barczyńska R, Litwin M, Sliżewska K, Szalecki M, Berdowska A, Bandurska K, et al. Bacterial microbiota and fatty acids in the faeces of overweight and obese children. Polish Journal of Microbiology. 2018;**67**(3):339-345

[148] Ashaolu TJ. Immune boosting functional foods and their mechanisms: A critical evaluation of probiotics and prebiotics. Biomedicine & Pharmacotherapy. 2020;**130**:110625

[149] Chambers ES, Viardot A, Psichas A, Morrison DJ, Murphy KG, Zac-Varghese SEK, et al. Effects of targeted delivery of propionate to the human colon on appetite regulation, body weight maintenance and adiposity in overweight adults. Gut. 2015;**64**(11):1744-1754

[150] Pessione E. Lactic acid bacteria contribution to gut microbiota complexity: Lights and shadows. Frontiers in Cellular and Infection Microbiology. 2012;**2**:86

[151] Brahe LK, Astrup A, Larsen LH. Is butyrate the link between diet, intestinal microbiota and obesity-related metabolic diseases? Obesity Reviews. 2013;**14**(12):950-959

[152] Isolauri E. Microbiota and obesity. Intestinal Microbiome: Functional Aspects in Health and Disease. 2017;**88**:95-106

[153] Kumar A, Wu H, Collier-Hyams LS, Kwon YM, Hanson JM, Neish AS. The bacterial fermentation product butyrate influences epithelial signaling via reactive oxygen species-mediated changes in cullin-1 neddylation. The Journal of Immunology. 2009;**182**(1):538-546

[154] Louis P, Flint HJ. Diversity, metabolism and microbial ecology of butyrate-producing bacteria from the human large intestine. FEMS Microbiology Letters. 2009;**294**(1):1-8

[155] Han MM, Sun JF, Su XH, Peng YF, Goyal H, Wu CH, et al. Probiotics improve glucose and lipid metabolism in pregnant women: A meta-analysis. Annals of Translational Medicine. 2019;**7**(5):99-111

[156] Tabrizi R, Moosazadeh M, Lankarani KB, Akbari M, Heydari ST, Kolahdooz F, et al. The effects of synbiotic supplementation on glucose metabolism and lipid

profiles in patients with diabetes: A systematic review and meta-analysis of randomized controlled trials. Probiotics and Antimicrobial Proteins. 2018;**10**(2):329-342

[157] He J, Zhang F, Han Y. Effect of probiotics on lipid profiles and blood pressure in patients with type 2 diabetes: A meta-analysis of RCTs. Medicine. 2017;**96**(51):e9166

[158] Sahhaf Ebrahimi F, Homayouni Rad A, Mosen M, Abbasalizadeh F, Tabrizi A, Khalili L. Effect of *L. acidophilus* and *B. lactis* on blood glucose in women with gestational diabetes mellitus: A randomized placebo-controlled trial. Diabetology & Metabolic Syndrome. 2019;**11**(1):1-7. Available from: https://dmsjournal.biomedcentral.com/articles/10.1186/s13098-019-0471-5

[159] Huang R, Wang K, Hu J. Effect of probiotics on depression: A systematic review and meta-analysis of randomized controlled trials. Nutrients. 2016;**8**(8):483

[160] Liu RT, Walsh RFL, Sheehan AE. Prebiotics and probiotics for depression and anxiety: A systematic review and meta-analysis of controlled clinical trials. Neuroscience and Biobehavioral Reviews. 2019;**102**:13-23

[161] Reis DJ, Ilardi SS, Punt SEW. The anxiolytic effect of probiotics: A systematic review and meta-analysis of the clinical and preclinical literature. PLoS One. 2018;**13**(6):e0199041

[162] Huang R, Ning H, Yang L, Jia C, Yang F, Xu G, et al. Efficacy of probiotics on anxiety: A meta-analysis of randomized controlled trials. Neuropsychiatry. 2017;**07**(06):862-871

[163] Liu B, He Y, Wang M, Liu J, Ju Y, Zhang Y, et al. Efficacy of probiotics on anxiety-a meta-analysis of randomized controlled trials. Depression and Anxiety. 2018;**35**(10):935-945

[164] Zhang N, Liao X, Zhang Y, Li M, Wang W, Zhai S. Probiotic supplements for relieving stress in healthy participants: A protocol for systematic review and meta-analysis of randomized controlled trials. Medicine. 2019;**98**(20):e15416

[165] Nikolova V, Zaidi SY, Young AH, Cleare AJ, Stone JM. Gut feeling: Randomized controlled trials of probiotics for the treatment of clinical depression: Systematic review and meta-analysis. Therapeutic Advances in Psychopharmacology. 2019;**9**:2045125319859963

[166] Ng QX, Peters C, Ho CYX, Lim DY, Yeo WS. A meta-analysis of the use of probiotics to alleviate depressive symptoms. Journal of Affective Disorders. 2018;**228**:13-19

[167] Rahimlou M, Hosseini SA, Majdinasab N, Haghighizadeh MH, Husain D. Effects of long-term administration of multi-strain probiotic on circulating levels of BDNF, NGF, IL-6 and mental health in patients with multiple sclerosis: A randomized, double-blind, placebo-controlled trial. Nutritional Neuroscience. 2020;**25**(2):411-422. DOI: 101080/1028415X20201758887. Available from: https://www.tandfonline.com/doi/abs/10.1080/1028415X.2020.1758887

[168] Wallace CJK, Milev R. The effects of probiotics on depressive symptoms in humans: A systematic review. Annals of General Psychiatry. 2017;**16**(1):14

[169] Miller AH, Maletic V, Raison CL. Inflammation and its discontents: The role of cytokines in the pathophysiology

of major depression. Biological Psychiatry. 2009;**65**(9):732-741

[170] Anisman H, Merali Z, Hayley S. Neurotransmitter, peptide and cytokine processes in relation to depressive disorder: Comorbidity between depression and neurodegenerative disorders. Progress in Neurobiology. 2008;**85**(1):1-74

[171] Dunn AJ. Effects of cytokines and infections on brain neurochemistry. Clinical Neuroscience Research. 2006;**6**(1-2):52-68

[172] Paterson LM, Nutt DJ, Wilson SJ. NAPSAQ-1: National Patient Sleep Assessment Questionnaire in depression. International Journal of Psychiatry in Clinical Practice. 2009;**13**(1):48-58

[173] Jackson ML, Butt H, Ball M, Lewis DP, Bruck D. Sleep quality and the treatment of intestinal microbiota imbalance in chronic fatigue syndrome: A pilot study. Sleep Science. 2015;**8**(3):124-133

[174] McEwen BS. Physiology and neurobiology of stress and adaptation: Central role of the brain. Physiological Reviews. 2007;**87**(3):873-904

[175] Luo J, Wang T, Liang S, Hu X, Li W, Jin F. Ingestion of Lactobacillus strain reduces anxiety and improves cognitive function in the hyperammonemia rat. Science China. Life Sciences. 2014;**57**(3):327-335

[176] Ait-Belgnaoui A, Durand H, Cartier C, Chaumaz G, Eutamene H, Ferrier L, et al. Prevention of gut leakiness by a probiotic treatment leads to attenuated HPA response to an acute psychological stress in rats. Psychoneuroendocrinology. 2012;**37**(11):1885-1895

Chapter 5

Adherence of *Candida albicans* on Polymethyl Methacrylate in Probiotics Solution

Arezoo Aghakouchakzadeh, Niayesh Daneshvarpour and Ahmadreza Mirzaei

Abstract

Probiotics are living microorganisms that induce health benefits and advantages on the host, especially when it is used in an adequate amount. Over the years, different definitions of probiotics are established based on their mechanisms, site of action, delivery format, method, or host. As probiotics have various effects, they are used in different areas and one of them is dentistry. Approximately 150 species of yeast are referred to as Candida. Normally, Candida lives without causing harm to its environment which in the most cases is the mucus membranes of various parts of the body, including the ears, eyes, gastrointestinal tract, mouth, nose, reproductive organs, sinuses, skin, stool, and vagina. These mucus membranes are known as beneficial flora and the yeast component in the flora performs important functions in the human body. However, an overgrowth of *Candida albicans* results from an imbalance in the body's normal flora. The term is Candidiasis or Thrush. Most common way to treat this condition is by using Nystatin solution. According to new studies, probiotic solutions can be used to reduce the number of *Candida albicans* adherence and thereby treat Candidiasis or Thrush. We aim to discuss the actual role of probiotic solutions in oral cavity and treatment of Candidiasis.

Keywords: probiotics, probiotic solutions, dentistry, candidiasis, thrush, oral cavity, normal flora, denture stomatitis

1. Introduction

The term probiotic comes from the Greek language meaning "for life." It was first introduced by Lilly and Stillwell in 1965 to describe substances that stimulate the growth of microorganisms. In 1971, Sperti used the probiotic term to define substances secreted by tissue, which have the ability to stimulate microbial growth. Parker first used the term probiotic in relation to its modern usage, defining it as "organisms and substances that contribute to intestinal microbial balance." Later, Fuller amended this definition by emphasizing the important role of probiotics in establishing the balance of intestinal microbial. This reformed definition emphasizes on the requirement of viability for probiotics and introduces the aspect of a beneficial effect on the host. Havenaar et al. expanded the definition further to include mono or mixed cultures of microorganisms applied to animals or humans that improve the properties of the indigenous microflora. Salminen and Schaafsma further broadened the definition of probiotics to include dairy products such as fermented cereals, sauerkraut, and salami that contain viable probiotic microorganisms. This definition showed that probiotics benefit, effect health and nutrition of the host. Salminen and Schaafsma broadened the definition of probiotics even further by no longer limiting the proposed health effects to influences on the indigenous microflora.

Today, we know that unlike Salminen definition probiotic microorganisms are also can be find in nondairy products [1].

Candida is actually another name for fungi that define over 150 yeast species that exists harmlessly in healthy individuals. An imbalance in normal flora may lead to an overgrowth of one of these species named as *Candida albicans*, which can cause candidiasis or thrush, a fungal infection that has a widespread impact on the body's overall health and well-being. Candida is one of the normal flora substances, which is known as "beneficial flora" and also has a useful purpose in the body. When there is an imbalance in the normal flora, it can cause an overgrowth in the number of *Candida albicans*. The expression used for the overgrowth of *Candida albicans* that may lead to an infection is Candidiasis or Thrush. This is a fungal infection which is also called Mycosis through any of the species of Candida; however, *Candida albicans* is the most common one. When this infection happens, it can cause a widespread deterioration to our overall health and well-being of the body.

Oral candidiasis is a common fungal infection in the oral mucosa, caused by *Candida albicans*. Many people have this organism, and the rate of carriage increases with age [2]. Denture stomatitis, an inflammation of the denture-bearing mucosa affecting two-thirds of elderly denture wearers, is often associated with Candida. It is more common on the palatal mucosa and in female patients [3].

There are different types of denture materials and one of the most common of them is polymethyl methacrylate. Polymethyl methacrylate is a lightweight, synthetic polymer that is an economical alternative to polycarbonate. Unlike polycarbonate, polymethyl methacrylate (PMMA) does not contain potential harmful subunits, such as bisphenol-A, and is easier to handle, process, and less expensive. This chapter aims to discuss the effect of probiotic solutions on the adherence of *Candida albicans* to polymethyl methacrylate dentures.

In this chapter, we aim to talk about the effect of probiotic solutions on adherence of *candida albicans* to polymethyl methacrylate dentures.

2. Probiotic bacteria

The international definition of probiotics is "a living microorganisms that induce health benefits and advantages on the host, especially when it is used in an adequate amount." Over the years, different definitions of probiotics are established based on their mechanisms, site of action, delivery format, method, or host. As probiotics have various effects, they are used in different areas [1].

2.1 History

The term probiotic comes from the Greek language meaning "for life." It was first introduced by Lilly and Stillwell in 1965 to describe substances that stimulate the growth of microorganisms. In 1971, Sperti used the probiotic term to define substances secreted by tissue which have the ability to stimulate microbial growth. Parker first used the term probiotic in relation to its modern usage, defining it as "organisms and substances that contribute to intestinal microbial balance." Later, Fuller amended this definition by emphasizing the important role of probiotics in establishing the balance of intestinal microbial. This reformed definition emphasizes on the requirement of viability for probiotics and introduces the aspect of a beneficial effect on the host. Havenaar et al. expanded the definition further to include mono or mixed cultures of microorganisms applied to animals or humans that improve the properties of the indigenous microflora. Salminen and Schaafsma further broadened the definition of probiotics to include dairy products such as fermented cereals, sauerkraut, and salami that contain viable probiotic microorganisms. This definition showed that probiotics benefit, effect health and nutrition of the host. Salminen and Schaafsma broadened the definition of probiotics even further by no longer limiting the proposed health effects to influences on the indigenous microflora.

According to today's definition, probiotics are called "healthy bacteria" with many health benefits such as preventing intestinal infections, improving immunity, lactose intolerance and intestinal microbial balance, and anti-hypercholesterolemia and antihypertensive effect, and reduces traveler's diarrhea. Recent research has also focused on their use in the treatment of skin and mouth diseases [2].

2.2 Probiotics and oral cavity

Because oral cavity is the first section of the gastrointestinal tract, it is logical to think that some probiotics may affect the oral microbiota. The most commonly used probiotic bacterial strains are the *genera Lactobacillus* and *Bifidobacterium*. Specific *lactobacilli* species are yet to be identified as exclusively in oral microbiota, although some common ones include *L. paracasei, L. plantarum, L. rhamnosus, and L. salivarius. Bifidobacteria* is among the first anaerobic bacteria to colonize in the oral cavity, and possible species isolated from oral samples are *B. bifidum, B. dentium, and B. longum*. Culture-based studies confirm that *bifidobacteria* is among the first anaerobes in the oral cavity. Indeed, both *lactobacilli* and *bifidobacteria* can be found in breast milk, suggesting early exposure of the oral cavity to these bacteria [4].

2.3 Potential mechanisms of probiotic effects in the oral cavity

Probiotics can improve oral health through three main mechanisms: normalization of oral microbiota, modulation of the immune response, and metabolic effects. By inhibiting harmful bacteria and promoting beneficial bacteria, probiotics can help restore balance in the mouth and reduce the risk of gum disease and tooth decay. Probiotics can also modulate the immune response and prevent inflammation, particularly in individuals with compromised immune systems. Lastly, probiotics can have metabolic effects that improve overall oral health by breaking down food particles and preventing the buildup of plaque and tartar. In summary, the potential mechanisms of probiotic action in the oral cavity resemble those in the intestine and can benefit oral health significantly [5].

2.4 Observed effects of probiotics on oral health

- Oral candida
- Caries and caries-associated microbes

- Periodontal disease
- Halitosis

(Focus of this chapter is on the effect of probiotic bacteria on adherence of *Candida albicans* on polymethacrylate denture. However, we will talk about other titles briefly).

3. Candida

Candida refers to a type of fungi that includes over 150 species of yeast. Typically, Candida exists without causing harm in healthy individuals who are not immunosuppressed. It is present in various mucosal areas, such as the ears, eyes, gastrointestinal tract, mouth, nose, reproductive organs, sinuses, skin, stool, and vagina, and is referred to as the "beneficial flora" due to its useful purpose in the body. However, an imbalance in the normal flora can cause *Candida albicans*, among other species, to overgrow and cause a fungal infection called Candidiasis or Thrush.

If Candidiasis occurs, it can lead to significant negative impacts on overall health and well-being it and can create a widespread impairment to our overall health and well-being of body.

Oral candidiasis is one of the fungal diseases affecting the oral mucosa. This infection is caused by the yeast *Candida albicans*. As explained, *Candida albicans* is one of the normal substances of oral microflora, found in approximately 30 to 50% of people. The carrier increased with the age of the patient. One of the conditions associated with Candida is denture stomatitis [2].

3.1 Denture stomatitis

Denture stomatitis is a term that has been applied to an inflammation of the denture-bearing mucosa, which may affect as many as two-thirds of an elderly population of denture wearers. It is more common on the palatal mucosa and in female patients.

3.1.1 Classification

Classification of denture stomatitis is usually based on the clinical appearance of inflamed mucosa observed beneath maxillary complete dentures. The most commonly used classification system is the one proposed by Newton in 1962. He suggested three different types of denture stomatitis: (1) pinpoint hyperemic foci, (2) diffuse hyperemia of the denture-supporting tissues, and (3) papillary hyperplasia. However, Budtz-Jorgensen and Bertram (1970) used different terms: (1) simple localized inflammation, (2) simple diffuse (generalized) inflammation, and (3) granular inflammation.

3.1.2 Symptoms

Denture stomatitis is a condition that often presents without noticeable symptoms. However, some patients may experience mucosal bleeding and swelling, as well as a burning or painful sensation, halitosis, an unpleasant taste, and dryness in the mouth. Studies have estimated that 28–70% of patients with denture stomatitis may report some levels of oral discomfort.

3.1.3 Etiology

The large majority of scientists believe that the cause of denture stomatitis is multifactorial, some stating that no primary etiological factor exists. However, specific factors have been considered to be more important:

- Denture trauma (including continuous denture wearing);
- Denture cleanness (including reaction to denture plaque);
- Allergic and primary irritant reactions to denture base materials;
- Dietary factors (including resultant hematological deficiencies);
- Candida infection;
- Systemic factors (including predisposing factors);
- Miscellaneous factors.

Regarding that using denture is one of the important causes of denture stomatitis, using specific kind of denture base materials can prevent this disease [6].

4. Different bases of denture

Dentistry as a profession we are familiar with now a day is considered to have begun about 3000 BC. About 2500 BC, the first dental prosthesis has been constructed in Egypt. But by 700 BC, professional dentures were made and during medieval times, dentures were rarely considered as a treatment option. From past to present, different materials have been used to fabricate dentures which are as follows:

- wood
- bone
- ivory
- porcelain (1774)
- gold (1794)
- vulcanite dentures (1839)
- tortoise shell (1850)

- gutta-percha (1851)
- cheoplastic (1856)
- aluminum (1867)
- celluloid (1869)
- bakelite (1909)
- vinyl resin (1930)
- stainless steel and base metal alloys (1937)
- polymethyl methacrylate (1937)

They are some features that are desired for a denture to contain. Dentures should be biocompatible, nontoxic, noncarciogenic, and translucent. The color of the denture should match color of teeth and gums [7].

4.1 Polymethyl methacrylate (PMMA)

Polymethyl methacrylate (PMMA) is a synthetic polymer that is used as an economical alternative to polycarbonate when extremely high strength is not necessary. Unlike polycarbonate, PMMA does not contain potentially harmful subunits like bisphenol-A. Moreover, it is easier to handle, process, and less expensive than polycarbonate, as illustrated in **Figure 1**.

In clinical practice, PMMA is mostly used as prosthesis for craniofacial tissue defects such as dentures. PMMA has great mechanical properties and low toxicity. PMMA is the most regular substance used to design complete and partial dentures. Despite its great features, it cannot accomplish all mechanical necessities of prosthesis. Flexural fatigue due to repeated masticatory and high-impact forces caused by dropping are the major causes of denture fractures. Features of PMMA denture are summarized in **Figure 2** [8].

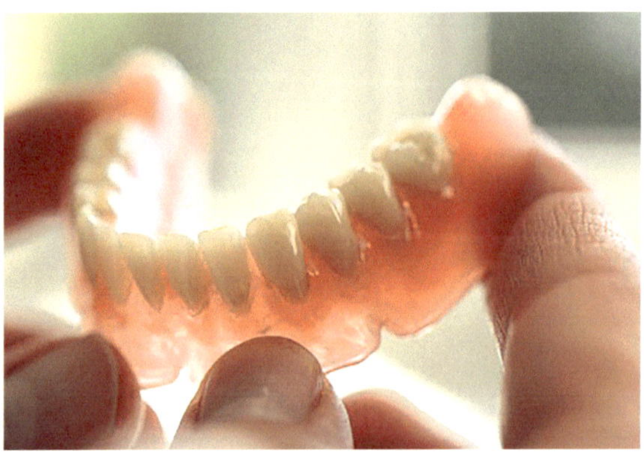

Figure 1.
Sample of polymethyl methacrylate denture.

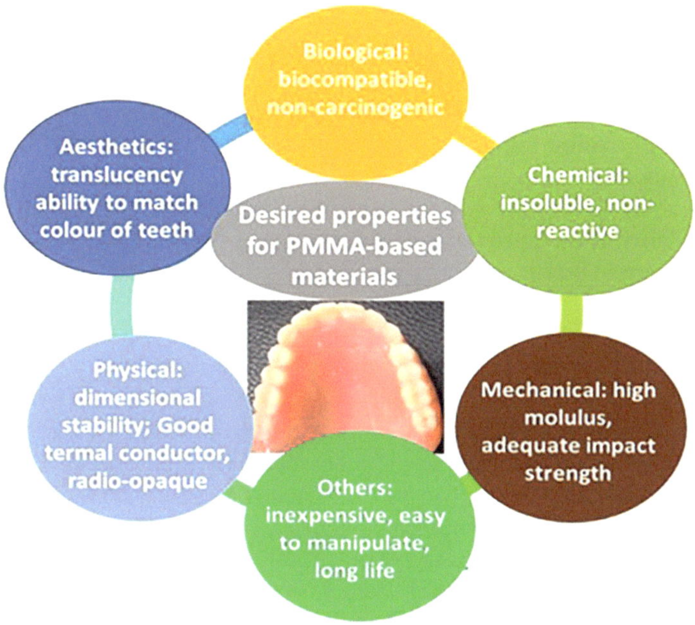

Figure 2.
PMMA features.

Polymethyl methacrylate (PMMA) is a popular material used in the fabrication of complete dentures, accounting for 95% of cases. This is due to its ease of processing, repair, and polishing, as well as favorable physicochemical properties and acceptable esthetics. For over 80 years, different processing techniques, such as pouring or mold filling (compression and injection molding), have been used to create dentures from PMMA. Each of these techniques presents its own benefits and drawbacks, making them more suitable for certain clinical procedures. Despite these differences, PMMA remains a versatile and popular option in complete denture fabrication because it is light weighted, easy to fabricate, and affordable. However, PMMA has some limitations, including low fracture resistance, poor physical properties in oral fluids, and potential allergic reactions. These limitations can impact clinical performance and denture longevity.

To overcome these drawbacks, several attempts have been made to improve the physical and mechanical properties of PMMA, such as material reinforcements, alternative material use with different compositions, and polymerization techniques, all of which aim to enhance the properties of PMMA to improve the clinical outcomes.

Digital denture fabrication has advanced with the use of computer-aided design and computer-aided manufacturing (CAD-CAM) technology. Two common methods used in this process include subtractive (milled) and additive (3D-printing) approaches.

In the milled method, a pre-polymerized PMMA disc is used to mill the denture base, resulting in high strength and adequate surface properties due to its fabrication under high temperatures and pressures. Compared to conventional fabrication methods, milled denture bases have no polymerization shrinkage and less residual monomer, providing significant advantages.

However, the performance of 3D-printed resins is currently lower than milled and conventional resins. The 3D-printing method builds the denture base layer-by-layer using photo-polymerized fluid resins, which leads to noticeable impacts on the strength and surface properties of the material after thermal cycling. Furthermore, 3D-printed resins exhibit higher levels of water sorption and solubility compared to traditional resins.

Although there are advantages and drawbacks to both the milled and 3D-printed denture base fabrication methods, further research is needed to improve the performance of 3D-printed resins and enhance their potential for use in dentistry [9, 10].

5. Adherence of *Candida albicans* on PMMA mechanisms

According to hydrophobic proteins on the surface of *Candida albicans*, this fungus is considered to be a highly hydrophobic substance. The adherence of *Candida albicans* to denture base surfaces has been associated closely with the hydrophobicity of the microorganism as a significant contributory physiochemical force.

For hydrophobic surfaces such as PMMA, monomer units exposed on the surface have interaction with the hydrophobic domains on a protein of *Candida albicans* by means of sturdy hydrophobic bonds. Therefore, the attractive hydrophobic interactions could bring about an inclination for *Candida albicans* to adhere greater with ease to hydrophobic surfaces than to hydrophilic surfaces. The contribution of electrostatic interplay between *Candida albicans* and polymeric surfaces is secondary to the hydrophobic force, due to the fact the adherence manner takes region in the presence of repulsive pressure [11].

6. Adherence of *Candida albicans* on PMMA in probiotics solution

It has been strongly counseled that probiotic consumption improves oral healthiness. However, the impact of probiotics at the microbial fame of denture wearers remains blurring. The acrylic prosthesis dentures in edentulous people possess a non-dropping, tough floor thereby facilitating candida adhesion and subsequent fungal colonization. The ability of the yeast to stick to the epithelial cells superficially and to the fitting denture floor remains as the essential key requirement for colonization of candida species and outcomes in making the denture as a store of contamination.

To evaluate the adherence of *Candida albicans* on PMMA denture base materials, many *in vitro* studies were conducted. In one study, two groups of PMMA dentures were experimented. First group of PMMA dentures was coated with probiotic solution at varying concentrations dipped in saliva containing candida species, and the other PMMA denture group was dipped in saliva containing candida species without probiotics. The result of this study is shown in **Figures 3** and **4**, and **Tables 1** and 2.

This study had two important result:

1. Probiotic application on denture base resin (PMMA) did decrease the *Candida albicans* count compared to the denture base without probiotic application.

2. As the concentration of probiotic over the denture base increases, the candida cell count decreased respectively [12].

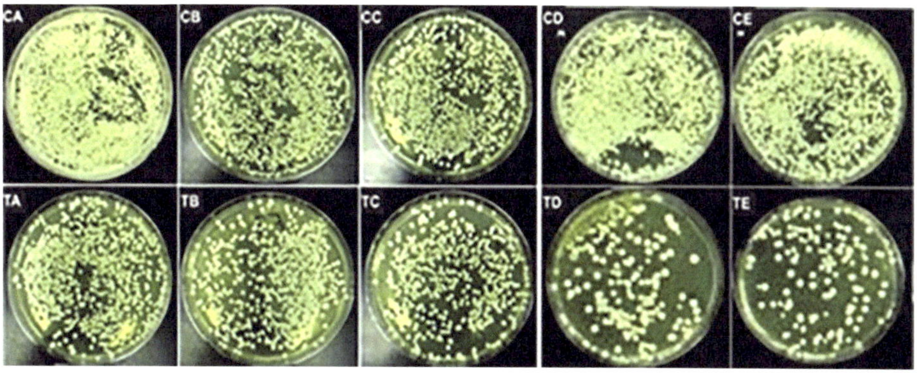

Figure 3.
The detection rate of candid species was 92.0% in the control group and it was reduced to 16.2% in the test group [12].

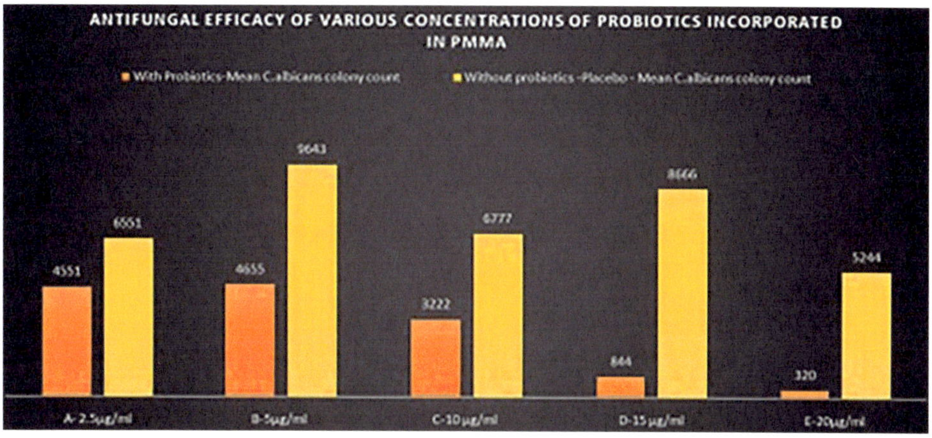

Figure 4.
Depicting the comparison of probiotics in varying concentrations against candida species [12].

DISKS	Mean value of *C. albicans* colony count—without probiotics	Probiotic concentration (Ilg/ml)	Mean value of *C. albicans* colony count—with probiotics
DISK 1	6551	2.5	4551
DISK2	9643	5	4655
DISK3	6777	10	3222
DISK4	8666	15	844
DISK5	5244	20	320

Table 1.
Depicting the comparison of probiotics in varying concentrations against candida species [12].

One other study showed that adhesion and colonization of probiotic bacteria on PMMA dentures prevent attachment of *Candida albicans* through competition for adhesion sites, nutrients, and products of environmental change. In this study, five groups containing 20 PMMA dentures were examined. Each of these groups was

Probiotic concentration (πg/ml)	2.5	5	10	15	20
Mean value of *C. albicans* colony count	4551	4655	3222	844	320

Table 2.
Depicting the comparison of Candida albicans *colony count in varying probiotic concentrations [12].*

dipped in Candida species and then exposed to different substance including the following: (1) probiotic solution of *L. rhamnosus GG*, (2) probiotic solution of k12 *Streptococcus salivarius*, (3) sodium hypochlorite solution, (4) normal saline, and (5) nystatin solution. According to the results of this study, probiotic solutions can be used to reduce the number of *Candida albicans* adhering to the PMMA denture base [13].

7. Probiotic bacteria and oral hygiene

Oral diseases like caries, gingivitis, or periodontitis are associated with a shift in bacterial biofilm composition and subsequent host reactions. Probiotics have been found to be beneficial in preventing or treating these conditions. *In vitro* studies have demonstrated that probiotic species can have potential effects on cariogenic or periodontal pathogens.

A meta-analysis of studies on the clinical effectiveness of probiotics in treating gingivitis has suggested that probiotics can significantly improve gum condition during therapy. When used regularly during orthodontic treatment, probiotics can reduce the number of bacteria from the *Streptococcus mutans* group in a patient's saliva and inhibit the expression of inflammatory mediators and an excessive immune response.

Probiotics eliminate and inhibit the growth of pathogenic microorganisms by competing for receptor sites and secreting metabolites with antibacterial activity. They also stimulate specific and non-specific immune responses by activating T lymphocytes and producing cytokines, allowing their effective use in oral diseases.

Probiotics offer several advantages over conventional antibiotics, including the ability to specifically target harmful bacteria without affecting beneficial bacteria. They restore balance to the oral microbiome and reduce the risk of oral diseases. Regular use of probiotics can be safe and effective for maintaining oral health, particularly in conditions such as gingivitis and periodontitis. However, more research is needed to determine the optimal strains, doses, and duration of probiotic use for specific oral health conditions [14, 15].

7.1 Caries and caries-associated microbes

Dental caries is a complex disease that arises mostly from bacterial infection, resulting in tooth demineralization and destruction (as shown in **Figure 5**). Tooth decay is a gradual process that occurs when acidogenic bacteria in the bacteria-laden biofilm and remnants of food accumulate on the tooth surface and eventually leads to tooth damage, loss, and infection. These bacteria thrive in microbial communities that form dental plaque accumulating on the tooth surface. Among the bacterial species found in the biofilm are *Streptococcus mutans, Streptococcus sobrinus*, and *Lactobacillus,* which produce organic acids as they metabolize fermentable carbohydrates. Organic acid production leads to the undesired low pH levels in the tooth environment, causing

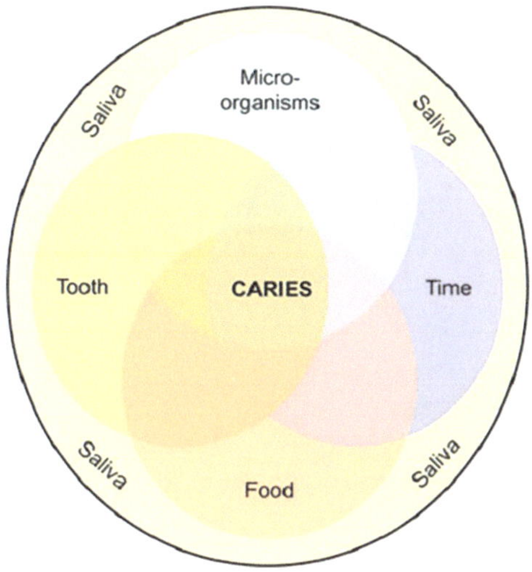

Figure 5.
Dental caries, a multifactorial disease.

demineralization of the tooth structure. Oral bacteria are vital etiological factors in caries development, with *S. mutans*, the primary causative microorganism discovered in a caries lesion, being the most prominent in dental caries pathogenesis.

There is evidence from multiple studies that prebiotic bacteria can inhibit caries development and probiotic supplements seem to reduce caries incidence in preschool children and schoolchildren with a high caries risk. Several studies suggest that consumption of products containing probiotic bacteria (*lactobacilli or bifidobacteria*) reduces the number of *mutans streptococci* in saliva causing reduction of dental caries [16–18].

7.2 Periodontal diseases

Periodontal diseases are prevalent among adults and are divided into two stages: gingivitis and periodontitis based on the presence or absence of attachment loss. Gingivitis is characterized by the presence of gingival inflammation with no loss of connective tissue attachment (as shown in **Figure 6**). Meanwhile, periodontitis is characterized by gingival inflammation accompanied by attachment loss and the resorption of coronal portions of tooth-supporting alveolar bone (also shown in **Figure 6**). Plaque bacteria are responsible for both conditions, inducing pathological changes in the tissues, either directly or indirectly. Although conventional therapies are effective, research continues through complementary therapies to improve periodontal treatments. Recently, probiotics have gained considerable interest as a possible management option against periodontal diseases, with several clinical trials conducted to investigate their impact on oral health.

A new approach of treating gingivitis and periodontitis that has been tried during the last few years is to control a number of infectious diseases through using and consuming of probiotics, so that the disease-causing pathogens are eliminated, promoting the development of a healthy flora, thus leading to restoration of health. Probiotic bacteria, especially lactobacilli, were effective adjunct for treating periodontal disease, particularly when combined with mechanical removal of pathogenic

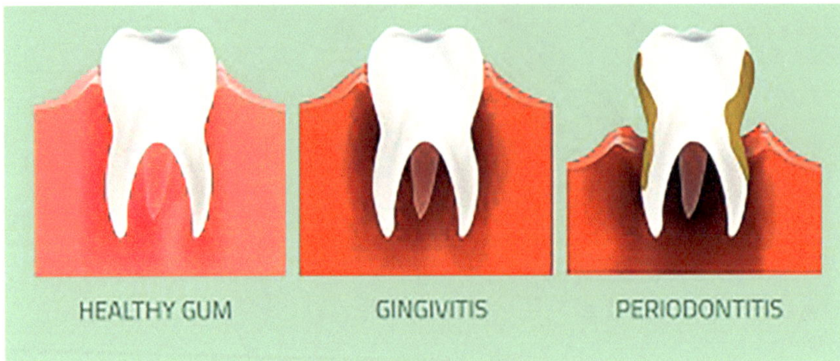

Figure 6.
Normal periodontium, gingivitis, periodontitis.

biofilms. Studies indicate that adjunctive use of specific probiotic supplements leads to significant amelioration of disease indices (probing pocket depth, gingival index, plaque index, bleeding on probing, and clinical attachment level), and reduces the need for antibiotics and surgery procedures [19].

7.3 Halitosis

Halitosis is a challenging chronic problem to address in the dental field. Aside from its apparent social impact, it also affects patients psychologically, leading to an increase in demand for dental treatments. Halitosis usually has an oral cause, originating from the breakdown of sulfur-containing amino acids on the tongue and in the periodontal sulcus, leading to the release of volatile sulfur compounds (VSC). Traditional methods such as scaling or root planning and chemotherapeutic solutions like chlorhexidine have shown some effectiveness, but their results are short-lived, and they have negative side effects, such as disrupting the oral cavity's homeostasis. Therefore, probiotics have emerged as a promising alternative with inhibitory effects on oral halitosis and without any of the side effects associated with the conventional treatments.

A single study suggests that the oral probiotic *Streptococcus salivarius*, which is found early in healthy individuals as a colonizer of oral surfaces and represents the primary microorganism in the tongue microbiota, has limited capacity to produce volatile sulfur compounds responsible for halitosis. On the other hand, other research advocates for the use of probiotics in managing halitosis. However, the existing evidence is not persuasive enough to support the efficacy of using probiotics for halitosis management. For more effective future studies, standardized recruitment protocols for halitosis subjects and organoleptic measurements are necessary when using probiotics as an intervention for managing halitosis [20, 21].

8. Conclusions

This chapter was written with the goal of evaluating the effect of probiotic solution on the adherence of *candida albicans*, the most common cause of candidiasis or thrush, on the polymethyl methacrylate denture in patients using partial or complete denture.

Based on the results of this chapter, following conclusion can be drawn:

1. Probiotic solutions can be used to reduce the number of *C. albicans* adhering to the removable denture base.

2. Probiotic application on PMMA dentures decreased the *C. albicans* count compared to the denture base without probiotic application.

3. As the concentration of probiotic over the denture base increase, the candida cell count decreased, respectively.

Author details

Arezoo Aghakouchakzadeh[1]*, Niayesh Daneshvarpour[2] and Ahmadreza Mirzaei[2]

1 Department of Oral and Maxillofacial Pathology, School of Dentistry, Alborz University of Medical Science, Karaj, Iran

2 Faculty of Dentistry, Alborz University of Medical Sciences, Karaj, Iran

*Address all correspondence to: a.aghakouchakzadeh@gmail.com

References

[1] Schrezenmeir J, de Vrese M. Probiotics, prebiotics, and synbiotics—Approaching a definition. The American Journal of Clinical Nutrition. 2001;**73**(2):361s-364s

[2] Singh A, Verma R, Murari A, Agrawal A. Oral candidiasis: An overview. Journal of Oral and Maxillofacial Pathology. 2014;**18**(Suppl. 1):S81

[3] Arendorf TM, Walker DM. Denture stomatitis: A review. Journal of Oral Rehabilitation. 1987;**14**(3):217-227

[4] Bizzini B, Pizzo G, Scapagnini G, Nuzzo D, Vasto S. Probiotics and oral health. Current Pharmaceutical Design. 2012;**18**(34):5522-5531

[5] Plaza-Diaz J, Ruiz-Ojeda FJ, Gil-Campos M, Gil A. Mechanisms of action of probiotics. Advances in Nutrition. 2019;**10**:S49-S66

[6] Figueiral MH, Azul A, Pinto E, Fonseca PA, Branco FM, Scully C. Denture-related stomatitis: Identification of aetiological and predisposing factors–a large cohort. Journal of Oral Rehabilitation. 2007;**34**(6):448-455

[7] Tandon R, Gupta S, Agarwal SK. Denture base materials: From past to future. Indian Journal of Dental Sciences. 2010;**2**(2):33-39

[8] Nowacka M. Biomaterials for tissue engineering and regenerative medicine. Wiadomosci Chemiczne. 2012;**66**:909-933

[9] Alshahrani FA, AlToraibily F, Alzaid M, Mahrous AA, Al Ghamdi MA, Gad MM. An updated review of salivary pH effects on Polymethyl methacrylate (PMMA)-based removable dental prostheses. Polymers (Basel). 2022;**14**(16):3387

[10] Park SE, Periathamby AR, Loza JC. Effect of surface-charged poly (methyl methacrylate) on the adhesion of Candida albicans 1. Journal of Prosthodontics. 2003;**12**(4):249-254

[11] Goswami RR, Pohare SD, Raut JS, Karuppayil SM. Cell surface hydrophobicity as a virulence factor in Candida albicans. Biosciences, Biotechnology Research Asia. 2017;**14**(4):1503

[12] Shankar RK, Balaji H, Shanmuganathan N, Parthasarathy N, Athiban I, Thirumalaikumaran R. Anti-fungal efficacy of probiotics in heat cure Dentures Base resin: An In-vitro study. Journal of Pharmaceutical Research International. 2022;**34**(49A):1-6

[13] Mirzaei A, Aghakouchakzadeh A, Mehrabani M, Khodaii Z. Evaluation adherence of Candida Albicans on Polymethacrylate in probiotics Soloution. Alborz University Medical Journal. 2020;**9**(4):53-58

[14] Gruner D, Paris S, Schwendicke F. Probiotics for managing caries and periodontitis: Systematic review and meta-analysis. Journal of Dentistry. 2016;**48**:16-25

[15] Kaźmierczyk-Winciorek M, Nędzi-Góra M, Słotwińska SM. The immunomodulating role of probiotics in the prevention and treatment of oral diseases. Central European Journalof Immunology. 2021;**46**(1):99-104

[16] Lin TH, Lin CH, Pan TM. The implication of probiotics in the

prevention of dental caries. Applied Microbiology and Biotechnology. 2018;**102**:577-586

[17] Zaura E, Twetman S. Critical appraisal of oral pre-and probiotics for caries prevention and care. Caries Research. 2019;**53**(5):514-526

[18] Wang B, Yao M, Lv L, Ling Z, Li L. The human microbiota in health and disease. Engineering. 2017;**3**(1):71-82

[19] Matsubara VH, Bandara H, Ishikawa KH, Mayer MPA, Samaranayake LP. The role of probiotic bacteria in managing periodontal disease: A systematic review. Expert Review of Anti-Infective Therapy. 2016;**14**(7):643-655

[20] Bustamante M, Oomah BD, Mosi-Roa Y, Rubilar M, Burgos-Díaz C. Probiotics as an adjunct therapy for the treatment of halitosis, dental caries and periodontitis. Probiotics Antimicrob Proteins. 2020;**12**:325-334

[21] Yoo JI, Shin IS, Jeon JG, Yang YM, Kim JG, Lee DW. The effect of probiotics on halitosis: A systematic review and meta-analysis. Probiotics Antimicrob Proteins. 2019;**11**:150-157

Chapter 6

Advances on Probiotics Utilization in Poultry Health and Nutrition

Janvi Hemant Kadam, Rasika Sagar Pawar, Mohd Fadhil Md. Din and Vasudeo Zambare

Abstract

Poultry is one of the most rapidly expanding food production sectors, especially in developing countries. The poultry birds are safe and in good health due to the antibiotic supplemented feeds. However, the increasing awareness regarding antibiotic resistance has led to a dire need for the development of antibiotic-free poultry. Therefore, in addition to the daunting challenge of sufficing the need for poultry food of the increasing population, the industry should also ensure that the production is based on sustainable practices. In poultry farming there are several alternatives to the antibiotics, and one of them is probiotics. Probiotics are beneficial and safe microorganisms for preservation of the host's health and well-being. There are convincing experimental shreds of evidence that discuss the impact of probiotics on the positive modulation of poultry's immunity, growth performance, feed utilization and general health condition. Therefore, this review shed light on the concept, impact and mode of action of probiotics in sustainable poultry production. By discussing the results obtained from the recent studies about the ability of probiotics to maintain the poultry animal's performance level, this chapter condensed the valuable information and open several avenues for further investigation and development of the probiotic applications in the poultry industry with a special focus on its effect in improving poultry's' health and nutritional value.

Keywords: poultry, probiotics, growth promoters, mode of action, immunity

1. Introduction

Poultry is crucial in supplying the burgeoning urban population's growing need for protein rich foods and is one of the young and quickly expanding subsets of animal husbandry [1]. The significance of raising poultry in enhancing the socio-economic conditions of regions that lack sufficient resources cannot be exaggerated. This is due to its features like swift bird generation, concentrated expansion, remarkable efficiency, reduced labor expenses, and minimal resource needs [2]. However, with increasing commercialization, poultry production continues to shift from subsidence agricultural practices to intensive food production, which has consequently increased the occurrence of diseases [3].

Antibiotics (when administered at sub-therapeutic levels) have been shown to be a successful method for illness control, growth enhancement, and feed conversion efficiency during the last several decades [4]. However, unrestricted use of antimicrobial drugs has resulted in their accumulation in terrestrial habitat, which has led to extensively documented adverse outcomes, including the rise of antibiotic-resistant bacterial strains, the accumulation of antibiotic remnants in the meat, and changes to the beneficial microbiota of the poultry [5]. There is always a risk associated with transmittance of resistant bacterial genes from poultry animals to humans via non-pathogenic bacteria to human pathogens. Therefore, the use of antibiotics in poultry has become risky [6].

Antibiotic resistance and concerns about food safety associated with overusing antibiotics prompted the European Union in 2006 to prohibit their use in animal feed [7, 8]. As a result, there has been a rise in the search for and use of alternatives to antibiotics, in order to safeguard poultry and human health.

The use of probiotics, often known as beneficial bacteria, suppress diseases in a number of ways, and is increasingly viewed as a substitute for antibiotics [9]. However, the significance of probiotics employed in poultry is not confined to the gastrointestinal system; they also play a noteworthy part in the enhancement of the organism's overall health. This study therefore compiles and assesses the current state of knowledge on probiotics for poultry's health and nutrition.

2. Probiotics

Probiotics are "live organisms and its substances that contribute to gut's microbial equilibrium," as Parker put it in 1974. Definition of probiotics as "a live microbial feed additive that beneficially impacts the host animal by enhancing its gut microbial balance" was established in 1989. More recently, "live microorganisms that when administered in suitable proportions impart a health benefit on the host" has been used to characterize probiotics [10].

Probiotics that are regularly utilized include strains of *Bacillus subtilis, Lactobacillus, Saccharomyces cerevisiae*, *Bifidobacterium, Aspergillus*, and *Streptococcus* all of which are capable of growth promotion and antimicrobial activity against pathogenic bacteria like *Escherichia coli, Salmonella typhimurium, Clostridium perfringens*, *Staphylococcus aureus*, etc. [11]. These strains can be isolated from fermented products or animal body such as breast milk, gut, fecal matter. *Lactobacillus plantarum* and *Leuconostoc mesenteroides* probiotics from some non-conventional sources of vegetables and fruits are also reported [12].

In the past, the probiotic market was predominantly led by the Asia Pacific region, with Europe following suit. The worldwide probiotic market's estimated worth is approximately USD 57.8 billion in 2022, and projections indicate a compound annual growth rate (CAGR) of 7.5% [13]. Apart from being consumed by humans, probiotics are also experiencing a growing application in animals, particularly in the context of poultry farming. The rising demand for poultry probiotic components in poultry diet can be attributed to the growing interest of consumers in eating more protein-rich meals like eggs. Probiotics employed in poultry farming may consist of a solitary strain or a blend of two or more strains, serving the purpose of disease prevention, health enhancement, and the augmentation of poultry growth and efficiency. It is widely recognized that utilizing a combination of multiple strains of probiotics can yield synergistic advantages [14]. Probiotics exist in different forms such as granules, powder, liquid paste and gel out of which dry forms are better for gastric environment and longer shelf life [11]. Several review articles have reported that probiotic use in poultry has provided various benefits such as improvement in growth performance, along with immune enhancement, and sustainability of gut microbes.

3. Mode of action

There is no one method via which probiotics exert their benefits; nevertheless, they are essential to the health of the host immune system and the interaction involving the gut microbiota and the immune system of the host. Probiotic microorganisms used in poultry production should fulfill several requirements to be considered effective, including being indigenous to the host, adhering to the intestinal epithelium, surviving gastric juices and mucous, engaging in competition for colonization within the gastrointestinal tract alongside other microorganisms, and exhibiting high viability under storage conditions [15].

Probiotics have been shown to improve digestion, increase the production of digestive enzymes, and even detoxify substances in the diet, resulting in improved growth and performance in poultry. Next possible action is: by prevention of pathogens via competition for adhesion sites; producing organic acids which can alter gut pH (predominantly probiotics containing *Lactobacillus* strains), which can promote absorption of minerals and protein, volatile fatty acids and antibacterial substances like bacteriocins, hydrogen peroxide, defensins, etc.; and physiological effect by regenerating intestinal mucosa, and immunological effects by modulating antigen presenting cells, regulatory T and B cells, and regulation of pro-inflammatory cytokines [16].

Furthermore, probiotics might alter the development and composition of the microbiota in the gut by restraining the impact of harmful bacteria, as well as bolster the body's natural defense mechanism through the synthesis of inhibitory substances. The adhesion of specific probiotics to the gut mucin, a glycoprotein, suggested the competitive suppression or colonization resistance of infectious pathogens adhering

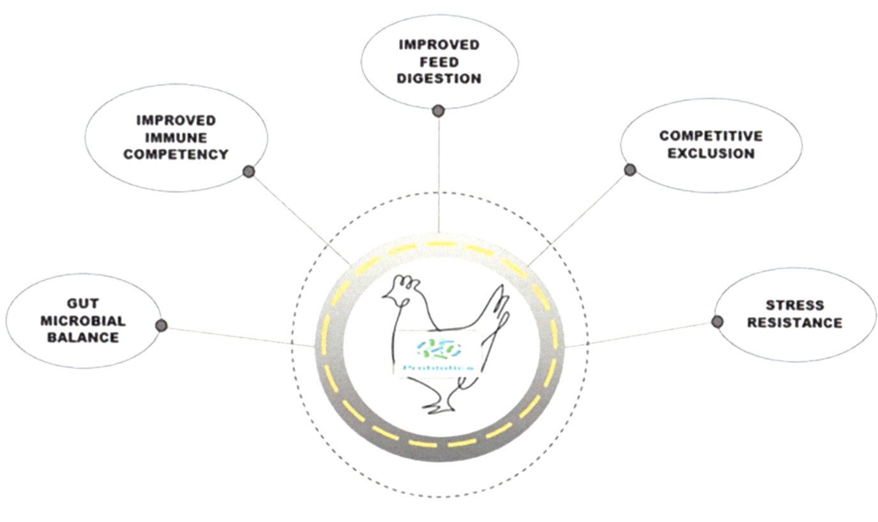

Figure 1.
Mode of action and impact of probiotics in poultry.

to the shared route/site [17]. Thus, it out competes the proliferation of opportunistic pathogenic microbes. Lastly, increasing the resistance of poultry animals against stress caused by temperature as a potent environmental factor.

The aforementioned mechanism of action provided foundational data for understanding the positive benefits on the poultry animals (**Figure 1**). However, transcriptome and proteomic analyses are needed in future studies of probiotic and host interaction to better understand probiotic activity.

4. Effect on growth performance

It has been theorized that probiotics can help poultry birds continue their typical development and functioning by serving as a source of vitamins, nutrients, and digestive enzymes that have a beneficial impact on feed utilization, nutrient absorption, and growth rates. Various commercial probiotic supplements have been tested for their growth-promoting effects in poultry. Studies have demonstrated that probiotics such as *Bacillus subtilis* and Lactobacillus species have the potential to improve feed conversion ratios (FCR) and increase body weight gain in broilers. These effects are attributed to the mechanisms mentioned earlier, which collectively lead to optimized nutrient utilization and enhanced growth rates. Zymospore® (Vetanco Brazil, *B. subtilis*), a commercially available direct-fed microbe, increased the bacterial variety of the broiler's gut microflora evidenced by heightened levels of lactic acid bacteria and clostridiales, thereby promoting feed digestion and growth, even under experimentally challenging conditions [18]. Broiler chickens given commercial probiotics (Lacto sacc, Alltech, Inc.) showed a considerable feed conversion ratio, as determined by Georgieva et al. [19].

In addition to single-strain probiotic supplements, herbal probiotic additives have also been explored for their growth-enhancing properties. These additives often combine beneficial microorganisms with herbal extracts, creating a synergistic effect on growth performance. For example, a study reported significant effect on weight gain in broilers provided with diet supplemented with Promix® (*B. subtilis*, *Bifidobacterium bifidum*, *Bifidobacterium longum*, *Lactobacillus acidophilus*, *S. cerevisiae*) and herbs (*Curcuma xanthorriza*, *Curcuma aeruginosa*, *Zingiber offocinale*, *Curcuma domestica*, *Kaempferia galanga*), a commercial herbal probiotic feed additive [20]. When challenged with Salmonella pullorum, a recent study observed significant effect ($P \leq 0.05$) on feed intake, mortality, and gut microflora in dwarf male chicks fed with basal diet supplemented with probiotic fermented herbal blend [21].

Nutrient adequacy and nutrient deficiency conditions controlling the probiotic growth. In cases of nutrient deficiency, probiotics assist in enhancing nutrient absorption and utilization, effectively compensating for reduced nutrient availability in the diet. This suggests that probiotics could play a crucial role in improving growth rates even in challenging dietary situations. A study observed, significant improvement in Feed conversion ratio (FCR), Feed intake (FI) and on weight gain (WG) in broiler hens fed with triticalate-based diet enriched with probiotics and enzymes [22]. The ileal digestibility coefficient of proteins, starch, and gross energy all improved significantly ($P \leq 0.05$) when the probiotic (*Bacillus subtilis*) was added to the broiler diets of both nutrient-adequate and nutrient-deficient birds [23]. Similarly, significant ($P \leq 0.01$) increased in body weight and decreased FCR was observed in chicks fed with meal supplemented with *Bacillus subtilis* probiotic, the results were in comparison with conventional feed additive—bacitracin methylene disalicylate (BMD). However, when challenged with *E. coli*, both *B. subtilis* and BMD did not compensate for the growth deterioration in chicks [24]. A study showed that the overall performance of white Pekin ducks was enhanced when a probiotic combination of *L. acidophilus* and *Lactobacillus casei* was added to a diet low in protein [25]. Bidura et al. reported that enrichment of basal diet with probiotics, *Saccharomysces sp.* Increased growth performances along with decreased levels in serum and meat cholesterol in male duckling [26]. It has been found out that dietary supplementation with probiotics, *Pediococcus acidilactici* and *B. subtilis* in water, improves the intestinal health and resistance of chickens against coccidiosis-causing *Eimeria species* [27].

In contrast, as in Ref. [28], it was discovered that supplementing with probiotics had no discernible effect on chicken carcass, growth performance or meat quality. Recently, endeavors have been directed towards the identification and isolation of lactic acid bacteria possessing probiotic capabilities, to engage in interactions, whether direct or indirect, with aflatoxin-producing fungi, or to detoxify aflatoxins themselves. A study reported beneficial effect of probiotic, *Lactobacillus plantarum* 299v in subsiding the toxic effect of poultry fed contaminated by aflatoxins [29]. According to research, supplementing the diets of dual-purpose hens with the probiotics *Lactobacillus paracasei sparacasei* and *Lactobacillus rhamnosus* significantly ($P < 0.05$) increased both body weight gain and FCR [30]. Khabirov et al. postulated that supplementing broiler feed with Normosil, i.e., live cultures of *Lactobacillus* and *Enterococcus* strains improved overall growth, nutrient digestibility and hematological characteristics [31]. Another study reported that *Bacillus licheniformis* as probiotic in basal diet showed better improvement in broiler chickens' body weight gain and production efficiency factor in comparison with *Bacillus subtilis* [32].

The effects of Probiotics on poultry's growth performance are summarized in **Table 1**.

Probiotics	**Effect**	**References**
Effect on growth performance		
Zymospore® Direct feed microbials, *Bacillus subtilis*	Improvement in feed intake, feed conversion ratio and body weight	[18]
Bacillus based triticale diet	Increased feed intake, feed conversion ratio and weight gain along with cellular immunity	[22]
B. subtilis	Improvement in intestinal digestibility coefficients for starch, crude protein, and overall gross energy	[23]
B. subtilis	Positive impact on growth performance, improved gut health	[24]
L. plantarum and *L. paracasei* fermented herbal blend	Avoid death, improved growth performance, enhanced immunity and controlled intestinal flora	[21]
L. plantarum	Protective effect against hepatotoxicity and oxidative stress caused by aflatoxin along with improvement in growth performance	[29]
L. paracaseis sparacasei, L. rhamnosus	Improvement in the growth performances	[30]
Lactobacillus, Enterococcus strains	Improved overall growth, nutrient digestibility and hematological characteristics	[31]
B. licheniformis	Improvement in body weight gain and overall production	[32]
L acidophilus, L. casei	Compensated for protein deficient diet	[25]

Probiotics	Effect	References
Saccharomysces sp	Increased growth performances along with decreased levels in serum and meat cholesterol	[26]
P. acidilactici, B. subtilis	Improvement in intestinal health and resistance against *Eimeria sp*.	[27]
Promix®	Excellent effect on weight gain	[20]
B. subtilis PB6 (CLOSTAT)®	Improvement in skeletal health and meat quality	[33]
Effect during stress conditions		
S. cerevisiae	Reduction in erythrocyte osmotic fragility, lipid peroxidation and higher expressionof superoxide dismutase activity	[34]
B. subtilis	Reduce breast muscle oxidative degeneration and improved meat quality	[35]
B. subtilis	Immunity suppression both in thermoneutral and heat-stimulated situations, improved food conversion ratio	[36]
Lactobacillus strains	Prevalence of *Lactobacillus sp*. on heat stressing	[37]
S. cerevisiae, L. acidophilus selenium enriched	Inhibited hepatic oxidation	[38]
L. acidophilus, S. cerevisiae selenium enriched	Improved body weight gain and bone health	[39]
L. casei, L. acidophilus, and *Bifidobacterium lactis*	Gene regulation for immunity, and metabolism of glucose and lipid	[40]
Lactobacillus acidophilus, Lactobacillus plantarum, and *Enterococcus faecalis* (RUYIRUYI) ®	Improved intestinal integrity, ameliorated inflammatory response	[41]
Effect on immune modulation		
Lactobacillus sp.	Effective against reducing pathogenic enterobacterial colonization, downregulation of pro inflammatory cytokines	[42]
L. acidophilus, S. cerevisiae selenium enriched	Upregulation of IFN-gamma mRNA genes thus protecting against *E. tenella* infection	[43]
L. fermentum, L. plantarum, S. cerevisiae, Enterococcus faecium, Pediococcus acidilactici	Upregulation of mRNA anti-inflammatory genes thus protecting against *P. multocida*	[44]
L. fermentum, L. acidophilus	Downregulation of pro inflammatory cytokines	[45]
L. acidophilus, L. casei	Improvement in overall immunity	[25]
L. plantarum	Improvement in both cell mediated and humoral immune response	[46]
Probiotic with diclazuril	Increase in the levels of interleukin and immunoglobulin	[47]

Table 1.
Probiotics' effects on poultry.

5. Effect during stressful conditions

The term "stress" is used to refer to the body's reactions to extrinsic or environmental factors that threaten homeostasis, or the body's normal state of physiological equilibrium. Environmental stressor normally weakens the immune system of animals and increases their susceptibility to disease occurrence. Poultry birds respond to stress by modifying their behavior, biochemistry, and physiology in an effort to restore body's equilibrium. Based on the above, poultry animals normally suffer from one important stressful condition i.e., heat stress.

The deleterious effects of heat stress on the immunology, physiology, and microbiology of birds leads to negative impact on poultry industry. Genes like heat shock protein (HSP) are likely to have their expression altered in response to heat stress. Various studies have confirmed effective use of probiotics to supplementation in eliminating poultry heat stress. Ogbuagu et al. reported that combination of fisetin and probiotics, decreased erythrocyte osmotic fragility, lipid peroxidation and increased superoxide dismutase, thus reducing the effects of oxidative stress alterations in broiler chickens exposed to heat stress [34].

During chronic heat stress supplementing broiler with dietary probiotic of *B. subtilis* improved meat quality and alleviate oxidative deterioration of breast muscles [35]. A study similarly reported dietary *B. subtilis* (1×10^6 CFU/g feed) significantly improved broiler performance with respect to FCR and alleviation of immune response under both thermoneutral and heat stimulated conditions [36]. Terminal-RFLP analysis was used in another study to see how probiotic. The Cecal and jejunal microbiota of broiler chickens under heat stress is affected *Lactobacillus* strains. The study found out that there was no significant abundance in the microbial population but the supplementation did show higher prevalence of *Lactobacillus sp*. in heat stressed chickens in comparison with the controls [37].

Oxidative stress is a common consequence of heat stress in poultry. The combination of antioxidant compounds and probiotics offers a multifaceted approach to combating oxidative stress. One of the trace elements, selenium, is essential for the body's functioning. It shields red blood cells against the detrimental impacts of free radicals and constitutes a component of the robust antioxidant known as glutathione peroxidase. In summary, the normal development of enzymatic systems like superoxide dismutase and glutathione peroxidase is reliant on its presence. Khan et al. postulated that supplementing basal diet of broiler with selenium enriched probiotics (SP) (*S. cerevisiae* and *L. acidophilus*) enhanced antioxidant system to effectively inhibit hepatic oxidation during heat stress; probiotics alone were not as effective [38]. In another study SP, significantly improved body weight gain and bone health by up-regulating the expression of DIO2 and T3 in heat stressed broiler [39]. The effect of probiotic use in stressed poultry are summarized in **Table 1**.

Moreover, stress can disrupt the balance of the gut microbiota, affecting nutrient absorption and overall gut health. The role of probiotics in moderating this impact is explored in the following section.

6. Immuno-modulatory effect of probiotics

The gut of poultry serves as a critical interface where the immune system interacts with the external environment, including ingested feed and potential pathogens. This dynamic environment houses a diverse microbial community that plays a pivotal role in shaping the host's immune responses. Probiotics, as beneficial members of the gut microbiota, have gained attention for their immunomodulatory effects, influencing the intricate relationship between the gut and the immune system.

Certain probiotic strains have the ability to stimulate immune cells in the gut-associated lymphoid tissue (GALT), including dendritic cells, macrophages, and T cells. This activation enhances the recognition and response to pathogens while preventing excessive immune activation [48]. Moreover, Probiotics have been explored as potential adjuvants to enhance the efficacy of vaccines in poultry. By promoting a balanced immune response, probiotics can improve the recognition and memory formation of vaccine antigens. This leads to increased vaccine effectiveness and protection against pathogens. In a study conducted by Sarwar, it was observed that the vaccination against infectious bursal disease (IBDV) and Newcastle disease (ND) in combination with probiotic strains of *L. paracasei*, *L. casei*, *L acidophilus, Bifidobacterium*, *Streptococcus thermophiles* showed antibody titer improvement when compared control broiler groups administered with only with vaccine and probiotic alone [49].

Numerous studies have put forth the hypothesis that probiotics could potentially function as a viable substitute for antibiotics in the diets of poultry and are anticipated to boost animal immunity and health status. In a study, Penha Filho et al. presented that *Lactobacillus*-based probiotics proved to be effective against heavy infection of pathogenic enterobacterial infection of *Salmonella enteritidis* (SE) in chickens, by reducing SE's colonization in chicks. Study reported immunomodulatory effect of the probiotic such as, decrease in the levels of pro-inflammatory cytokines. It further showed stimulation of TLR2 expression in caecal tonsils which can further pay way to consider this probiotic as TLR2 based adjuvant with injectable vaccines [42]. On the other hand, a study observed upregulation of IFN-gamma mRNA genes in selenium enriched probiotic supplemented chickens when challenged with *E. Tenella*, thus providing protection against infection. Here the immunomodulatory response was linked with the increased antioxidant capacities [43]. Similarly, another research observed elevation of mRNA anti-inflammatory genes HIF1A (hypoxia inducible factor 1 alpha) and TSG-6 (tumor necrosis factor- (TNF) in the caecal mucosa of broilers fed with dietary probiotics when they were challenged with *P. multocida* [44]. *Lactobacillus fermentum* and *L. acidophilus* decrease the expression of pro-inflammatory cytokines in broilers affected with necrotic enteritis [45].

White pekin ducks' nonspecific immune responses were greatly boosted when their diets were supplemented with probiotics. Additionally, incorporation of probiotics to a low crude protein diet increased duck immunity to the same levels as those on a high crude protein diet [25]. Dietary addition of *L. plantarum* probiotic (1×10^8 CFU) showed significant ($p < 0.05$) improvement in both cell mediated and humoral immune response thus protecting the chickens against coccidiosis [46]. Additionally, rise in the levels of interleukin and immunoglobulin was observed by Memon et al. in broiler chicks thus explaining the synergistic activity of probiotic with synthetic drugs such as diclazuril, under induced Eimeria infection [47]. **Table 1** highlights the influence of probiotics on the immunity of poultry.

7. Metagenomics and metaproteomics in poultry

The gut microbiota of birds plays a pivotal role in various aspects of their health and performance. Advances in metagenomic and metaproteomic techniques have enabled scientists to delve deeper into the complex microbial communities residing within the avian gut. Metagenomics involves analyzing the genetic material present in a sample to identify and characterize the diversity of microorganisms. On the other hand, metaproteomic focuses on the proteins expressed by these microorganisms, providing insights into their functional roles [50].

In a study, the fecal microbiota of broiler growers with varying FCR was analyzed using shotgun sequencing. The analysis revealed distinct microbial compositions between low and high FCR birds, with differences in phylum-level abundances and gene proportions related to metabolism, stress response, and virulence. Notably, certain genes associated with improved feed efficiency were found to be overrepresented in low FCR birds, providing insights for enhancing poultry feed efficiency and formulation strategies [51]. Yet another study, investigated the influence of heat stress on the gut microbiota of caged laying hens using metagenomics sequencing. Firmicutes, Bacteroidetes, and Proteobacteria were dominant phyla. Heat stress reduced Firmicutes and increased Bacteroidetes, leading to altered metabolic pathways like cysteine and methionine metabolism. The findings provide insights into potential interventions for mitigating heat stress effects in poultry [52]. Moreover, a study explored how diet affects the protein content of chicken gastrointestinal tract (GIT) using label-free metaproteomics. The crop section showed Lactobacillaceae dominance, irrespective of diet, while Veillonellaceae increased with phosphorus supplementation. In the ceca, Bacteroidaceae proteins rose with phosphorus, and Eubacteriaceae decreased; protein patterns indicated thriving communities with supplementation, highlighting GIT dynamics [53].

Thus, metagenomic and metaproteomic analyses can assist in the selection of probiotic strains with specific functional attributes. By identifying strains that promote beneficial metabolic pathways or produce bioactive compounds, researchers can tailor probiotic formulations to address particular challenges, such as enhancing nutrient absorption or modulating immune system.

8. Limitations on the use of probiotics in poultry

Because the potential of probiotics supplements varies depending on the species and is not shared between different genera and species of microbes, the widespread adoption of probiotics as part of poultry diets has brought it with some unique difficulties. Furthermore, there is always the possibility that the probiotics will be inadequately handled after they have reached the market, rendering them ineffective. Loss of viability of probiotics may occur when they come into touch with disinfectants in water or other interacting compounds in feed during oral administration. The probiotics' lack of availability until they reach the site of action in the host body is another potential barrier [54].

9. Conclusion

The studies discussed above indicate that probiotics may play a significant role in sustainable poultry farming. In all likelihood, they will serve as the superior replacement for antibiotics in poultry industries. Significant work and studies have proved that probiotics help in maintaining health status in poultry animals as they improve gut conditions and enhance nutrient absorption, thus overall improving the growth performance. Probiotics provide protective effect against stress conditions by enhancing antioxidant potential of enzymes. Probiotics also modulate immune response and provide protecting against infections through various mechanism of action. In future, probiotics in poultry feed should continue to determine the optimal conditions and standard methodology under which their application will have the greatest possible beneficial impact on meat quality. Additionally, more clinical trials may be conducted to investigate other potential areas of benefit.

Acknowledgements

There is no acknowledgement for this chapter.

Conflict of interest

The authors declare no conflict of interest.

Author details

Janvi Hemant Kadam[1], Rasika Sagar Pawar[2], Mohd Fadhil Md. Din[3] and Vasudeo Zambare[3,4]*

1 Department of Biotechnology, KET's V.G. Vaze College, Mumbai, India

2 Department of Microbiology, SMT Chandibai Himathmal Mansukhani College, Mumbai, India

3 Center for Environmental Sustainability and Water Security (IPASA), Department of Water and Environmental Engineering, School of Civil Engineering, Universiti Teknologi Malaysia, Bahru, Malaysia

4 R&D Department, Balaji Enzyme and Chemical Pvt. Ltd., Mumbai, Maharashtra, India

*Address all correspondence to: vasuzambare@gmail.com

References

[1] Kumar M, Dahiya SP, Ratwan P. Backyard poultry farming in India: A tool for nutritional security and women empowerment. Biological Rhythm Research. 2019;**52**(10):1476-1491. DOI: 10.1080/09291016.2019.1628396

[2] Kalia VC, Shim WY, Patel SK, Gong C, Lee J-K. Recent developments in antimicrobial growth promoters in chicken health: Opportunities and challenges. Science of The Total Environment. 2022;**834**:155300. DOI: 10.1016/j.scitotenv.2022.155300

[3] Suleman S, Yasmin F, Farooq W, Rasheed M, Qureshi JA. Poultry feed contamination and its potential hazards on human health. Biomedical Letters. 2022;**8**(1):70-81. DOI: 10.47262/bl/8.1.20210901

[4] Mungroo N, Neethirajan S. Biosensors for the detection of antibiotics in poultry industry—A review. Biosensors. 2014;**4**(4):472-493. DOI: 10.3390/bios4040472

[5] Tabidi MH, Mukhtar AM, Mohammed HI. Effects of probiotic and antibiotic on performance and growth attributes of broiler chicks. Global Journal of Medicinal Plant Research. 2013;**1**(1):136-142

[6] Singer RS, Hofacre CL. Potential impacts of antibiotic use in poultry production. Avian Diseases. 2006;**50**(2):161-172. DOI: 10.1637/7569-033106r.1

[7] Castanon JIR. History of the use of antibiotic as growth promoters in European poultry feeds. Poultry Science. 2007;**86**(11):2466-2471. DOI: 10.3382/ps.2007-00249

[8] Pawar R, Zambare V, Nabar B. Comparative assessment of antibiotic resistance in lactic acid bacteria isolated from healthy human adult and infant feces. Nepal Journal of Biotechnology. 2020;**8**(2):69-65

[9] Kazemi SA, Ahmadi H, Karimi Torshizi MA. Evaluating two multistrain probiotics on growth performance, intestinal morphology, lipid oxidation and ileal microflora in chickens. Journal of Animal Physiology and Animal Nutrition. 2019;**103**(5):1399-1407. DOI: 10.1111/jpn.13124

[10] FAO/WHO. Report of a Joint FAO/WHO Expert Consultation on Evaluation of Health and Nutritional Properties of Probiotics in Food Including Powder Milk with Live Lactic Acid Bacteria. 2001; October 1-4, 2001; Córdoba, Argentina

[11] Iannitti T, Palmieri B. Therapeutical use of probiotic formulations in clinical practice. Clinical Nutrition. 2010;**29**(6):701-725. DOI: 10.1016/j.clnu.2010.05.004

[12] Pawar R, Dhawal P, Nabar B, Barve S, Zambare V. Mechanisms and applications of probiotics in healthcare industry. Biotechnology in Healthcare. 2022:225-257. DOI: 10.1016/b978-0-323-90042-3.00002-5

[13] Probiotics in Animal Feed Market Analysis|Markets and Markets [Internet]. Available from: https://www.marketsandmarkets.com/Market-Reports/probiotics-animal-feed-market-85832335.html [Accessed: January 15, 2023]

[14] Choudhari G, Zambare V, Pawar R. Screening, isolation and characterization of probiotically safe lactic acid bacteria from human faeces for biofilm

formation. International Journal of Research in BioSciences. 2018;**7**(2):10-18

[15] Tiwari G, Tiwari R, Pandey S, Pandey P. Promising future of probiotics for human health: Current scenario. Chronicles of Young Scientists. 2012;**3**(1):17. DOI: 10.4103/2229-5186.94308

[16] Cox CM, Dalloul RA. Immunomodulatory role of probiotics in poultry and potential in ovo application. Beneficial Microbes. 2015;**6**(1):45-52. DOI: 10.3920/bm2014.0062

[17] Tsirtsikos P, Fegeros K, Balaskas C, Kominakis A, Mountzouris KC. Dietary probiotic inclusion level modulates intestinal mucin composition and mucosal morphology in broilers. Poultry Science. 2012;**91**(8):1860-1868. DOI: 10.3382/ps.2011-02005

[18] De Souza OF, Vecchi B, Gumina E, Matté F, Gazoni FL, Hernandez-Velasco X, et al. Development and evaluation of a commercial direct-fed microbial (Zymospore®) on the fecal microbiome and growth performance of broiler chickens under experimental challenge conditions. Animals. 2022;**12**(11):1436. DOI: 10.3390/ani12111436

[19] Georgieva V, Denev ST, Marinov B. Effect of some probiotic and nutritive means on chicken broiler productivity. Zhivotnovdni Nauki. 2000;**37**:19-23

[20] Wahyuni AETH, Prakasita VC, Nahak TEM, Tae AV, Chandra J, Ajiguna A, et al. Peluang Imbuhan Pakan Herbal-Probiotik Komersial "Promix®" Sebagai pengganti antibiotic growth promoter (AGP) pada ayam Pedaging yang Diberi Vaksin ND. Jurnal Sain Veteriner. 2019;**37**(2):180. DOI: 10.22146/jsv. 40375

[21] Wang Y, Li J, Xie Y, Zhang H, Jin J, Xiong L, et al. Effects of a probiotic-fermented herbal blend on the growth performance, intestinal flora and immune function of chicks infected with salmonella pullorum. Poultry Science. 2021;**100**(7):101196. DOI: 10.1016/j.psj.2021.101196

[22] Hosseini SM, Chamani M, Mousavi SN, Hosseini SA, Sadeghi AA. Effects of dietary physical form and dietary inclusion of probiotic and enzyme on growth performance, cellular and humoral immunity, and relative weights of lymphoid organs at early period of broiler chickens fed triticale-based diets. South African Journal of Animal Science. 2017;**47**(6):776. DOI: 10.4314/sajas.v47i6.5

[23] Goodarzi Boroojeni F, Vahjen W, Männer K, Blanch A, Sandvang D, Zentek J. *Bacillus subtilis* in broiler diets with different levels of energy and protein. Poultry Science. 2018;**97**(11):3967-3976

[24] Manafi M, Khalaji S, Hedayati M, Pirany N. Efficacy of *Bacillus subtilis* and bacitracin methylene disalicylate on growth performance, digestibility, blood metabolites, immunity, and intestinal microbiota after intramuscular inoculation with escherichia coli in broilers. Poultry Science. 2017;**96**(5):1174-1183. DOI: 10.3382/ps/pew347

[25] Khattab AAA, El Basuini MFM, El-Ratel IT, Fouda SF. Dietary probiotics as a strategy for improving growth performance, intestinal efficacy, immunity, and antioxidant capacity of white Pekin ducks fed with different levels of CP. Poultry Science. 2021;**100**(3):100898. DOI: 10.1016/j.psj.2020.11.067

[26] Bidura IGNG, Siti NW, Partama IBG. Effect of probiotics, *saccharomyces* spp. kb-5 and KB-8, in diets on growth

performance and cholesterol levels in ducks. South African. Journal of Animal Science. 2019;**49**(2):219. DOI: 10.4314/sajas.v49i2.2

[27] Erdoğmuş SZ, Gülmez N, Findik A, Sah H, Gülmez M. Probiyotiklerin Eimeria tenella İle Enfekte Broiler Piliçlerin Sağlık Durumu ve Verim Performansı Üzerine Etkileri. Kafkas Universitesi Veteriner Fakultesi Dergisi. 2018;**25**(3):311-320. DOI: 10.9775/kvfd.2018.20889

[28] Kim HW, Yan FF, Hu JY, Cheng HW, Kim YHB. Effects of probiotics feeding on meat quality of chicken breast during postmortem storage. Poultry Science. 2016;**95**(6):1457-1464. DOI: 10.3382/ps/pew055

[29] Khanian M, Karimi-Torshizi M-A, Allameh A. Alleviation of aflatoxin-related oxidative damage to liver and improvement of growth performance in broiler chickens consumed *Lactobacillus plantarum* 299v for entire growth period. Toxicon. 2019;**158**:57-62. DOI: 10.1016/j.toxicon.2018.11.431

[30] Fesseha H, Demlie T, Mathewos M, Eshetu E. Effect of *Lactobacillus* species probiotics on growth performance of dual-purpose chicken. Veterinary Medicine: Research and Reports. 2021;**12**:75-83. DOI: 10.2147/vmrr.s300881

[31] Khabirov A, Khaziakhmetov F, Kuznetsov V, Tagirov H, Rebezov M, Andreyeva A, et al. Effect of NORMOSIL probiotic supplementation on the growth performance and blood parameters of broiler chickens. Indian Journal of Pharmaceutical Education and Research. 2020;**54**(4):1046-1055. DOI: 10.5530/ijper.54.4.199

[32] Zaghari M, Sarani P, Hajati H. Comparison of two probiotic preparations on growth performance, intestinal microbiota, nutrient digestibility and cytokine gene expression in broiler chickens. Journal of Applied Animal Research. 2020;**48**(1):166-175. DOI: 10.1080/09712119.2020.1754218

[33] Mohammed AA, Zaki RS, Negm EA, Mahmoud MA, Cheng HW. Effects of dietary supplementation of a probiotic (*Bacillus subtilis*) on bone mass and meat quality of broiler chickens. Poultry Science. 2021;**100**(3):100906. DOI: 10.1016/j.psj.2020.11.073

[34] Ogbuagu NE, Aluwong T, Ayo JO, Sumanu VO. Effect of fisetin and probiotic supplementation on erythrocyte osmotic fragility, malondialdehyde concentration and superoxide dismutase activity in broiler chickens exposed to heat stress. Journal of Veterinary Medical Science. 2018;**80**(12):1895-1900. DOI: 10.1292/jvms.18-0477

[35] Cramer TA, Kim HW, Chao Y, Wang W, Cheng HW, Kim YH. Effects of probiotic (*Bacillus subtilis*) supplementation on meat quality characteristics of breast muscle from broilers exposed to chronic heat stress. Poultry Science. 2018;**97**(9):3358-3368. DOI: 10.3382/ps/pey176

[36] Wang WC, Yan FF, Hu JY, Amen OA, Cheng HW. Supplementation of *Bacillus subtilis*-based probiotic reduces heat stress-related behaviors and inflammatory response in broiler Chickens1. Journal of Animal Science. 2018;**96**(5):1654-1666. DOI: 10.1093/jas/sky092

[37] Lan PT, Sakamoto M, Benno Y. Effects of two probiotic *Lactobacillus* strains on jejunal and cecal microbiota of broiler chicken under acute heat stress condition as revealed by molecular analysis of 16S rRNA genes.

Microbiology and Immunology. 2004;**48**(12):917-929. DOI: 10.1111/j.1348-0421.2004.tb03620.x

[38] Khan A, Khan I, Khan S, Afzal S, Hamid M, Tariq M, et al. Selenium-enriched probiotics improve hepatic protection by regulating pro-inflammatory cytokines and antioxidant capacity in broilers under heat stress conditions. Journal of Advanced Veterinary and Animal Research. 2019;**6**(3):355. DOI: 10.5455/javar.2019.f354

[39] Khan AZ, Khan IU, Afzal S, Khan S, Khan MA, Altaf Hossain FM, et al. Effects of selenium-enriched probiotics on lameness and growth improvement in broiler chickens under heat stress condition. Acta Veterinaria Eurasia. 2021;**47**(1):19-18. DOI: 10.5152/actavet.2020.20044

[40] Zhang L, Wang Y, Jia H, Liu X, Zhang R, Guan J. Transcriptome and metabolome analyses reveal the regulatory effects of compound probiotics on cecal metabolism in heat-stressed broilers. Poultry Science. 2023;**102**(1):102323. DOI: 10.1016/j.psj.2022.102323

[41] Li Q, Wan G, Peng C, Xu L, Yu Y, Li L, et al. Effect of probiotic supplementation on growth performance, intestinal morphology, barrier integrity, and inflammatory response in broilers subjected to cyclic heat stress. Animal Science Journal. 2020;**91**(1):e13433. DOI: 10.1111/asj.13433

[42] Penha Filho RA, Díaz SJ, Fernando FS, Chang Y-F, Andreatti Filho RL, Berchieri JA. Immunomodulatory activity and control of *Salmonella enteritidis* colonization in the intestinal tract of chickens by *Lactobacillus* based probiotic. Veterinary Immunology and Immunopathology. 2015;**167**(1-2):64-69. DOI: 10.1016/j.vetimm.2015.06.006

[43] Mengistu BM, Bitsue HK, Huang K. The effects of selenium-enriched probiotics on growth performance, oocysts shedding, intestinal cecal lesion scores, antioxidant capacity, and mRNA gene expression in chickens infected with *Eimeria tenella*. Biological Trace Element Research. 2020;**199**(1):278-291. DOI: 10.1007/s12011-020-02118-7

[44] Reuben RC, Sarkar SL, Ibnat H, Setu MA, Roy PC, Jahid IK. Novel multi-strain probiotics reduces Pasteurella multocida induced fowl cholera mortality in broilers. Scientific Reports. 2021;**11**(1):8885. DOI: 10.1038/s41598-021-88299-0

[45] Wang H, Ni X, Qing X, Liu L, Xin J, Luo M, et al. Probiotic *Lactobacillus johnsonii* BS15 improves blood parameters related to immunity in broilers experimentally infected with subclinical necrotic enteritis. Frontiers in Microbiology. 2018:**9**:49. DOI: 10.3389/fmicb.2018.00049

[46] Mohsin M, Zhang Z, Yin G. Effect of probiotics on the performance and intestinal health of broiler chickens infected with *Eimeria tenella*. Vaccine. 2022;**10**(1):97. DOI: 10.3390/vaccines10010097

[47] Memon FU, Leghari IH, Rajput N, Gadahi JA, Sahito JZ, Yang Y, et al. Immunomodulatoryandameliorative effects of probiotic in combination with diclazuril on broilers under Coccidia infection. Journal of Applied Microbiology. 2022;**132**(4):3181-3188. DOI: 10.1111/jam.15380

[48] Śmiałek M, Kowalczyk J, Koncicki A. The use of probiotics in the reduction of campylobacter spp prevalence in poultry.

Animals. 2021;**11**(5):1355. DOI: 10.3390/ani11051355

[49] Sarwar N. Protective effect of probiotics in combination with vaccination on antibody response, biochemical and hematological indices in broilers. Pakistan Veterinary Journal. 2019;**39**(03):451-454. DOI: 10.29261/pakvetj/2019.023

[50] Borda-Molina D, Seifert J, Camarinha-Silva A. Current perspectives of the chicken gastrointestinal tract and its microbiome. Computational and Structural Biotechnology Journal. 2018;**16**:131-139. DOI: 10.1016/j.csbj.2018.03.002

[51] Singh KM, Shah TM, Reddy B, Deshpande S, Rank DN, Joshi CG. Taxonomic and gene-centric metagenomics of the fecal microbiome of low and high feed conversion ratio (FCR) broilers. Journal of Applied Genetics. 2013;**55**(1):145-154. DOI: 10.1007/s13353-013-0179-4

[52] Zhu L, Liao R, Wu N, Zhu G, Yang C. Heat stress mediates changes in fecal microbiome and functional pathways of laying hens. Applied Microbiology and Biotechnology. 2018;**103**(1):461-472. DOI: 10.1007/s00253-018-9465-8

[53] Tilocca B, Witzig M, Rodehutscord M, Seifert J. Variations of phosphorous accessibility causing changes in microbiome functions in the gastrointestinal tract of chickens. PLoS One. 2016;**11**(10):e0164735. DOI: 10.1371/journal.pone.0164735

[54] Bajagai YS, Klieve AV, Dart PJ, Bryden WL. Probiotics in animal nutrition – Production, impact and regulation. In: Makkar HPS, editor. Animal Production and Health. Paper No. 179. Rome, Italy: Food and Agriculture Organisation of the United Nations (FAO); 2016

Section 2

Probiotics in Nutrition

Chapter 7

Regular Physical Activity Influences Gut Microbiota with Positive Health Effects

Mihaela Jurdana and Darja Barlič Maganja

Abstract

The gut microbiota is believed to have a major impact on human health and disease. It is involved in barrier functions and maintenance of homeostasis. It provides nutrients and metabolites, participates in a signaling network, regulates epithelial development, and influences the immune system as well as protects the intestinal mucosa from the aggression of pathogenic microorganisms. There is growing evidence that physical activity has an impact on the gut microbiota. Recent studies in animals and humans suggest that regular physical activity increases the presence of beneficial microbial species and improves host health. However, some specific differences should be noted: different forms of physical activity, frequency or intensity, aerobic or resistance training, and benefits and consequences for amateur or competitive athletes. Because the positive role of physical activity can have an impact on health and various types of diseases, the results of research studies in this area are increasingly becoming the focus of scientific interest. In addition, probiotic supplements modulate intestinal microbial flora, and the ability of probiotics to modulate perturbations in immune function after exercise highlights their potential for use in individuals exposed to high levels of physical activity.

Keywords: gut microbiota, immune system, physical exercise, health, probiotics

1. Introduction

The human gastrointestinal tract is inhabited by hundreds of thousands of microorganisms that represent highly diverse microbiota. Gut microbiota comprises a metabolically active and complex ecosystem (bacteria, archaea, viruses, and unicellular eukaryotes) that colonizes the digestive tract soon after birth [1]. It has a crucial role in establishing a dynamic association with the human organism, having crucial roles in several physiological and pathological processes [2, 3]. It protects the host from the colonization of pathogens and is linked to nutrient digestion and absorption as well as to immunological, metabolic, and motor functions [4].

In the adult gut microbiota, four major microbial phyla are known to represent over 90% of the bacterial components: *Firmicutes*, *Bacteroides*, *Proteobacteria*, and *Actinobacteria* [5]. *Firmicutes* phyla mainly include *Ruminococcus*, *Clostridium*,

Lactobacillus, *Eubacterium*, *Faecalibacterium*, and *Roseburia*, while *Bacteroides* include *Prevotella* and *Xylanibacter*. Fewer representatives are from the phyla *Actinobacteria* and *Proteobacteria* [6].

The development and maturation of gut microbiota is a dynamic process that starts in early life. Its composition may be affected by several intrinsic and extrinsic factors, like mode of delivery, mother's age, diet and metabolic status, type of feeding, family genetics, lifestyle, exercise, immunological factors, drugs like antibiotics, and availability of nutrients [7–13]. Colonization of the infant's gut was thought to begin at birth, but scientific evidence has provided indications of bacterial presence in the placenta, umbilical cord, and amniotic fluid in healthy full-term pregnancies [14–16]. These findings suggest that microbial exposure may start before delivery, allowing colonization of the fetus with maternal microbiota. Another driver affecting the microbial colonization of the infant's intestine represents the delivery mode [17]. Vagina-associated microbes such as *Lactobacillus* and *Prevotella* colonize the neonatal gut of vaginally delivered infants [18, 19], while infants which are not directly exposed to maternal microbes during C-section become colonized by environmental microorganisms from maternal skin, the hospital staff, and the hospital environment [7, 11, 19–21]. The introduction of solid food to an infant's diet changes the microbiota, and by the age of three, it resembles a relatively stable adult-like profile with a dense microbial population [12]. The composition of the gut microbiota in the adult population is relatively stable and is only transiently altered by different external factors. It is now evidenced that dietary factors, particularly the amount, type, and balance of the main dietary macronutrients (carbohydrates, proteins, and fats), and different types and intensities of exercise play an important role in shaping the gut microbiota composition [22, 23]. The preservation of healthy gut microbiota has an important role in maintaining good health, with crucial effects on mucosal barrier fortification, motility of the gut, conversion of food into required nutrients, immune system homeostasis, and protection against pathogenic microorganisms [24].

2. Microbiota metabolites in health and disease

Exercise or physical activity can greatly affect the composition of the gut microbiota. It improves several metabolic and inflammatory parameters in chronic diseases and has been used as a therapeutic strategy in chronic diseases. In this chapter, we summarize several experimental findings on the possible mechanisms by which physical activity could influence gut microbiota. We also discuss the health benefits of physical activity, probiotic consumption, and microbiota diversity. The modification in the composition and function of the gut microbiota has an impact on intestinal permeability, digestion, metabolism, and immune responses. Many diseases, from digestive to metabolic problems as well as immunological and neuropsychiatric disorders, are linked to the pro-inflammatory state caused by the alternation of gut microbiota balance [13]. The gut microbiome contributes to digestion and promotes food absorption for host energy production. Its fermentation of non-digestible dietary residues leads to metabolites such as short-chain fatty acids (SCFAs, like butyrate, acetate, and propionate), which modulate the host energy balance increasing the availability of nutrients [25]. Fermented SCFAs, secreted into the gut lumen, exceed the epithelial barrier and are released into the bloodstream. They can be used as energy sources by the intestinal microbiota and by the host cells. They could provide nearly 10% of our daily energy requirements [26]. Butyrate is used as an energy source primarily by epithelial cells in the colon. Propionate is involved in liver gluconeogenesis [27]. It also decreases serum cholesterol levels, inhibits fatty-acid synthesis, and may be involved in weight control by stimulating satiety [28]. Acetate is metabolized in muscle tissue and can also cross the blood-brain barrier. It is used as a substrate for liver cholesterol and fatty acid synthesis [29, 30], increases colonic blood flow and oxygen uptake, and enhances ileal motility by affecting ileal contractions [31].

SCFAs can also contribute to shaping the gut environment and colon physiology, participating in different host-signaling mechanisms as well as possessing some anti-inflammatory effects [32–34]. Butyrate regulates the neutrophil function and migration, increases the expression of tight junction proteins in colon epithelia, enhances gut integrity, and activates intraepithelial lymphocytes (IELs), which express cytokines (IFN-γ and keratinocyte growth factor) to protect epithelial cells from injury [35, 36].

Besides producing SCFAs, bacterial species of the gut microbiota synthesize glycan, amino acids, and vitamins (K, B12, biotin, folate, and thiamine) and participate in the digestion of polysaccharides, increasing the amount of glucose in the liver and, therefore, increasing lipogenesis [33, 37–39].

Protective functions of microbiota are performed also through competition with pathogens for nutrients and receptors and the production of antimicrobial molecules and metabolites to avoid colonization by pathogens [40]. Through ligands from commensal bacteria (lipopolysaccharide, LPS), the gut microbiota influences the mucosal immune system development and function [41].

Gastrointestinal mucosa is a complex system acting as a physical barrier that regulates epithelial permeability. The regulation of trans-epithelial permeability allows the absorption of nutrients from the intestinal lumen through the cells lining the gut wall into the blood circulation [42]. Gut bacteria-epithelial cell interactions have been suggested as key contributors to epithelial permeability. Dysregulation of the gut microbiota and disruption of the gut mucosa enable harmful substances to pass through the barrier and can lead to the development of several chronic diseases [13, 43]. Gut dysbiosis, characterized by an imbalance in the composition and activity of gut microbial communities, has been linked to functional and inflammatory disorders [44, 45].

3. Gut microbiota composition and physical activity

Physical activity, especially moderate, has a positive effect on our body [34]. It can reduce metabolic and inflammatory diseases and influence the microbiota and health of humans and animals. Physical activity can be divided into the moderate level ($< 70\%$ VO_2 max) and high-intensity level ($> 70\%$ VO_{2max}). According to published studies, moderate physical activity has a positive effect on intestinal permeability, absorption and assimilation of food, and excretion of toxic metabolites [46]. In contrast, higher exercise intensity can negatively affect the digestive system and lead to the exercise-induced gastrointestinal syndrome, which affects 70% of athletes [47]. This may be the result of exercise-induced changes in the immune system of the digestive tract, leading to an increase in the inflammatory response and gastrointestinal symptoms [48].

The balance between exercise intensity, performance, and microbiota composition should be monitored for a long-time to optimize performance, health, and well-being and limit gastrointestinal syndromes.

3.1 Associations between physical activity and changes in gut microbiota in animal studies

Many animal experiments have been performed on mice and rodents, which are good models for mimicking human physiology. In animals, different forms of exercise, especially voluntary and forced, resulted in different effects on the composition of the microbiome. Many germ-free animal studies have indicated the relationship between gut microbiota and host function [49, 50]. Alteration in gut microbiota and its metabolites can affect the structure of the mucus layer and immune system after gut microbiota colonization in germ-free animals. It was demonstrated [50] that exercise training triggered changes in gut microbiota community structure in donor mice and in gut physiology in recipient mice after 5 weeks of gut microbiota transplantation and colonization. Thus, the composition of the gut microbiota of recipient mice is dependent on the physical activity of their respective donors. This suggests that physical training directly alters the host response through cytokines and the production of intestinal metabolites.

SCFAs upregulated after exercise contribute to improved energy production and reduce inflammation in the gut of physically active individuals [51]. In addition, voluntary exercise training increases host butyrate concentration and its bacterial genera, which is associated with an increase in fat-free mass in early life [52].

It is believed that an increase in butyrate levels after exercise protects against intestinal inflammation and colon cancer [53, 54]. The mechanism of these changes is not yet fully understood. However, voluntary and/or forced exercise certainly influences the composition of the gut microbiota in animals.

Maternal gut microbiota during pregnancy and lactation influences the gut microbiota of rat offspring. Physical activity during pregnancy affects maternal obesity in offspring and plasma insulin and glucose concentrations [55]. Exercises started in youth can influence the bacteria ratio. In some studies, a decrease in Firmicutes and/or an increase in Bacteroidetes was observed [56–58], while other studies showed the opposite effect [49, 59–61] or no effect [62].

Early childhood exercise can influence the composition of the gut microbiota in rats and improve the development of brain function [52]. The authors confirmed the anti-inflammatory effect of regular exercise, which protects from chronic inflammatory diseases [63].

In addition, recent studies have linked the microbiota to muscle function after antibiotic use. Depletion of the microbiota by antibiotic use resulted in decreased running performance and contractile muscle function [34, 46]. A similar effect was observed with low-carbohydrate diets, which decreased SCFA production.

3.2 Associations between physical activity and changes in gut microbiota in human studies

A positive effect of physical activity on the composition of the gut microbiota has been found in human studies and confirmed animal findings. A positive effect of moderate exercise on the gut was the shortening of stool time and contact time between pathogens and the gastrointestinal mucosa [64], so exercise prevents the risk of many inflammatory diseases and various cancers. Other possible beneficial effects of moderate exercise include reduction of LPS production, increased production of SCFAs and immunoglobulins, and increase of butyrate concentration with anticarcinogenic and anti-inflammatory properties [64].

Similar to animal studies, exercise-induced changes in microbiota diversity may reduce obesity-related complications in humans. The effect on the microbiota can be assessed by measuring diversity or functions. α-diversity represents the overall diversity of samples, while β-diversity compares how different bacterial species are distributed across different samples [42].

Based on the available studies, intense exercise, compared to moderate exercise, seems to cause more significant disturbances than moderate exercise on the human body's homeostasis [34]. High levels of inflammation (higher inflammatory interleukin-6 (IL-6)) and tumor necrosis factor-alpha (TNF-α), as well as gastrointestinal symptoms with increased intestinal permeability, were found in elite athletes [65, 66]. This may be related to diet as macronutrient intake before, during, and after exercise may influence performance and inflammatory responses in athletes [67]. Adequate carbohydrate intake after acute exercise lowers inflammatory cytokines. In addition, differences in fiber consumption impact the type and amount of SCFAs produced by microbiota [68]. Several studies have reported that fiber intake in athletes is low compared with dietary guidelines. In addition, special attention should be paid to protein supplementation in athletes. It has been demonstrated that long-term protein supplementation can have negative effects on the gut microbiota (abundance of *Bacteroidetes*) [69].

Importantly, the fitness status of participants also affects gut microbiota; individuals with good physical condition have more butyrate-producing bacterial taxa from the *Firmicutes* phylum, and 6-week intervention study in lean adults increased fecal SCFAs [34].

The World Health Organization (WHO) has published recommendations for physical activity in adults (150 minutes of moderate physical activity or at least 75 minutes of vigorous physical activity per week). The composition of the gut microbiota in women who exercised according to the recommendation of WHO was modified [70]. Similarly, in male participants with insulin resistance, both high-intensity and moderate-intensity continuous exercise resulted in an increase in *Bacteroidetes* and a decrease in inflammation [71]. A 6-month intervention with progressive exercise training leads to an increase in α-diversity as well as in the concentration of some physiologically relevant metabolites [72].

A large study conducted on 86 elite rugby athletes showed a greater gut microbiota richness/diversity compared to controls [73]. This study among elite rugby players provided evidence of the beneficial effect of exercise on gut microbiota diversity. However, the results indicated that these differences between the elite and control groups were associated with dietary extremes that could represent confounding factors.

Another study on international rugby players showed differences in the composition and functional capacity of gut microbiota as well as in microbial and human-derived metabolites [74].

In addition, a positive correlation was found between cardiorespiratory fitness (CRF), an indicator of physical fitness, and microbial diversity in 39 healthy individuals, especially in taxa that augmented the production of butyrate [75]. The authors concluded that exercise can be prescribed in patients with dysbiosis-associated diseases.

The microbiota of professional and amateur cyclists was studied by Petersen [64]. They found that the gut microbiota of professional cyclists differed from that of amateurs. In addition, a correlation between certain microorganisms in professional cyclists and high training intensities was confirmed. This study suggests that training intensity influences bacterial community structure.

Higher exercise intensity leads to changes in the gut microbiota (**Figure 1**). Exercise leads to a positive change in the bacterial composition of the gut microbiota. Higher exercise intensities require dietary intervention to prevent gastrointestinal dysfunction and inflammatory responses. Longitudinal studies monitoring exercise intensity, diet and other characteristics, and gut microbiota are still lacking. To express the intensity level of physical activity, the rate of energy expenditure expressed as metabolic equivalents (METs) is used: 1 MET is the rate of energy expenditure at rest, which for most people approximates an oxygen uptake of 3.5 milliliters per kilogram of body weight per minute (**Figure 1**).

Murtaza and coworkers [76] investigated the effects of different nutritional protocols on the fecal microbiota of elite endurance race walkers during an intense training program. This study showed that an intense training load with different dietary patterns had effects on the diversity of the gut microbiota. Specifically, it was found that a ketogenic, low-carbohydrate, and high-fat diet resulted in changes in the richness of some bacterial species [76].

Furthermore, the health benefits of physical activity in older adults have been established in several scientific studies. A relationship between physical activity and the diversity of the intestinal microbiota has been found in elderly people [77]. The abundance of *Bacteroides* significantly increased after aerobic exercise training in elderly women [78]. Results of many studies reported that gut microbiota composition does not change in some conditions, such as hypertension, obesity-associated inflammation, and gastrointestinal diseases [53, 79]. Exercise can modulate the gut microbiota diversity and could have positive effects on the pathogenesis of mentioned conditions. Since lower inflammation has been demonstrated, it is possible that exercise could decrease inflammatory markers in older adults. Exercise-induced changes in microbial composition are related to exercise duration. Recently, it has been confirmed that short-term endurance exercise in elderly men has little effect on the composition and diversity of the gut microbiota.

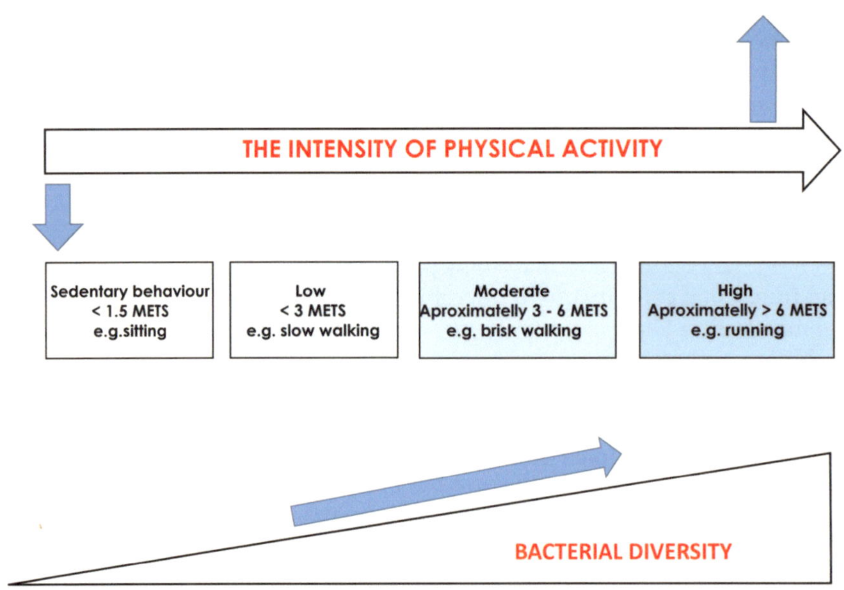

Figure 1.
Exercise can increase the number of beneficial microbial species and enrich the diversity of microflora.

However, small changes in the microbiota have been associated with lower cardiometabolic risk factors [79]. The study suggests that the gut microbiota is influenced by high-intensity exercise and diet and might play a crucial role in modulating cardiovascular disease development [80].

Overall, physical activity could be a strong modulator of gut microbiota composition. Experimental data showed that physical activity between 60 and 70% VO_{2max} affected β diversity; interestingly, exercise at 70% VO_{2max} resulted in an increase of α diversity or a decrease in *Clostridium difficile* [46].

Further studies need to clarify the effects of different types, intensities, and frequencies of physical activity on microbiota diversity and function. High intensity of physical activity decreases producers of SCFAs and increases pathogenic bacteria. This condition requires dietary supplementation [59] or a nutritional strategy [1] to maintain the structure and richness of the gut microbiota.

4. The beneficial effect of probiotics in physically active individuals

Probiotics are currently defined as live microorganisms that have a beneficial health effect on the host when consumed in adequate amounts [81, 82]. They have an impact on the intestinal ecosystem through interactions with the host cells as well as intestinal microbiota regulating gut mucosal immunity. Among others, these interactions can contribute to improving the intestinal microenvironment, strengthening the intestinal barrier, modulating mucus secretion and the secretion of immunoglobulins or cytokines, as well as activating the innate immune response.

The beneficial role of probiotics relies on their ability to modulate the host's microbiota and to improve the barrier function of the gut mucosa [83, 84]. Probiotics produce broad-spectrum inhibitory bacteriocins and metabolites such as SCFAs inducing a decrease of the pH less favorable for bacterial growth [85]. Higher SCFA concentrations also reduce the differentiation of dendritic cells, thus decreasing pro-inflammatory cytokines production [86–88].

Probiotics improve the barrier function and tight junctions (TJs) between intestinal epithelial cells at the level of signaling pathways leading to the increase of the mucus layer or to the production of defensins as well as proteins of TJs. They regulate the expression of the TJs, where cellular contacts occur and thus maintain cell morphology. As have already been reviewed, several probiotic strains, like *Lactobacillus rhamnosus* GG, *Lactobacillus casei* DN-114001, *Escherichia coli* Nissle 1917, and different strains of *Lactobacillus plantarum*, have a protective effect against pathogen infections via the regulation of TJ proteins [89].

Other important components that build a protective barrier and avoid the adhesion of harmful bacteria to the epithelial cells are the mucus layer and cells of the intestinal epithelium and underlying lamina propria [90]. Each of them consists of several cell types preventing any direct contact with bacteria in the intestinal lumen. The intestinal epithelium consists of enterocytes responsible for absorbing molecules from the intestinal lumen. Paneth cells specialized in synthesizing and secreting antimicrobial peptides (AMPs) upon contact with enteric bacteria, Goblet cells, and entero-endocrine cells [90–92]. Goblet cells produce mucus and are mainly composed of high molecular weight glycoproteins called mucins. They are of two types: secreted mucins are responsible for the formation of the mucus layer, while transmembrane mucins are likely involved in signaling pathways [93–95]. A healthy mucus layer plays an important role in preventing inflammatory and infectious diseases. Altered expression of specific mucins was associated with gastrointestinal diseases such as Crohn's disease [96] and ulcerative colitis [97] highlighting the importance of these proteins in the intestine. Several studies confirmed that specific strains of probiotic bacteria might affect the mucus barrier by regulating mucin expression. Thus, they can influence the properties of the mucus layer and indirectly regulate the gut immune system [89]. In multiple *in vitro* and in *vivo models*, it was shown that specific probiotic bacteria stimulate the gene expression levels of mucins. Among them, *L. plantarum* 299v, *E. coli* Nissle 1917, *L. casei* GG and *Lactobacillus acidophilus* LA1, and *Lactobacillus reuteri* R2LC or 4659 as well as probiotic mixture VSL#3 were confirmed to increase the level of mucins in the gut, therefore, influencing the properties of the mucus layer and indirectly regulate the gut immune system [95, 98–103]. It has also been evidenced that *Akkermancia muciniphila* increases the number of Goblet cells and the production of antimicrobial peptides, suggesting that it communicates with host cells and consequently stimulates the production of mucus [104].

Recent findings demonstrate that probiotics modulate the intestinal immune system by activating the immune response by recognizing specific receptors of innate immunity cells (epithelial cells, dendritic cells, and T cells). These receptors are called pattern recognition receptors (PRR) and include mostly Toll-like receptors (TLRs) and nucleotide-binding oligomerization domain agents (NODs) [105]. They are recognized by MAMPs (microbe-associated molecular patterns). Their interaction with the gut epithelium stimulates the cells of the gut immune system at the lamina propria [106]. Differentiation of T helper lymphocytes and the activation of regulatory T cells stimulate the pro- or anti-inflammatory cytokines production. Probiotic bacteria, especially various *Bifidobacterium* strains, can act differently depending on the cytokine profile [107]. The effects may be systemic or local and limited to the stimulation of IgA secretion by Peyer's patch cells [84, 108].

Several studies have shown that probiotics supplementation could improve immune function in athletes [109]; reduce upper respiratory tract illness (URTI) [110], gastrointestinal symptoms [111–113], and gut permeability [114, 115]; as well as increase physical performance in elite and competitive athletes [113, 116].

Existing studies have shown an association between intestinal microbiota composition and physical activity, suggesting that modifications in the gut microbiota composition may contribute to the physical performance and exercise capacity of the host [117]. Probiotics may promote health through the improvement of the immune system and indirectly influence the performance of athletes by preventing illnesses that negatively affect healthy training [109, 118]. Recently, the International Society of Sports Nutrition (ISSN) provided a position stand on probiotics, concluding that probiotics have strain-specific effects in athletes [119]. Specific probiotic strains can improve the integrity of the gut barrier function in athletes after prolonged exercise, especially in the heat, which has been shown to increase gut permeability potentially causing systemic toxemia. Administration of selected probiotic strains has been linked to improved body composition and lean body mass, improved recovery from muscle-damaging exercise, normalizing age-related declines in testosterone levels, reductions in cortisol levels indicating improved responses to a physical or mental stressor, reduction of exercise-induced lactate, and increased neurotransmitter synthesis, cognition, and mood [reviewed in 119].

Generally, mid to long-term benefits (supplementation periods varying from 2 weeks to 3 months) of probiotics on physical performance have been studied [117]. In different studies, various probiotic strains and doses were examined, so it is difficult to compare the obtained results. Among them, the most studied bacteria are members of *Lactobacillus* and *Bifidobacterium* genera.

Lactiplantibacillus plantarum TWK10 is among the most studied probiotic strains in terms of physical performance outcomes. A dose-dependent increase in muscle mass was observed in a preclinical animal study [120] and was further confirmed in clinical studies [121]. Endurance performance in an exhaustive treadmill exercise was improved in healthy, untrained adult males, who were supplemented daily with TWK10 for 6 weeks, compared with those who received a placebo [122]. The post-exercise blood glucose level was higher in TWK10 group compared with the control group suggesting improved energy harvest from gluconeogenic precursors during exhaustive exercise.

In male runners, supplementation with a multi-strain probiotic (*L. acidophilus*, *Lacticaseibacillus rhamnosus*, *Lacticaseibacillus casei*, *L. plantarum*, *Limosilactobacillus fermentum*, *Bifidobacterium lactis*, *B. breve*, *Bifidobacterium bifidum*, and *Streptococcus thermophilus*) for 4 weeks significantly increased the running time to fatigue [110].

Probiotic supplementation (*S. thermophilus* FP4 and *Bifidobacterium breve* BR03) was reported to likely enhance isometric average peak torque production, attenuating performance decrements and muscle tension in the days following a muscle-damaging exercise [123]. In a similar study design, *Bacillus coagulans* GBI-306086 significantly increased recovery at 24 and 72 h and decreased soreness at 72 h post-exercise [124]. Probiotic supplementation correlated with maintained performance and a small increase in creatine phosphokinase.

Probiotics, belonging to the *Veillonella* genus, isolated from a marathon runner, have recently shown promising results in mouse performance models [125]. These bacteria feed on lactic acid and produce propionate, which may increase endurance capacity.

In mice, oral administration of either *Bifidobacterium longum* subsp. longum OLP-01 [126] or *Ligilactobacillus salivarius* subsp. salicinius SA-03 [127], isolated from a female weightlifting Olympic medalist, was shown to significantly increase forelimb grip strength and endurance capacity in a swim-to-exhaustion test. Both bacterial strains significantly decreased blood lactate, ammonia, and creatine kinase levels after an acute exercise and increased hepatic and muscle glycogen stores, which indicated improved energy utilization and the attenuation of fatigue-related biomarkers in mice.

However, not all studies have shown enhancements in endurance performance following probiotic use in highly trained subjects or athletes [119]. It has been shown that the exhaustive endurance exercise was not affected in endurance-trained males after 4 weeks of *Lactobacillus fermentum* VRI-003 supplementation [128] or after *Lactobacillus helveticus* Lafti L10 in trained subjects [129]. Also, 3 months of supplementation with a probiotic formula containing bacteria of different species (*B. bifidum* W23, *B. lactis* W51, *Enterococcus faecium* W54, *L. acidophilus* W22, *Levilactobacillus brevis* W63, and *Lactococcus lactis* W58) did not have benefit in endurance performance in highly trained athletes [130]. However, after a 2-month intervention in female swimmers, probiotic yogurt with *L. acidophilus* SPP, *L. bulgaricus*, *B. bifidum*, and *S. thermophilus* improved the VO_{2max} but had no impact on the 400-m swimming time [131]. Also after a 6-week intervention in competitive, high-level, female swimmers *B. longum* 35,624 did not enhance aerobic or anaerobic swimming performance or improve power or force production measurements [132]. After a 12-week multi-strain probiotic or probiotic + glutamine supplementation, no effects were observed on the time to complete an ultra-marathon race compared with controls [133].

Multi-strain probiotic supplementation (*L. acidophilus* CUL60 and CUL21, *B. bifidum* CUL20, and *Bifidobacterium animalis* subs p. lactis CUL34) for 28 days prior to a marathon race was associated with a limited decrease in average speed in the probiotics group compared to the control group [134]. However, there were no significant differences in finish times between the groups. *Bacillus subtilis* supplementation during training soccer and volleyball female players, in conjunction with postworkout nutrition, had no effect on physical performance [135]. However, body fat percentages were significantly lower in the probiotic group. *B. subtilis* DE111 did not improve either strength or performance in male [136] or female athletes [137] when combined with a training protocol involving resistance exercises.

Multi-strain probiotic supplementation for 12 weeks, combined with circuit training, improved muscular performance to a similar degree as circuit training alone in healthy, sedentary males [138], confirming the positive effect of resistance training on muscular outcomes, demonstrated well by other probiotic and exercise interventions among athletes [136, 137].

The well-established probiotic effects on gut health and immune system function may benefit endurance athletes, who perform high-intensity training and often encounter physiological challenges associated with GI and immune health during and after a competition. However, high-quality clinical studies, with adequate power, is necessary to uncover the impacts of probiotics on physical performance and the mechanisms of action through which probiotics affect exercise outcomes.

5. Conclusions

In recent years, the research of human gut microbiota and their interaction with their human host has extensively increased. It has been shown that the composition of the gut microbiota is influenced by several factors such as diet, age, host genetics, drugs, as well as exercise and its level of activity. Animal and human studies have indicated that gut microbiota plays an important role in the occurrence of several diseases. Mainly, it has been evidenced that its composition and function have a direct effect on host physiology and can also affect physical performance.

Exercise improves the diversity of the gut microbiota, the maintenance of normal gut physiology, and contributes to the reduction of gastrointestinal symptoms and inflammatory markers in various pathological conditions as well as altering hundreds of metabolites.

Therefore, regular physical activity should be considered as a treatment to maintain the eubiosis of the microbiota, leading to an improvement in health status. Higher CRF levels lead to greater bacterial diversity, regardless of diet. Aerobic activities appear to be able to produce significant changes in the composition of the microbiota, although the modalities and intensity of exercise may affect the microbiota differently.

The amount and frequency recommended by WHO (the minimum dose of physical activity) for adults seem to cause some changes in the composition of the microbiota. Strenuous and/or excessively prolonged exercise with inadequate carbohydrate intake may have a negative impact on the microbiota due to inflammation and gastrointestinal symptoms. Nevertheless, further studies are needed to understand how physical activity and diet independently affect the microbiota.

The use of probiotics has recently received increasing attention. Probiotics have potential health benefits, generally improving or restoring the gut microbiota, and have been shown to modulate the immune system. Recent studies have shown that probiotics reduce upper respiratory tract illness (URTI) and the onset and severity of gastrointestinal symptoms as well as gut barrier function impairment during intense exercise. By improving the immune system, they indirectly influence the performance of athletes by preventing diseases that negatively affect healthy exercise. Through SCFAs produced by probiotic bacteria, they contribute to improved energy production and reduce inflammation in the gut of physically active individuals. Selected probiotic strains have been associated with improved body composition and lean body mass, improved recovery from muscle-damaging exercise, normalization of age-related decline in testosterone levels, and reduction in cortisol levels and exercise-induced lactate. The use of probiotics is a promising approach to improve the health, well-being, and performance of athletes.

Funding

The author(s) received no specific funding for this work.

Conflict of interest

The author has no competing interest to declare that may directly or indirectly affect the content of this article.

Appendices and nomenclature

AMPs	antimicrobial peptides
CRF	cardiorespiratory fitness
IELs	intraepithelial lymphocytes
IFN-γ	interferon gamma
IL-6	interleukin-6
ISSN	international society of sports nutrition
LPS	lipopolysaccharide
MAMPs	microbe-associated molecular patterns
MET	metabolic equivalents
NODs	nucleotide-binding oligomerization domain agents
SCFAs	short-chain fatty acids
TJs	tight junctions
TLRs	toll-like receptors
TNF-α	tumor necrosis factor-alpha
URTI	upper respiratory tract illness
WHO	world health organization

Author details

Mihaela Jurdana* and Darja Barlič Maganja
Faculty of Health Sciences, University of Primorska, Izola, Slovenia

*Address all correspondence to: mihaela.jurdana@fvz.upr.si

References

[1] Sekirov I, Russell SL, Antunes LC, Finlay BB. Gut microbiota in health and disease. Physiological Reviews. 2010;**90**(3):859-904. DOI: 10.1152/physrev.00045.2009

[2] Clemente JC, Ursell LK, Parfrey LW, Knight R. The impact of the gut microbiota on human health: An integrative view. Cell. 2012;**148**(6):1258-1270. DOI: 10.1016/j.cell.2012.01.035

[3] Goulet O. Potential role of the intestinal microbiota in programming health and disease. Nutrition Reviews. 2015;**73**:32-40. DOI: 10.1093/nutrit/nuv039

[4] Patel V. The gut microbiome. In: Short E, editor. A Prescription for Healthy Living. A Guide to Lifestyle Medicine. 2021. pp. 165-175. DOI: 10.1016/B978-0-12-821573-9.00015-1

[5] Spor A, Koren O, Ley R. Unraveling the effects of the environment and host genotype on the gut microbiome. Nature Reviews Microbiology. 2011;**9**:279-290. DOI: 10.1038/nrmicro2540

[6] Eckburg PB, Bik EM, Bernstein CN, Purdom E, Dethlefsen L, Sargent M, et al. Diversity of the human intestinal microbial flora. Science. 2005;**308**(5728):1635-1638. DOI: 10.1126/science.1110591

[7] Bokulich NA, Chung J, Battaglia T, Henderson N, Jay M, Li H, et al. Antibiotics, birth mode, and diet shape microbiome maturation during early life. Science Translational Medicine. 2016;**8**(343):343ra82. DOI: 10.1126/scitranslmed.aad7121

[8] Yatsunenko T, Rey FE, Manary MJ, Trehan I, Dominguez-Bello MG, Contreras M, et al. Human gut microbiome viewed across age and geography. Nature. 2012;**486**(7402):222-227. DOI: 10.1038/nature11053

[9] Kashtanova DA, Popenko AS, Tkacheva ON, Tyakht AB, Alexeev DG, Boytsov SA. Association between the gut microbiota and diet: Fetal life, early childhood, and further life. Nutrition (Burbank, Los Angeles County, Calif.). 2015;**32**(6):620-627. DOI: 10.1016/j.nut.2015.12.037

[10] Power SE, O'Toole PW, Stanton C, Ross RP, Fitzgerald GF. Intestinal microbiota, diet and health. British Journal of Nutrition. 2014;**111**(3):387-402. DOI: 10.1017/S0007114513002560

[11] Rodríguez JM, Murphy K, Stanton C, Ross RP, Kobe OI, Juge N, et al. The composition of the gut microbiota throughout life, with an emphasis on early life. Microbial Ecology in Health and Disease. 2015;**26**(1):26050. DOI: 10.3402/mehd.v26.26050

[12] Milani C, Duranti S, Bottacini F, Casey E, Turroni F, Mahony J, et al. The first microbial colonizers of the human gut: Composition, activities, and health implications of the infant gut microbiota. Microbiology and Molecular Biology Reviews. 2017;**81**(4):e00036-e00017. DOI: 10.1128/MMBR.00036-17

[13] Gomaa EZ. Human gut microbiota/microbiome in health and diseases: A review. Antonie Van Leeuwenhoek. 2020;**113**(12):2019-2040. DOI: 10.1007/s10482-020-01474-7

[14] Jiménez E, Fernández L, Marín ML, Martín R, Odriozola JM, Nueno-Palop C, et al. Isolation of commensal bacteria from umbilical cord blood of healthy

neonates born by cesarean section. Current Microbiology. 2005;**51**(4):270-274. DOI: 10.1007/s00284-005-0020-3

[15] DiGiulio DB, Romero R, Amogan HP, Kusanovic JP, Bik EM, Gotsch F, et al. Microbial prevalence, diversity and abundance in amniotic fluid during preterm labor: A molecular and culture-based investigation. PLoS One. 2008;**3**(8):e3056. DOI: 10.1371/journal.pone.0003056

[16] Aagaard K, Ma J, Antony KM, Ganu R, Petrosino J, Versalovic J. The placenta harbors a unique microbiome. Science Translational Medicine. 2014;**6**(237):237ra65-237ra65. DOI: 10.1126/scitranslmed.3008599

[17] Munyaka PM, Khafipour E, Ghia JE. External influence of early childhood establishment of gut microbiota and subsequent health implications. Frontiers in Pediatrics. 2014;**2**:109. DOI: 10.3389/fped.2014.00109

[18] Dominguez-Bello MG, Costello EK, Contreras M, Magris M, Hidalgo G, Fierer N, et al. Delivery mode shapes the acquisition and structure of the initial microbiota across multiple body habitats in newborns. Proceedings of the National Academy of Sciences. 2010;**107**(26):11971-11975. DOI: 10.1073/pnas.1002601107

[19] Biasucci G, Rubini M, Riboni S, Morelli L, Bessi E, Retetangos C. Mode of delivery affects the bacterial community in the newborn gut. Early Human Development. 2010;**86**(1):13-15. DOI: 10.1016/j.earlhumdev.2010.01.004

[20] Fouhy F, Ross RP, Fitzgerald GF, Stanton C, Cotter PD. Composition of the early intestinal microbiota: Knowledge, knowledge gaps and the use of high-throughput sequencing to address these gaps. Gut Microbes. 2012;**3**(3):203-220. DOI: 10.4161/gmic.20169

[21] Bäckhed F, Roswall J, Peng Y, Feng Q, Jia H, Kovatcheva-Datchary P, et al. Dynamics and stabilization of the human gut microbiome during the first year of life. Cell Host & Microbe. 2015;**17**(5):690-703. DOI: 10.1016/j.chom.2015.04.004

[22] Scott KP, Gratz SW, Sheridan PO, Flint HJ, Duncan SH. The influence of diet on the gut microbiota. Pharmacological Research. 2013;**69**(1):52-60. DOI: 10.1016/j.phrs.2012.10.020

[23] Milani C, Ticinesi A, Gerritsen J, Nouvenne A, Lugli GA, Mancabelli L, et al. Gut microbiota composition and Clostridium difficile infection in hospitalized elderly individuals: A metagenomic study. Scientific Reports. 2016;**6**(1):1-12. DOI: 10.1038/srep25945

[24] Aziz Q, Doré J, Emmanuel A, Guarner F, Quigley EMM. Gut microbiota and gastrointestinal health: Current concepts and future directions. Neurogastroenterology & Motility. 2013;**25**(1):4-15. DOI: 10.1111/nmo.12046

[25] Samuel BS, Shaito A, Motoike T, Rey FE, Backhed F, Manchester JK, et al. Effects of the gut microbiota on host adiposity are modulated by the short-chain fatty-acid binding G protein-coupled receptor, Gpr41. Proceedings of the National Academy of Sciences. 2008;**105**(43):16767-16772. DOI: 10.1073/pnas.0808567105

[26] Bergman EN. Energy contributions of volatile fatty acids from the gastrointestinal tract in various species. Physiological Reviews. 1990;**70**(2):567-590. DOI: 10.1152/physrev.1990.70.2.567

[27] LeBlanc JG, Chain F, Martín R, Bermúdez-Humarán LG, Courau S, Langella P. Beneficial effects on host

energy metabolism of short-chain fatty acids and vitamins produced by commensal and probiotic bacteria. Microbial Cell Factories. 2017;**16**(1):1-10. DOI: 10.1186/s12934-017-0691-z

[28] Hosseini E, Grootaert C, Verstraete W, Van de Wiele T. Propionate as a health-promoting microbial metabolite in the human gut. Nutrition Reviews. 2011;**69**(5):245-258. DOI: 10.1111/j.1753-4887.2011.00388.x

[29] Lin Y, Vonk RJ, Slooff MJ, Kuipers F, Smit MJ. Differences in propionate-induced inhibition of cholesterol and triacylglycerol synthesis between human and rat hepatocytes in primary culture. British Journal of Nutrition. 1995;**74**(2):197-207. DOI: 10.1079/BJN19950123

[30] Nishina PM, Freedland RA. Effects of propionate on lipid biosynthesis in isolated rat hepatocytes. The Journal of Nutrition. 1990;**120**(7):668-673. DOI: 10.1093/jn/120.7.668

[31] Scheppach W. Effects of short-chain fatty acids on gut morphology and function. Gut. 1994;**35**(Suppl. 1):S35-S38. DOI: 10.1136/gut.35.1_suppl.s35

[32] Hsu YJ, Chiu CC, Li YP, Huang WC, Te Huang Y, Huang CC, et al. Effect of intestinal microbiota on exercise performance in mice. The Journal of Strength & Conditioning Research. 2015;**29**(2):552-558. DOI: 10.1519/JSC.0000000000000644

[33] Wahlström A, Sayin SI, Marschall HU, Bäckhed F. Intestinal crosstalk between bile acids and microbiota and its impact on host metabolism. Cell Metabolism. 2016;**24**(1):41-50. DOI: 10.1016/j.cmet.2016.05.005

[34] Clauss M, Gérard P, Mosca A, Leclerc M. Interplay between exercise and gut microbiome in the context of human health and performance. Frontiers in Nutrition. 2021;**8**:637010. DOI: 10.3389/fnut.2021.637010

[35] Nicholson JK, Holmes E, Kinross J, Burcelin R, Gibson G, Jia W, et al. Host-gut microbiota metabolic interactions. Science. 2012;**336**(6086):1262-1267. DOI: 10.1126/science.1223813

[36] Shi N, Li N, Duan X, Niu H. Interaction between the gut microbiome and mucosal immune system. Military Medical Research. 2017;**4**(1):1-7. DOI: 10.1186/s40779-017-0122-9

[37] Flint HJ, Scott KP, Duncan SH, Louis P, Forano E. Microbial degradation of complex carbohydrates in the gut. Gut Microbes. 2012;**3**(4):289-306. DOI: 10.4161/gmic.19897

[38] Brahe LK, Astrup A, Larsen LH. Can we prevent obesity-related metabolic diseases by dietary modulation of the gut microbiota? Advances in Nutrition. 2016;**7**(1):90-101. DOI: 10.3945/an.115.010587

[39] Molinero N, Ruiz L, Sánchez B, Margolles A, Delgado S. Intestinal bacteria interplay with bile and cholesterol metabolism: Implications on host physiology. Frontiers in Physiology. 2019;**10**:185. DOI: 10.3389/fphys.2019.00185

[40] Akira S, Hemmi H. Recognition of pathogen-associated molecular patterns by TLR family. Immunology Letters. 2003;**85**(2):85-95. DOI: 10.1016/S0165-2478(02)00228-6

[41] Rakoff-Nahoum S, Paglino J, Eslami-Varzaneh F, Edberg S, Medzhitov R. Recognition of commensal microflora by toll-like receptors is required for intestinal homeostasis. Cell. 2004;**118**(2):229-241. DOI: 10.1016/j.cell.2004.07.002

[42] Bjarnason I, Macpherson A, Hollander D. Intestinal permeability: An overview. Gastroenterology. 1995;**108**(5):1566-1581. DOI: 10.1016/0016-5085(95)90708-4

[43] Vancamelbeke M, Vermeire S. The intestinal barrier: A fundamental role in health and disease. Expert Review of Gastroenterology & Hepatology. 2017;**11**(9):821-834. DOI: 10.1080/17474124.2017.1343143

[44] Natividad JM, Verdu EF. Modulation of intestinal barrier by intestinal microbiota: Pathological and therapeutic implications. Pharmacological Research. 2013;**69**(1):42-51. DOI: 10.1016/j.phrs.2012.10.007

[45] Allam-Ndoul B, Castonguay-Paradis S, Veilleux A. Gut microbiota and intestinal trans-epithelial permeability. International Journal of Molecular Sciences. 2020;**21**(17):6402. DOI: 10.3390/ijms21176402

[46] Dziewiecka H, Buttar HS, Kasperska A, Ostapiuk-Karolczuk J, Domagalska M, Cichoń J, et al. Physical activity induced alterations of gut microbiota in humans: A systematic review. BMC Sports Science, Medicine & Rehabilitation. 2022;**14**(1):122. DOI: 10.1186/s13102-022-00513-2

[47] Ribeiro FM, Petriz B, Marques G, Kamilla LH, Franco OL. Is there an exercise-intensity threshold capable of avoiding the leaky gut? Frontiers in Nutrition. 2021;**8**:627-289. DOI: 10.3389/fnut.2021.627289

[48] Camilleri M. Leaky gut: Mechanisms, measurement and clinical implications in humans. Gut. 2019;**68**(8):1516-1526. DOI: 10.1136/gutjnl-2019-318427

[49] Choi J, Eum SY, Rampersaud E, Daunert S, Abreu MT, Toborek M. Exercise attenuates PCB-induced changes in the mouse gut microbiome. Environmental Health Perspectives. 2013;**121**(6):725-730. DOI: 10.1289/ehp.1306534

[50] Allen JM, Mailing LJ, Cohrs J, Salmonson C, Fryer JD, Nehra V, et al. Exercise training-induced modification of the gut microbiota persists after microbiota colonization and attenuates the response to chemically-induced colitis in gnotobiotic mice. Gut Microbes. 2018;**9**(2):115-130. DOI: 10.1080/19490976.2017.1372077

[51] Turnbaugh PJ, Ley RE, Mahowald MA, Magrini V, Mardis ER, Gordon JI. An obesity-associated gut microbiome with increhased capacity for energy harvest. Nature. 2006;**444**(7122):1027-1031. DOI: 10.1038/nature05414

[52] Mika A, Van Treuren W, González A, Herrera JJ, Knight R, Fleshner M. Exercise is more effective at altering gut microbial composition and producing stable changes in lean mass in juvenile versus adult male F344 rats. PLoS One. 2015;**10**(5):e0125889. DOI: 10.1371/journal.pone.0125889

[53] Monda V, Villano I, Messina A, Valenzano A, Esposito T, Moscatelli F, et al. Exercise modifies the gut microbiota with positive health effects. Oxidative Medicine and Cellular Longevity. 2017;**2017**:3831972. DOI: 10.1155/2017/3831972

[54] Matsumoto M, Inoue R, Tsukahara T, Ushida K, Chij H, Matsubara N, et al. Voluntary running exercise alters microbiota composition and increases n-butyrate concentration in the rat cecum. Bioscience, Biotechnology and Biochemistry. 2008;**72**(2):572-576. DOI: 10.1271/bbb.70474

[55] Bhagavata Srinivasan SP, Raipuria M, Bahari H, Kaakoush NO, Morris MJ. Impacts of diet and exercise on maternal gut microbiota are transferred to offspring. Front Endocrinol (Lausanne). 2018;**9**:716. DOI: 10.3389/fendo.2018.00716

[56] Queipo-Ortuño MI, Seoane LM, Murri M, Pardo M, Gomez-Zumaquero JM, Cardona F, et al. Gut microbiota composition in male rat models under different nutritional status and physical activity and its association with serum leptin and ghrelin levels. PLoS One. 2013;**8**(5):e65465. DOI: 10.1371/journal.pone.0065465

[57] Denou E, Marcinko K, Surette MG, Steinberg GR, Schertzer JD. High-intensity exercise training increases the diversity and metabolic capacity of the mouse distal gut microbiota during diet-induced obesity. American Journal of Physiology-Endocrinology and Metabolism. 2016;**310**(11):E982-E993. DOI: 10.1152/ajpendo.00537.2015

[58] Brandt N, Kotowska D, Kristensen CM, Olesen J, Lützhøft DO, Halling JF, et al. The impact of exercise training and resveratrol supplementation on gut microbiota composition in high-fat diet fed mice. Physiological Reports. 2018;**6**(20):e13881. DOI: 10.14814/phy2.13881

[59] Kang SS, Jeraldo PR, Kurti A, Miller MEB, Cook MD, Whitlock K, et al. Diet and exercise orthogonally alter the gut microbiome and reveal independent associations with anxiety and cognition. Molecular Neurodegeneration. 2014;**9**:1. DOI: 10.1186/1750-1326-9-36

[60] Lambert JE, Myslicki JP, Bomhof MR, Belke DD, Shearer J, Reimer RA. Exercise training modifies gut microbiota in normal and diabetic mice. Applied Physiology Nutrition and Metabolism. 2015;**40**:749-752. DOI: 10.1139/apnm-2014-0452

[61] Feng X, Uchida Y, Koch L, Britton S, Hu J, Lutrin D, et al. Exercise prevents enhanced postoperative neuroinflammation and cognitive decline and rectifies the gut microbiome in a rat model of metabolic syndrome. Frontiers in Immunology. 2017;**8**:1768. DOI: 10.3389/fimmu.2017.01768

[62] Okamoto T, Morino K, Ugi S, Nakagawa F, Lemecha M, Ida S, et al. Microbiome potentiates endurance exercise through intestinal acetate production. The American Journal of Physiology-Endocrinology and Metabolism. 2019;**316**:E956-E966. DOI: 10.1152/ajpendo.00510.2018

[63] Cook MD, Allen JM, Pence BD, Wallig MA, Gaskins HR, White BA, et al. Exercise and gut immune function: Evidence of alterations in colon immune cell homeostasis and microbiome characteristics with exercise training. Immunology and Cell Biology. 2016;**94**(2):158-163. DOI: 10.1038/icb.2015.108

[64] Petersen LM, Bautista EJ, Nguyen H, Hanson BM, Chen L, Lek SH, et al. Community characteristics of the gut microbiomes of competitive cyclists. Microbiome. 2017;**5**(1):98. DOI: 10.1186/s40168-017-0320-4

[65] Castell LM, Poortmans JR, Leclercq R, Brasseur M, Duchateau J, Newsholme EA. Some aspects of the acute phase response after a marathon race, and the effects of glutamine supplementation. The European Journal of Applied Physiology. 1996;**75**:47-53. DOI: 10.1007/s004210050125

[66] Suzuki K, Yamada M, Kurakake S, Okamura N, Yamaya K, Liu Q, et al. Circulating cytokines and hormones with immunosuppressive but

neutrophil-priming potentials rise after endurance exercise in humans. The European Journal of Applied Physiology. 2000;**81**:281-287. DOI: 10.1007/s004210050044

[67] Jurdana M, Jenko Pražnikar Z, Jakus T. Macronutrient intake and energy availability in young male elite cyclists: The importance of adequate CHO intake: CHO intake in young elite cyclists. Progress in Nutrition [Internet]. 2022;**24**(3):e2022096. Available from: https://mattioli1885journals.com/index.php/progressinnutrition/article/view/12439

[68] Besten G den, Eunen K van, Groen AK, Venema K, Reijngoud D-J, Bakker BM. The role of short-chain fatty acids in the interplay between diet, gut microbiota, and host energy metabolism. The Journal of Lipid Research. 2013; 54: 2325-2340. DOI: 10.1194/jlr.R036012

[69] Moreno-Pérez D, Bressa C, Bailén M, Hamed-Bousdar S, Naclerio F, Carmona M, et al. Effect of a protein supplement on the gut microbiota of endurance athletes: A randomized, controlled, double-blind pilot study. Nutrients. 2018;**10**(3):337. DOI: 10.337.10.3390/nu10030337

[70] Bressa C, Bailén-Andrino M, Pérez-Santiago J, González-Soltero R, Pérez M, Montalvo-Lominchar MG, et al. Differences in gut microbiota profile between women with active lifestyle and sedentary women. PLoS One. 2017;**12**:e0171352. DOI: 10.1371/journal.pone.0171352

[71] Motiani KK, Collado MC, Eskelinen JJ, Virtanen KA, Löyttyniemi E, Salminen S, et al. Exercise training modulates gut microbiota profile and improves endotoxemia. Medicine and Science in Sports and Exercise. 2020;**52**:94-104. DOI: 10.1249/MSS.0000000000002112

[72] Barton W, Cronin O, Garcia-Perez I, Whiston R, Holmes E, Woods T, et al. The effects of sustained fitness improvement on the gut microbiome: A longitudinal, repeated measures case-study approach. Translational Sports Medicine. 2021;**4**:174-192. DOI: 10.1002/tsm2.215

[73] Clarke SF, Murphy EF, O'Sullivan O, Lucey AJ, Humphrey M, Hogan A, et al. Exercise and associated dietary extremes impact on gut microbial diversity. Gut. 2014;**63**(12):1913-1920. DOI: 10.1136/gutjnl-2013-306541

[74] O'Donovan CM, Madigan SM, Garcia-Perez I, Rankin A, O'Sullivan O, Cotter PD. Distinct microbiome composition and metabolome exists across subgroups of elite Irish athletes. The Journal of Science and Medicine in Sport. 2020;**23**:63-68. DOI: 10.1016/j.jsams.2019.08.290

[75] Estaki M, Pither J, Baumeister P, et al. Cardiorespiratory fitness as a predictor of intestinal microbial diversity and distinct metagenomic functions. Microbiome. 2016;**4**(1):42. Published 2016 Aug 8. DOI: 10.1186/s40168-016-0189-7

[76] Murtaza N, Burke LM, Vlahovich N, Little JP, Gill SK, Ghosh S, et al. The effects of dietary pattern during intensified training on stool microbiota of elite race walkers. Nutrients. 2019;**11**(2):261. DOI: 10.3390/nu11020261

[77] Jackson MA, Jeffery IB, Beaumont M, Bell JT, Clark AG, Ley RE, et al. Signatures of early frailty in the gut microbiota. Genome Medicine. 2016;**8**(1):8. DOI: 10.1186/s13073-016-0262-7

[78] Morita E, Yokoyama H, Imai D, Takeda R, Ota A, Kawai E, et al. Aerobic exercise training with brisk walking increases intestinal bacteroides in healthy elderly women. Nutrients. 2019;**11**:868. DOI: 10.3390/nu11040868

[79] Taniguchi H, Tanisawa K, Sun X, Kubo T, Hoshino Y, Hosokawa M, et al. Effects of short-term endurance exercise on gut microbiota in elderly men. Physiological Reports. 2018;**6**(23):e13935. DOI: 10.14814/phy2.13935

[80] Juneau M, Hayami D, Gayda M, Lacroix S, Nigam A. Provocative issues in heart disease prevention. The Canadian Journal of Cardiology. 2014;**30**(12Suppl):S401-S409. DOI: 10.1016/j.cjca.2014.09.014

[81] Anonyme. Report of a joint FAO/WHO expert consultation. Guidelines for the evaluation of probiotics in food. London, Canada. April 2002. Available from: http://www.fda.gov/ohrms/dockets/dockets/95s0316/95s-0316-rpt0282-tab-03-ref-19-joint-faowho-vol219.pdf

[82] Pawar R, Dhawal P, Nabar B, Barve S, Zambare V. Mechanism and applications of probiotics in healthcare industry. In: Biotechnology in Healthcare: Applications and Initiative, Volume 2, D. Barh (ed), Elsevier: London, UK. 2022; pp. 225-245. DOI: 10.1016/B978-0-323-90042-3.00002-5. ISBN: 978-0-323-90042-3

[83] Hill C, Guarner F, Reid G, Gibson GR, Merenstein DJ, Pot B, et al. The international scientific association for probiotics and prebiotics consensus statement on the scope and appropriate use of the term probiotic. Nature Reviews Gastroenterology & Hepatology. 2014;**11**:506-514. DOI: 10.1038/nrgastro.2014.66

[84] Kim SK, Guevarra RB, Kim YT, Kwon J, Kim H, Cho JH, et al. Role of probiotics in human gut microbiome-associated diseases. Journal of Microbiology and Biotechnology. 2019;**29**:1335-1340. DOI: 10.4014/jmb.1906.06064

[85] Butel M-J. Probiotics, gut microbiota and health. Médecine et Maladies Infectieuses. 2014;**44**(1):1-8. DOI: 10.1016/j.medmal.2013.10.002

[86] Liu L, Li L, Min J, Wang J, Wu H, Zeng Y, et al. Butyrate interferes with the differentiation and function of human monocyte-derived dendritic cells. Cellular Immunology. 2012;**277**(1-2):66-73. DOI: 10.1016/j.cellimm.2012.05.011

[87] Corrêa-Oliveira R, Fachi JL, Vieira A, Sato FT, Vinolo MAR. Regulation of immune cell function by short-chain fatty acids. Clinical & Translational Immunology. 2016;**5**:e73. DOI: 10.1038/cti.2016.17

[88] Martin-Gallausiaux C, Marinelli L, Blottière HM, Larraufie P, Lapaque N. SCFA: Mechanisms and functional importance in the gut. Proceedings of the Nutrition Society. 2021;**80**(1):37-49. DOI: 10.1017/S0029665120006916

[89] La Fata G, Weber P, Mohajeri MH. Probiotics and the gut immune system: Indirect regulation. Probiotics and Antimicrobial Proteins. 2018;**10**:11-21. DOI: 10.1007/s12602-017-9322-6

[90] De Santis S, Cavalcanti E, Mastronardi M, Jirillo E, Chieppa M. Nutritional keys for intestinal barrier modulation. Frontiers in Immunology. 2015;**6**:612. DOI: 10.3389/fimmu.2015.00612

[91] Lievin-Le Moal V, Servin AL. Anti-infective activities of lactobacillus strains in the human intestinal microbiota: From probiotics to gastrointestinal

anti-infectious biotherapeutic agents. Clinical Microbiology Reviews. 2014;**27**:167-199. DOI: 10.1128/CMR.00080-13

[92] Vaishnava S, Behrendt CL, Ismail AS, Eckmann L, Hooper LV. Paneth cells directly sense gut commensals and maintain homeostasis at the intestinal host-microbial interface. PNAS. 2008;**105**:20858-20863. DOI: 10.1073/pnas.0808723105

[93] Corfield AP, Myerscough N, Longman R, Sylvester P, Arul S, Pignatelli M. Mucins and mucosal protection in the gastrointestinal tract: New prospects for mucins in the pathology of gastrointestinal disease. Gut. 2000;**47**:589-594. DOI: 10.1136/gut.47.4.589

[94] Cornick S, Tawiah A, Chadee K. Roles and regulation of the mucus barrier in the gut. Tissue Barriers. 2015;**3**:e982426. DOI: 10.4161/21688370.2014.982426

[95] Mack DR, Michail S, Wei S, McDougall L, Hollingsworth MA. Probiotics inhibit enteropathogenic *E. Coli* adherence in vitro by inducing intestinal mucin gene expression. American Journal of Physics. 1999;**276**:G941-G950. DOI: 10.1152/ajpgi.1999.276.4.G941

[96] Buisine MP, Desreumaux P, Leteurtre E, Copin MC, Colombel JF, Porchet N, et al. Mucin gene expression in intestinal epithelial cells in Crohn's disease. Gut. 2001;**49**:544-551. DOI: 10.1136/gut.49.4.544

[97] Rhodes JM. Colonic mucus and ulcerative colitis. Gut. 1997;**40**:80-808. DOI: 10.1136/gut.40.6.807

[98] Bernet MF, Brassart D, Neeser JR, Servin AL. *Lactobacillus acidophilus* LA 1 binds to cultured human intestinal cell lines and inhibits cell attachment and cell invasion by enterovirulent bacteria. Gut. 1994;**35**:483-489. DOI: 10.1136/gut.40.6.807

[99] Hafez MM. Upregulation of intestinal mucin expression by the probiotic bacterium *E. coli* Nissle 1917. Probiotics and Antimicrobial Proteins. 2012;**4**:67-77. DOI: 10.1007/s12602-012-9092-0

[100] Hardy H, Harris J, Lyon E, Beal J, Foey AD. Probiotics, prebiotics and immunomodulation of gut mucosal defences: Homeostasis and immunopathology. Nutrients. 2013;**5**:1869-1912. DOI: 10.3390/nu5061869

[101] Mattar AF, Teitelbaum DH, Drongowski RA, Yongyi F, Harmon CM, Coran AG. Probiotics up-regulate MUC-2 mucin gene expression in a Caco-2 cell-culture model. Pediatric Surgery International. 2002;**18**:586-590. DOI: 10.1007/s00383-002-0855-7

[102] Caballero-Franco C, Keller K, De Simone C, Chadee K. The VSL#3 probiotic formula induces mucin gene expression and secretion in colonic epithelial cells. American Journal of Physiology. Gastrointestinal and Liver Physiology. 2007;**292**:G315-G322. DOI: 10.1152/ajpgi.00265.2006

[103] Ahl D, Liu H, Schreiber O, Ross S, Phillipson M, Holm L. *Lactobacillus reuteri* increases mucus thickness and ameliorates dextran sulphate sodium-induced colitis in mice. Acta Physiologica. 2016;**217**:300-310. DOI: 10.1111/apha.12695

[104] van der Lugt B, van Beek AA, Aalvink S, et al. Akkermansia muciniphila ameliorates the age-related decline in colonic mucus thickness and attenuates immune activation in

accelerated aging Ercc1−/Δ7 mice. Immunity and Ageing. 2019;**16**:6. DOI: 10.1186/s12979-019-0145-z

[105] Wu H, Chen X, Zhang S, Li J. Gut microbiota, the potential biological medicine for prevention, intervention and drug sensitization to fight diseases. Nutrients. 2022;**14**:4220. DOI: 10.3390/nu14204220

[106] Round JL, Mazmanian SK. The gut microbiome shapes intestinal immune responses during health and disease. Nature Reviews Immunology. 2009;**9**(5):313-323. DOI: 10.1038/nri2515

[107] Menard O, Butel MJ, Gaboriau-RouthiauV,Waligora-DuprietAJ. Gnotobiotic mouse immune response induced by *Bifidobacterium* sp. strains isolated from infants. Applied and Environmental Microbiology. 2008;**74**:660-666. DOI: 10.1128/AEM.01261-07

[108] Shang J, Wan F, Zhao L, Meng X, Li B. Potential immunomodulatory activity of a selected strain Bifidobacterium bifidum H3-R2 as evidenced in vitro and in immunosuppressed mice. Frontiers in Microbiology. 2020;**11**:2089. DOI: 10.3389/fmicb.2020.02089

[109] Leite GSF, Resende AS, West NP, Lancha AH. Probiotics and sports: A new magic bullet? Nutrients. 2019;**60**:152-160. DOI: 10.1016/j.nut.2018.09.023

[110] Shing CM, Peake JM, Lim CL, Briskey D, Walsh NP, Fortes MB, et al. Effects of probiotics supplementation on gastrointestinal permeability, inflammation and exercise performance in the heat. European Journal of Applied Physiology. 2014;**114**:93-103. DOI: 10.1007/s00421-013-2748-y

[111] Łagowska K, Bajerska J, Kamiński S, Del Bo' C. Effects of probiotics supplementation on gastrointestinal symptoms in athletes: A systematic review of randomized controlled trials. Nutrients. 2022;**14**:2645. DOI: 10.3390/nu14132645

[112] Quero CD, Manonelles P, Fernández M, Abellán-Aynés O, López-Plaza D, Andreu-Caravaca L, et al. Differential health effects on inflammatory, immunological and stress parameters in professional soccer players and sedentary individuals after consuming a synbiotic. A triple-blinded, randomised, placebo-controlled pilot study. Nutrients. 2021;**13**:1321. DOI: 10.3390/nu13041321

[113] Maughan RJ, Burke LM, Dvorak J, Larson-Meyer DE, Peeling P, Phillips SM, et al. IOC consensus statement: Dietary supplements and the high-performance athlete. International Journal of Sport Nutrition and Exercise Metabolism. 2018;**28**:104-125. DOI: 10.1123/ijsnem.2018-0020

[114] Kekkonen RA, Vasankari TJ, Vuorimaa T, Haahtela T, Julkunen I, Korpela R. The effect of probiotics on respiratory infections and gastrointestinal symptoms during training in marathon runners. International Journal of Sport Nutrition and Exercise Metabolism. 2007;**17**:352-363. DOI: 10.1123/ijsnem.17.4.352

[115] Schreiber C, Tamir S, Golan R, Weinstein A, Weinstein Y. The effect of probiotic supplementation on performance, inflammatory markers and gastrointestinal symptoms in elite road cyclists. Journal of International Society of Sports Nutrition. 2021;**18**:36. DOI: 10.1186/s12970-021-00432-6

[116] Roberts J, Suckling C, Peedle G, Murphy J, Dawkins T, Roberts M. An exploratory investigation of endotoxin

levels in novice long distance triathletes, and the effects of a multi-strain probiotic/prebiotic, antioxidant intervention. Nutrients. 2016;**8**:733. DOI: 10.3390/nu8110733

[117] Marttinen M, Ala-Jaakkola R, Laitila A, Lehtinen MJ. Gut microbiota, probiotics and physical performance in athletes and physically active individuals. Nutrients. 2020;**12**(10):2936. DOI: 10.3390/nu12102936

[118] Colbey C, Cox AJ, Pyne DB, Zhang P, Cripps AW, West NP. Upper respiratory symptoms, gut health and mucosal immunity in athletes. Sports Medicine. 2018;**48**(Suppl. 1):65-77. DOI: 10.1007/s40279-017-0846-4

[119] Jäger R, Mohr AE, Carpenter KC, Kerksick CM, Purpura M, Moussa A, et al. International society of sports nutrition position stand: Probiotics. Journal of International Society of Sports Nutrition. 2019;**16**(1):62. DOI: 10.1186/s12970-019-0329-0

[120] Chen YM, Wei L, Chiu YS, Hsu YJ, Tsai TY, Wang MF, et al. *Lactobacillus plantarum* TWK10 supplementation improves exercise performance and increases muscle mass in mice. Nutrients. 2016;**8**(4):205. DOI: 10.3390/nu8040205

[121] Huang WC, Lee MC, Lee CC, Ng KS, Hsu YJ, Tsai TY, et al. Effect of *Lactobacillus plantarum* TWK10 on exercise physiological adaptation, performance, and body composition in healthy humans. Nutrients. 2019;**11**:2836. DOI: 10.3390/nu11112836

[122] Huang WC, Hsu YJ, Li H, Kan NW, Chen YM, Lin JS, et al. Effect of *Lactobacillus plantarum* TWK10 on improving endurance performance in humans. Chinese Journal of Physiology. 2018;**61**:163-170. DOI: 10.4077/CJP.2018.BAH587

[123] O'Brien KV, Stewart LK, Forney LA, Aryana KJ, Prinyawiwatkul W, Boeneke CA. The effects of postexercise consumption of a kefir beverage on performance and recovery during intensive endurance training. Journal of Dairy Science. 2015;**98**:7446-7449. DOI: 10.3168/jds.2015-9392

[124] Salehzadeh K. The effects of probiotic yogurt drink on lipid profile, CRP and record changes in aerobic athletes. International Journal of Life Sciences. 2015;**9**:32-37. DOI: 10.3126/ijls.v9i4.12672

[125] Peake JM, Neubauer O, Della Gatta PA, Nosaka K. Muscle damage and inflammation during recovery from exercise. Journal of Applied Physiology. 2017;**122**:559-570. DOI: 10.1152/japplphysiol.00971.2016

[126] Lee MC, Hsu YJ, Chuang HL, Hsieh PS, Ho HH, Chen WL, et al. *In vivo* ergogenic properties of the *Bifidobacterium longum* OLP-01 isolated from a weightlifting gold medalist. Nutrients. 2019;**11**:2003. DOI: 10.3390/nu11092003

[127] Lee MC, Hsu YJ, Ho HH, Hsieh SH, Kuo YW, Sung HC, et al. *Lactobacillus salivarius* subspecies salicinius SA-03 is a new probiotic capable of enhancing exercise performance and decreasing fatigue. Microorganisms. 2020;**8**:545. DOI: 10.3390/microorganisms8040545

[128] Cox AJ, Pyne DB, Saunders PU, Fricker PA. Oral administration of the probiotic *Lactobacillus fermentum* VRI-003 and mucosal immunity in endurance athletes. British Journal of Sports Medicine. 2010;**44**:222-226. DOI: 10.1136/bjsm.2007.044628

[129] Michalickova D, Minic R, Dikic N, Andjelkovic M, Kostic-Vucicevic M, Stojmenovic T, et al. *Lactobacillus helveticus* Lafti L10 supplementation reduces respiratory infection duration in a cohort of elite athletes: A randomized, double-blind, placebo-controlled trial. Applied Physiology, Nutrition and Metabolism. 2016;**41**:782-789. DOI: 10.1139/apnm-2015-0541

[130] Strasser B, Geiger D, Schauer M, Gostner JM, Gatterer H, Burtscher M, et al. Probiotic supplements beneficially affect tryptophan-kynurenine metabolism and reduce the incidence of upper respiratory tract infections in trained athletes: A randomized, double-blinded, placebo-controlled trial. Nutrients. 2016;**8**:752. DOI: 10.3390/nu8110752

[131] Salarkia N, Ghadamli L, Zaeri F, Sabaghian RL. Effects of probiotic yogurt on performance, respiratory and digestive systems of young adult female endurance swimmers: A randomized controlled trial. Medical Journal of the Islamic Republic of Iran. 2013;**27**:141-146

[132] Carbuhn AF, Reynolds SM, Campbell CW, Bradford LA, Deckert JA, Kreutzer A, et al. Effects of probiotic (*Bifidobacterium longum* 35624) supplementation on exercise performance, immune modulation, and cognitive outlook in division I female swimmers. Sports. 2018;**6**:116. DOI: 10.3390/sports6040116

[133] Marshall H, Chrismas BCR, Suckling CA, Roberts JD, Foster J, Taylor L. Chronic probiotic supplementation with or without glutamine does not influence the eHsp72 response to a multi-day ultra-endurance exercise event. Applied Physiology, Nutrition and Metabolism. 2017;**42**:876-883. DOI: 10.1139/apnm-2017-0131

[134] Pugh JN, Sparks AS, Doran DA, Fleming SC, Langan-Evans C, Kirk B, et al. Four weeks of probiotic supplementation reduces GI symptoms during a marathon race. European Journal of Applied Physiology. 2019;**119**(7):1491-1501. DOI: 10.1007/s00421-019-04136-3

[135] Inoue T, Kobayashi Y, Mori N, Sakagawa M, Xiao JZ, Moritani T, et al. Effect of combined bifidobacteria supplementation and resistance training on cognitive function, body composition and bowel habits of healthy elderly subjects. Beneficial Microbes. 2018;**9**:843-853. DOI: 10.3920/BM2017.0193

[136] Townsend JR, Bender D, Vantrease WC, Sapp PA, Toy AM, Woods CA, et al. Effects of probiotic (*Bacillus subtilis* DE111) supplementation on immune function, hormonal status, and physical performance in division I baseball players. Sports. 2018;**6**:70. DOI: 10.3390/sports6030070

[137] Toohey JC, Townsend JR, Johnson SB, Toy AM, Vantrease WC, Bender D, et al. Effects of probiotic (*Bacillus subtilis*) supplementation during offseason resistance training in female division I athletes. Journal of Strength and Conditioning Research. 2020;**34**(11):3173-3181. DOI: 10.1519/JSC.0000000000002675

[138] Ibrahim NS, Muhamad AS, Ooi FK, Meor-Osman J, Chen CK. The effects of combined probiotic ingestion and circuit training on muscular strength and power and cytokine responses in young males. Applied Physiology, Nutrition and Metabolism. 2018;**43**:180-186. DOI: 10.1139/apnm-2017-0464

Chapter 8

Probiotics in the Management of Diabetes

Akash Kumar, Jhilam Pramanik, Nandani Goyal, Bhupendra G. Prajapati and Dimple Chauhan

Abstract

Gut microflora that has been present in our bodies since infancy are known to influence health, metabolism, and disease. Diabetes is a developing epidemic, and treatment that cures diabetes has yet to be discovered. Probiotics are living bacteria that may colonize the human gastrointestinal system and help to maintain a healthy microbiome and help normalize disrupted metabolism in diabetic patients. Lipopolysaccharides, trimethylamine, and imidazole propionate seem to hinder insulin signaling, whereas secondary bile acids, short-chain fatty acids (SCFAs), and tryptophan metabolites seem to enhance it. This chapter emphasizes the relationship between gut microflora and impaired glucose metabolism. This chapter also covers the mechanisms through which probiotics alleviate diabetes by addressing the gut microflora from the perspectives of amino acid metabolism, intestinal permeability, immunological responses, oxidative stress, and SCFAs.

Keywords: diabetes, probiotics, gut microflora, short-chain fatty acids (SCFAs), *Lactobacillus*, *Bifidobacterium*

1. Introduction

Diabetes mellitus (DM), often known as diabetes, is a metabolic syndrome caused by abnormalities in the body's capacity to generate insulin and/or activate insulin, or both. Hyperglycemia and glucose intolerance are the symptoms of diabetes mellitus [1]. Hyperglycemia increases the complications in the microvascular system (neuropathy, retinopathy, and nephropathy) as well as in the macrovascular system (stroke, ischemic heart disease, and peripheral vascular disease). As a result, there is a marked increase in morbidity and a significant decline in the quality of life [2–4]. According to the World Health Organization (WHO), 420 million people worldwide have diabetes, and the prevalence was estimated to be 2.8% in 2000, rising to 4.8% by 2030. Over the last two decades, the disease has been more prevalent than expected [5]. DM is seen as a huge global health and economic burden in the aging population and is now the eighth biggest cause of mortality globally [6]. The number of diabetics in India alone is already over 40 million, and by 2030, the country will have the biggest diabetic population in the world with a population of over 90 million [7, 8].

Diabetes has three basic subtypes: type 1, type 2, and gestational diabetes [9–11]. About 10% of all cases of diabetes are type 1 diabetes (T1DM), which is characterized by the impairment of insulin-secreting B-cells and needs daily insulin therapy for survival [12, 13]. T1DM is becoming more common in the world as a result of ineffective preventative and treatment approaches. Therefore, a thorough understanding of T1DM's pathophysiology is necessary. Environmental factors and genetic factors play a crucial role in the progression of T1DM [14, 15]. Most people with diabetes (90–95%) have type 2 diabetes (T2DM), which is defined by impaired lipid and glucose metabolism brought on by insufficient insulin production or by its insensitivity [1]. Although T2DM is mostly diagnosed in older persons, the frequency of the condition in youngsters has been shown to rise as a result of obesity and physical inactivity [16]. Smoking, hereditary factors, excessive calorie consumption, and sedentary lifestyle are the main risk factors for T2DM, with alteration in gut microbiota as one of the causes and associated comorbidities [17]. A common problem that affects roughly 2–5% of all pregnancies, gestational diabetes mellitus (GDM) is characterized by high glucose levels in the second and third trimesters of pregnancy. It may manifest as either type I or type II diabetes in persons who have an inherited tendency to have the disease [18]. In the future, T2DM is more likely to occur in women with GDM due to their increased risk of pregnancy problems and premature birth [19, 20].

As per epidemiological observations, one of the characteristics of diabetic patients is changes in the diversity of intestinal microflora. Additionally, there is increasing evidence that diabetes and intestinal microflora are closely related. The microflora, host cells, and nutrients make a complex ecosystem that creates up the human gut. The alimentary canal contains about 100 trillion bacteria, which together make up the intestinal flora [21]. The bacteria that make up the intestinal flora are numerous and diverse. Genus, family, order, and phylum classifications are used to taxonomically group these. In healthy adults, the six phyla *Firmicutes, Proteobacteria, Bacteroidetes, Actinobacteria, Fusobacteria*, and *Verrucomicrobia* make up most of the intestinal microflora [22]. Researchers have shown that gut microbiota in diabetics is less reliable than in healthy individuals. In a sick condition functionality of gut microbiota changes, a human metagenome-wide association study conducted in Europe and China found surprising connections between specific bacterial genes, gut microbes, and the digestive system in T2DM patients [23]. These individuals showed greater levels of *Lactobacillus* spp. than nondiabetics, and fasting glucose and glycated hemoglobin (HbA1c) levels are positively connected with these levels [24]. *Clostridium* spp. had a negative relationship with fasting blood sugar and plasma triglycerides [25]. According to one investigation, it has been found that the number of *Prevotella* and *Faecalibacterium* decreased in diabetic conditions and demonstrated that the microbiome impacts both T1DM and T2DM [26]. In the mucous layer, there is an increase in *Akkermansia muciniphila* after metformin therapy [27]. It has been hypothesized that type 1 diabetes (T1DM) and autoimmune diabetes may both develop due to inflammation [28]. Autoimmune diabetes has been related to the microbiota of the gut because of the common receptors in the inflamed pancreas and the gut [29].

Diabetes interventions include medication [30], nutritional care [31, 32], physical activity [32], or weight control [33, 34]. They might also involve education, coaching, or social support [35]. As stated above, diabetes affects the gut microbiome; therefore, probiotics can be employed as one of the nutritional interventions. These are live bacteria that are given in sufficient amounts and continue to remain in the gut bionetwork to have a beneficial impact on one's health [36]. Lilly and Stillwell used the word "probiotics" to refer to "organisms and substances which contribute to intestinal microbial balance" [37]. Probiotics are "organisms and compounds that help to gut microbial equilibrium," according to Parker [38]. The International Scientific Association for Probiotics and Prebiotics (ISAPP), which was supported by the Food and Agriculture Organization of the United Nations/World Health Organization (FAO/WHO, 2001), defined probiotics as "Live microorganisms which, when administered in adequate amounts, confer a health benefit on the host" [39]. Probiotics are defined by the World Health Organization (WHO) as "products or preparations containing live, designated microorganisms in appropriate quantities that give positive effects on the host by altering its gut microbiota" [40].

Probiotics play an important role in immune system development, immune system homeostasis, and epithelial cell differentiation and proliferation [41]. Probiotics are not a recent discovery but have been present in many of our traditional foods for a long time, including drinks, salty fish, yogurt, various types of cheese, and so forth. Before the invention of the microscope, people were able to prepare a variety of milk products with various flavors and structures [42]. This is the result of various microbial reactions brought on by various microbes [43]. We really had no idea how probiotic-containing foods were first used, especially for therapeutic purposes. It is possible that Ilya Ilyich Metchnikoff, who won the Nobel Prize in Medicine in 1908, was the first to notice the effects of what is now known as probiotics while working at the Pasteur Institute. He correlated the consumption of yogurt's microorganisms with good health. He proposed in 1907 that the bacteria *Lactobacillus bulgaricus* and *Streptococcus thermophilus*, which are involved in yogurt fermentation, block the putrefactive-type fermentations of the intestinal flora. He linked the consumption of yogurt containing the *Lactobacillus* species to the longevity and good health of Bulgarian peasants, and he presented his findings to the public in a manner that was easily understood [44].

The ISAPP consensus panel explained the concept that some probiotic mechanisms may be expressed by most strains of a larger taxonomic group, which is an evolving idea regarding the strain specificity of probiotic effects [45]. Lactic acid bacteria (LAB) are a group of predominant gut-friendly bacteria found in the digestive tract [46] and suppress pathogens through their secretions [47]. For instance, the majority of *Bifidobacterium* and *Lactobacillus* species both produce organic acids like lactate and acetate. There are several potential advantages for the gastrointestinal system. The inhibition of harmful microbes and the cross-feeding of other advantageous gut microbes result in the production of butyrate, which plays a significant role in cultivating a healthier gut environment [48]. The types of microbes from the genera *Lactobacillus, Bifidobacterium*, and *Saccharomyces* that are most frequently used as probiotics include these. Other genera of probiotics include *Escherichia, Propionibacterium, Streptococcus*, and *Bacillus*. Probiotics are poised to be an important tool for influencing the gut ecosystem's function to enhance the nutritional status and health [49, 50]. The mechanisms of action that researchers have identified in various probiotic strains against diabetes are shown in **Figure 1**. However, there are still a lot of gaps in our understanding of the mechanisms underlying health benefits.

Modification of the gut microbiota's composition is one alleged probiotic effect that has been challenging to prove in healthy humans. Although it is widely believed that probiotics "support a healthy intestinal flora," [51], probiotic organisms seldom survive for longer than a few weeks after consumption [52]. Alpha diversity, richness, and evenness of the fecal microbiota were examined in a systematic review of studies looking at the effects of probiotics [51].

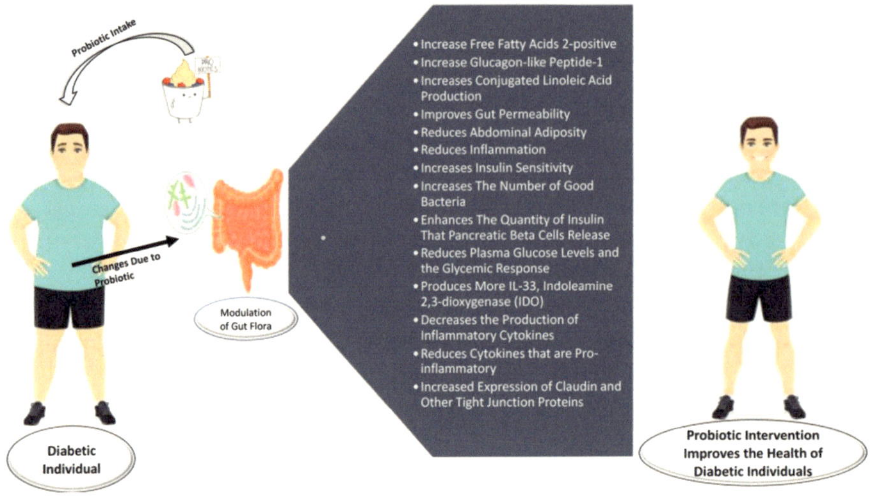

Figure 1.
Potential mechanisms linking probiotics to diabetes.

Research is still finding links between the microbiota and diabetes, and these seem to involve a variety of metabolic and immune response processes, most of which are linked to more specific mechanisms. Future investigations into the relationship between variations in the gut microbiota balance and diabetes may result in new interventional studies. This review provides an overview of the role of probiotics in diabetes management.

2. Probiotic interventions to ameliorate T1DM

Probiotics may, thus, be useful in T1DM prevention and management. By altering the gut microbiota, certain probiotic strains exhibit a positive impact on host health by boosting the synthesis of advantageous metabolites [53]. Additionally, by activating free fatty acid receptor 2 (FFAR2) and free fatty acid receptor 3 (FFAR3), which are involved in the regulation of the immune system and the pathogenesis of autoimmune diseases like T1DM, the administration of probiotic strains may increase the production of SCFAs (such as butyrate) and thereby balance the intestinal cellular homeostasis [54]. Additionally, intestinal L-cells' ability to produce glucagon-like peptide-1 (GLP-1) might be improved by the activation of FFAR2/3 by SCFAs. The hormone GLP-1 is known as the "incretin effect" because it promotes the release of insulin from pancreatic beta-cells, lowering blood sugar levels [55, 56]. These findings show how probiotics may prevent or manage T1DM by preserving or re-establishing the gut microbiota-immune axis' equilibrium. **Figure 2** shows an overview of potential mechanisms of probiotics against type 1 diabetes.

2.1 Animal studies

Lactobacillus brevis strains protect mice (streptozotocin [STZ]-induced T1DM) and lower blood glucose levels via the action of gamma-aminobutyric acid (GABA) [57]. It has been shown that probiotic strains from the families *Bifidobacteriaceae* and *Lactobacillaceae* and the genus *Streptococcus thermophilus* reduce intestinal

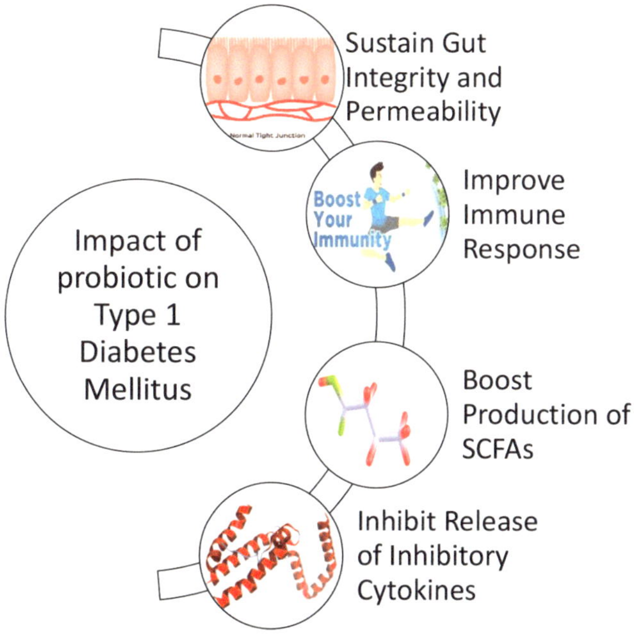

Figure 2.
Potential mechanisms of probiotics against type 1 diabetes.

inflammation, alleviate T1DM, and maintain gut immunological homeostasis by blocking IL-1 expression in nonobese diabetic (NOD) mice [58]. The feeding of a *Lactobacillus lactis* strain has also been demonstrated to have preventative benefits against T1DM development in NOD mice by the activation of the production of anti-inflammatory cytokines. Interestingly, the combination of the *L. lactis* strain with modest dosages of anti-CD3 boosted the production of IL-10. The intervention also led to the formation of antigen-specific Foxp3+ Tregs, which preserves pancreatic islets [59, 60]. *Bifidobacterium* species change the cytokine secretion pattern in gut-associated lymphatic tissue (GALT) from a proinflammatory condition to an anti-inflammatory. Controlling the preservation of the variety of B-cells and lowering insulitis reduced the likelihood of developing an islet-specific autoimmune disease and offered protection against autoimmune T1DM [61]. **Table 1** shows an overview of important studies demonstrating the effect of probiotics on an animal model with type 1 diabetes mellitus.

Biobreeding diabetes resistant (BBDR) rats are more likely to develop T1DM when exposed to Kilham rat virus (KRV) infectious disease [67]. Similar results have also been seen in LEW.1WR1 rats that have had viral infections; these animals acquire autoimmune T1DM as a result of the infection of their cells. It has been shown experimentally that the oral administration of the *Lactobacillus johnsonii* strain develops resistance to the onset of T1DM in BBDR rats [67]. Consequently, *L. johnsonii* was linked to TH17 lymphatic cell predilection inside the mesenteric lymph nodes (MLNs) and might lower the incidence of T1DM in the bio-breeding diabetes-prone (BBDP) rat model. Increasing the level of the intestinal tight-junction protein claudin, *L. johnsonii*, also reduced the likelihood of developing T1DM [66]. In another experiment, probiotic-fermented milk was fed to diabetic rats induced by STZ. Consuming probiotic-fermented milk also reduced oxidative stress, inflammation, blood sugar

Probiotics	Model type	Mechanism of action	Major findings	References
Oral probiotics VSL#3	Nonobese diabetic mouse model	Producing more IL-33, indoleamine 2,3-dioxygenase (IDO) Decreasing the production of inflammatory cytokines Encouraging differentiation of CD103+ Lowering Teff/Treg cell ratios in MLNs, PLNs, and gut mucosa	Alteration of the microbial ecology in the gut Altering the pathophysiology of T1DM	[58]
Streptococcus salivarius, *Lactobacilli*, and *Bifibobacteria*	Nonobese diabetic mouse model	Slowing down the rate of cellular disruption Pancreatic pseudocysts, the pancreas, and the spleen produce more IL-10.	Preventing autoimmune diabetes	[61]
Probiotic fermented milk with 1% of *Lactobacillus* species	Streptozotocin-induced albino Wistar rat model	A substantial reduction in the liver's ability to express genes involved in gluconeogenesis Significant reductions in IL-6 and TNF- levels in the serum; Declines in blood sugar levels, HbA1c, and blood lipid profiles.	Raising insulin levels while significantly lowering blood sugar levels Enhancement of glucose metabolism Reduction of oxidative stress, inflammation, and hepatic gluconeogenesis	[62]
Lactobacillus brevis	Streptozotocin-induced diabetic Mouse Model	High ability to produce GABA because of the gad gene Significant reduction in plasma insulin levels or blood glucose levels	Preventing T1DM from developing in mice	[57]
Bifidobacterium spp.	Streptozotocin-induced diabetic Mouse Model	A dramatic drop in levels of blood sugar Enhancing insulin receptor substrate, insulin receptor substrate 1, and expression of insulin receptor β Reducing the expression of IL-6 and macrophage chemoattractant protein-1	Manage diabetes	[63]
Lactobacillus reuteri	Streptozotocin-induced diabetic Mouse Model	Inhibition of osteoblast TNF-signaling results in the development of anti-inflammatory properties	The administration of probiotics may help T1DM patients' bones	[64]
Lactobacillus kefiranofaciens and Lactobacillus kefiri	Streptozotocin-induced diabetic Mouse Model	Pancreatic IL-10 level dramatically increased More IL-10 prevents the production of TNF-α and TH1 and other pro-inflammatory cytokines	Capacity to induce GLP-1 release	[65]

Probiotics	Model type	Mechanism of action	Major findings	References
Lactobacillus johnsonii N6.2	T1DM biobreeding diabetes-prone rats model	Modifications to the gut's natural microbiome Induced oxidative stress response and alterations in host mucosal protein Lowering intestinal mucosal oxidative response protein Reducing cytokines that are proinflammatory Increasing expression of claudin and other tight junction proteins	Delaying or preventing the onset of T1DM.	[66]

Table 1.
Overview of important studies demonstrating the effect of probiotics on an animal model with type 1 diabetes mellitus.

levels, and the rate of gluconeogenesis [62]. Another investigation employing probiotic strain *Lactobacillus plantarum* in diabetic rats concluded that taking probiotics significantly decreased the serum α-amylase's activity, favoring the glycemic index mechanism by limiting the digestion and hydrolysis of carbohydrates [68].

2.2 Human studies

Early exposure to probiotic supplements may reduce the incidence of islet-cell autoimmunity in relation to the increased risk of T1DM [69–71]. Additionally, probiotic usage has been linked to improved glucose control, increased GLP-1 production, and decreased TLR4 signaling in T1DM adults [72–74]. T1DM occurrences have reduced as a result of these modifications. Children with T1DM may benefit from taking *Lactobacillus rhamnosus* and *Bifidobacterium lactis* at a dosage of 10^9 colony-forming units (CFUs) once a day for six months regulates gut microbiota disturbances. Results indicated the modification of immune cells in a positive way and maintaining the quantity and proliferation of pancreatic β-cells [75]. Additionally, it has been suggested that adult human subjects consuming *Lactobacillus johnsonii* N6.2 (10^8 CFUs) in one capsule per day for eight weeks can control the natural killer cells and infiltration of monocytes. These modifications may help to prevent the development of T1DM. Furthermore, probiotic therapy has been linked to an increase in TH17 and TH1/TH17 cells. However, the probiotics-treated group showed a substantial rise in IgA concentration as compared to the placebo group [71]. **Table 2** shows an overview of important studies demonstrating the effect of probiotics on human subjects with type 1 diabetes mellitus.

By using probiotics products, T1DM adult patients might improve their glycemic control and manage symptoms associated with metabolic syndromes, such as hypertension, elevated level of triglyceride, and decreased HDL levels. These findings together imply that probiotic intake may lower the likelihood of T1DM progression. Other research on young children with a genetic risk of T1DM consumed a probiotic strain during the first two years of life and the risk of the onset of islet autoimmunity

Probiotics	Model type	Mechanism of action	Major findings	References
Lactobacillus johnsonii	Adult humans	Increasing tryptophan levels in the serum Lowering the plasma kynurenine to tryptophan ([Kyn]/[Trp]) ratio Delaying or lessening the memory of CD8+ T-cell apoptosis	Lowering the risk of developing T1DM.	[71]
Bifidobacterium lactis and Lactobacillus rhamnosus	Children (age range of 8–17)	Enhancing the barrier property of the gastrointestinal mucosa Decreasing autoimmunity risk Altering the local and systemic immunological responses	Retaining the function of the—β-cell while inhibiting the proliferation of infections	[75]
Probiotics and vitamin D	Children (age range of 4 to 10 years)	Reducing the risk of islet autoimmunity	Early probiotic supplementation may reduce the risk of islet autoimmunity	[70]
Probiotics	Adult human	Decreasing waist-to-hip ratio, body mass index, and obesity Controlling triglyceride levels, HDL cholesterol, and blood pressure Strongly linked to improve glycemic management	Beneficial impact on a range of variables connected to diabetes problems	[76]

Table 2.
Overview of important studies demonstrating the effect of probiotics on human subjects with type 1 diabetes mellitus.

and progression of T1DM was increased [77]. This suggests that all probiotic strains do not have the same effects, although the cause of the results from these studies is still unknown.

3. Probiotic interventions to ameliorate T2DM

Currently, probiotics from the former genera of *Lactobacillus* and *Bifidobacterium* are the major focus of most therapeutic investigations. However, specific bacterial strains are linked to the amelioration of disorders linked with inflammation. It is anticipated that some of the newly identified strains will become probiotics in the future [78]. **Figure 3** shows the overview of potential mechanisms of probiotics against type 2 diabetes. Numerous studies have utilized probiotics in T2DM patients to manage or treat the disease, but the number of studies is still less. When analyzing these studies, it is necessary to use caution because it is well known that the effectiveness of probiotics depends on various factors such as:

- The strain of microorganism (single or multistrain)
- Pathophysiology of the disease

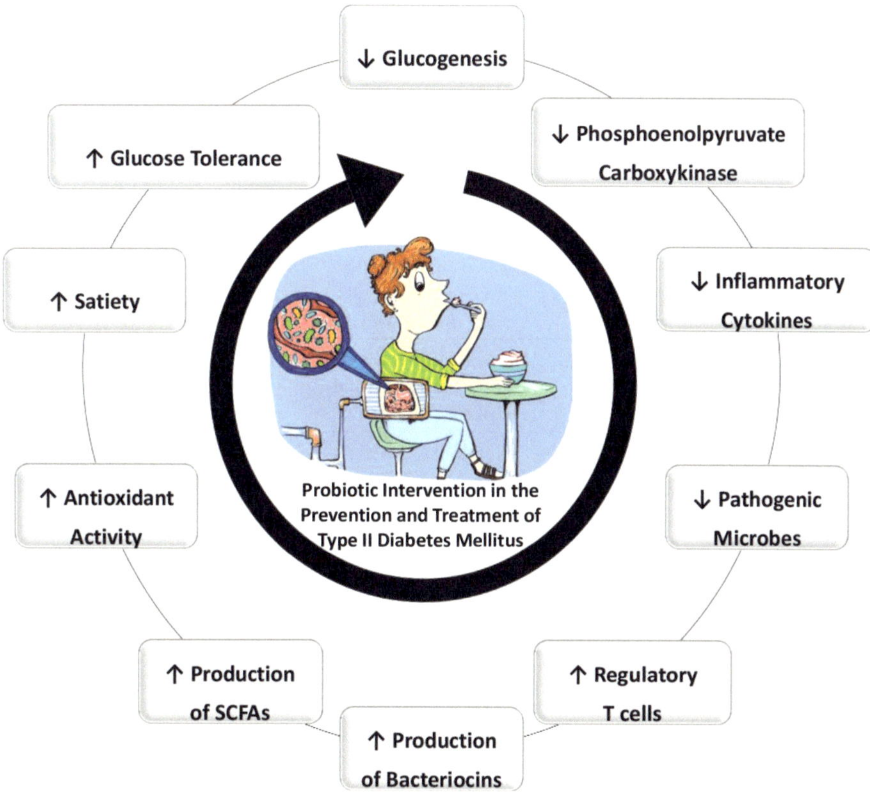

Figure 3.
Potential mechanisms of probiotics against type 2 diabetes.

- Subject of study
- Type and quantity of dosage
- Time period of intervention.

3.1 Animal model study

Probiotics have been proven in studies to reduce insulin resistance (IR) in diabetic animal models (see **Table 3**). Probiotics like *Lactobacillus* spp. and *Bifidobacterium* spp. have been widely studied in diabetic animal models for their biological effects on glucose intolerance and insulin resistance (IR). *Lactobacillus plantarum* was given to the rats (which consume high-fat-diet [HFD]- and STZ-induced diabetes). It has been observed that *L. plantarum* reduces pancreatic beta-cell dysfunction, systemic inflammation, and insulin resistance [79]. *L. plantarum* reduced the weight and relieved IR in mice fed on the HFD [80]. In mice with diabetes generated by HFD, therapy with *Lactobacillus fermentum* has been demonstrated to reduce IR and stop the progression of diabetes [81]. The injection of *Lactobacillus paracasei* TD062 increased the insulin signaling pathway and improved glucose homeostasis, delaying the onset of T2DM [82]. In STZ-induced diabetic rats, a multiprobiotic formula, including *Lactobacillus reuteri*,

Probiotics	Model used	Mechanism	Outcomes	References
Lactobacillus plantarum	HFD- and STZ-induced T2DM mice	Reducing systemic inflammation and insulin resistance	Ameliorate T2DM	[79]
L. plantarum Ln4	Mice fed on HFD	Modifications in hepatic gene expression that control lipid and glucose metabolism (reduced CD36 and increased mRNA levels for IRS2, Akt2, AMPK, and LPL)	Reducing biomarkers for T2DM and obesity caused by diet	[80]
L. plantarum and *Lactobacillus fermentum*	Mice fed with HFD	Preventing the onset of insulin resistance and diabetes.	Seem to be effective against T2DM	[81]
Lactobacillus paracasei	HFD and STZ-induced T2DM mice	Controlling the levels of hepatic glycogen, lipid metabolism, glucose tolerance, postprandial blood glucose (PBG), and fasting blood glucose (FBG). Additionally, the antioxidant capability was enhanced	Preventing the development of T2DM	[82]
Lactobacillus reuteri, Lactobacillus crispatus, and *Bacillus subtilis*	STZ-induced diabetes	After the intervention period, Glut-4 and PPAR-γ gene expression improved Considerable elevation in insulin levels and a large reduction in plasma glucose and HbA1c values	Probiotics may help to manage diabetes and its complications if taken regularly	[83]
Nano-selenium-enriched *B. longum*	Streptozotocin-induced diabetes	The expression of insulin signaling pathway-related proteins was upregulated in the Nano-Se-B longum-treated groups	Preventive effect of Nano-Se-B longum on the onset of diabetes and renal damage	[84]
Lactobacillus plantarum	Mice fed with HFD	Significantly reduced the mRNA expression of interleukin-1β in adipose tissue and serum levels of nonesterified fatty acids in mice	Significant reduction of blood glucose levels	[85]
Lactobacillus casei	HFD- and STZ-induced T2DM mice	Decreased levels of the inflammatory markers, tumor necrosis factor-α and interleukin-6 and increased intestinal glucagon-like peptide-1 (GLP-1) levels, which are associated with the production of short-chain fatty acids (SCFAs)	Modifying the gut microbiota, increasing the production of SCFAs, and ameliorating type 2 diabetes	[86]

Probiotics	Model used	Mechanism	Outcomes	References
Lactobacillus paracasei	HFD- and STZ-induced T2DM mice	Reducing the level of oxidative stress and insulin resistance, while also safeguarding beta-cell function and inhibiting the expansion of alpha-cell	Indicating that the pancreatic islets as the key target tissues for the probiotic strain's ameliorative action against T2DM	[87]
Clostridium butyricum	HFD- and STZ-induced T2DM mice	Increased insulin signaling molecules, and peroxisome proliferator-activated receptor (PPAR), as well as altered intestinal flora diversity	Treating and preventing metabolic impairment caused by T2DM	[88]

Table 3.
Overview of important studies demonstrating the effect of probiotics on an animal model with type 2 diabetes mellitus.

Lactobacillus crispatus, and *Bacillus subtilis*, was studied. This research revealed that the daily consumption of probiotics may reduce glucose intolerance and increase insulin production [83]. By lowering fasting blood glucose (FBG), the oral glucose tolerance test (OGTT), and the HbA1c indices and increasing GLP-1 secretion, a composite probiotic made up of 10 *Lactobacillus* strains and four yeast strains were reported to improve T2DM in db/db mice [89]. Nano-selenium-enriched *Bifidobacterium longum* reduced the renal complication of T2DM in STZ-induced diabetes rats [84]. *B. longum* DD98 reduced the fasting blood glucose and HbA1c in HFD- and STZ-induced diabetic mice [90]. In diabetic rats caused by HFD and STZ, *Bifidobacterium animalis* administration increased oral glucose tolerance test and homeostatic model assessment for insulin resistance (HOMA-IR) indices and decreased proinflammatory cytokines [91].

3.2 Human studies

Sabico et al. examined the effects of consuming 10^{10} CFU/day of a multistrain probiotic regarding metabolic endotoxemia levels and cardiometabolic parameters in adult patients recently diagnosed with T2DM. It has been found that the waist-hip ratio decreased across groups, while HOMA-IR was increased. The fasting blood glucose (FBG) level is less in the probiotic group when compared with the control group, while there are no substantial changes in the endotoxin levels [92]. In further research, the effect of the same probiotic mixture was examined for six months while using the same dosage and criteria as the earlier study. Again, a clinically substantial change in the HOMA-IR was noted, and the probiotic group's insulin levels showed a borderline significant improvement [93]. When the flow of lipopolysaccharides (LPS) is decreased, it is anticipated that low-grade inflammation would decrease and insulin signaling will improve. Karczewski et al. assessed the effects of the probiotic *Lactobacillus plantarum*. The probiotic was injected directly into the duodenum of a group of people and followed by a tissue biopsy after 6 hours. According to the authors' observations, zonula occludens-1 and occludin are translocated more often near tight junctions [94]. Similar results for various strains of the *Lactobacillus* genus were obtained in cell cultures [95]. In a nine-month double-blinded, randomized, placebo-controlled research, Hsieh et al.

Probiotics	Model type	Mechanism of action	Major findings	References
Bifidobacterium animalis A6	28 type II diabetic patients	Significant decrease in fasting blood glucose, serum content of total cholesterol, the cardiovascular risk index (TC/HDL-C), the pro-inflammatory cytokines (IL-6, MCP-1) and adipokines (adiponectin, resistin, lipocalin-2, adipsin). Myokines (irisin, osteocrin) increased significantly, indicating possible improvement in skeletal muscle function	Probiotic camel milk powder twice a day for a consecutive four weeks can significantly decrease fasting blood glucose of type 2 diabetic patients	[98]
probiotic supplements including *Bifidobacterium bifidum* 2×10^9, *Lactobacillus casei* 2×10^9, *Lactobacillus acidophilus* 2×10^9 CFU/day (n = 30)	60 diabetic patients with CHD, aged 40–85 years	Decreasing inflammatory cytokines and suppressing the nuclear factor-κB pathway, their impact on gene expression and the activation of gut microbiota short-chain fatty acids (SCFA)-hormone axis	Probiotic supplementation for 12 weeks had beneficial effects on glycemic control, HDL-cholesterol, total-/HDL-cholesterol ratio, biomarkers of inflammation and oxidative stress in diabetic patients with CHD	[99]
Lactobacillus reuteri	68 T2DM patients	*L. reuteri* may influence changes in intestinal flora, which may lead to different outcomes after probiotic intake.	Significant reductions in HbA1c and serum cholesterol *Bifidobacterium* spp. were significantly increased	[96]
Symbiter	53 patients	Significant reduction of HOMA-IR from 6.85 ± 0.76 to 5.13 ± 0.49 (p = 0.047), but remained static in the placebo group. With respect to our secondary outcomes, HbA1c	Modestly improved insulin resistance	[100]
Ecologic®Barrier	patients with type 2 diabetes mellitus	significant decrease in circulating levels of endotoxin by almost 70% over six months, as well as glucose (38%), insulin (38%), HOMA-IR (64%), triglycerides (48%), total cholesterol (19%), total/HDL-cholesterol ratio (19%), TNF-α (67%), IL-6 (77%), CRP (53%), resistin (53%), and a significant increase in adiponectin (72%) as compared with baseline	multistrain probiotics is a promising adjuvant antidiabetes therapy	[93]

Table 4.
Overview of important studies demonstrating the effect of probiotics on human subjects with type 2 diabetes mellitus.

found that T2DM patients who consume capsules containing the probiotic *Lactobacillus reuteri* ADR-1 had lowered cholesterol and HbA1C level in their blood. The reduction in HbA1C was maintained even after three months of follow-up without probiotic treatment [96]. The effects of ingesting *Lactobacillus reuteri* for 12 weeks at various doses (low dose: 10^8 CFU/day vs. high dose: 10^{10} CFU/day) were examined by Mobini et al.; however, they were unable to detect a reduction in HbA1C in T2DM patients. In the group consuming high-dosage of probiotic, insulin sensitivity index (ISI) was high [97]. **Table 4** provides an overview of important studies demonstrating the effect of probiotics on human subjects with type 2 diabetes mellitus.

A 12-week probiotic therapy that comprised a multistrain probiotic was administered to 101 adults with T2DM. This intervention revealed that the probiotic intake lowers insulin resistance, fasting blood glucose, and HbA1C levels [101]. In an randomized controlled trial (RCT) by Palacios et al., patients with prediabetes and T2DM were enrolled to examine the outcomes of a probiotic multistrain. The only thing that separated the intervention and placebo groups was an increase in butyrate levels. It is noteworthy that those taking both metformin and a probiotic had decreased levels of insulin resistance, FBG, and HbA1c [102]. In a trial utilizing a single-strain probiotic (10^8 CFU/day of *Lactobacillus casei* for eight weeks), Khalili et al. discovered a decrease in FBG, insulin concentration, and insulin resistance [103].

4. Probiotic interventions to ameliorate gestational diabetes

Most of RCTs investigating the therapeutic benefits of probiotic supplementation in female GDM patients have been carried out in Iran; each study used a unique combination of microorganisms and examined a variety of outcomes in addition to glycemia such as gestational weight change [104], lipid profile [105], and inflammation [106]. Fasting blood sugar levels and insulin resistance dramatically decreased in the probiotic group in all these studies. Probiotics also decreased gestational weight

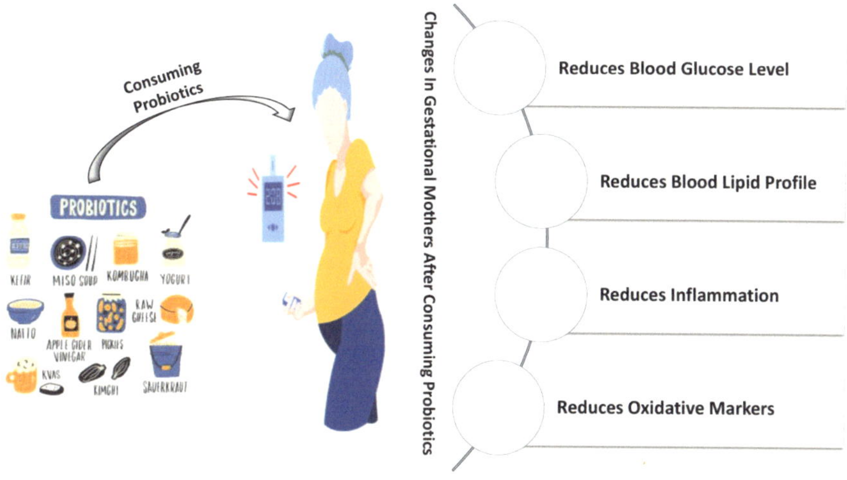

Figure 4.
Potential mechanisms of probiotics against gestational diabetes.

Probiotics	Model type	Major findings	References
Lactobacillus rhamnosus GG and *Bifidobacterium lactis* Bb12	Pregnant women; no chronic diseases apart from allergic diseases; less than 17 gw	Reducing prevalence of GDM	[109]
Lactobacillus salivarius UCC118	Women with GDM	No significant effect on the incidence of GDM	[107]
L. rhamnosus HN001	Pregnant women with a personal or partner history of atopic disease	Reducing the prevalence of GDM	[110]
myo-inositol 2 g + B. lactis and *L. rhamnosus*	Mexican women with three or more risk factors for developing GDM	Reducing the prevalence of GDM	[111]

Table 5.
Overview of important studies demonstrating the effect of probiotics on human subjects with gestational diabetes.

gain, serum very-low-density lipoprotein (VLDL) cholesterol, and triglyceride levels [104–106]. **Figure 4** shows an overview of potential mechanisms of probiotics against type 1 diabetes.

A recent study that randomly assigned GDM patients to receive probiotics (10^9 colony-forming units (CFU) per day of *Bifidobacterium bifidum* and *Lactobacillus acidophilus* or a placebo for four weeks also found significant improvement in glucose metabolism in the probiotic group, including fasting glucose, insulin, and HOMA-IR. An RCT conducted in Ireland randomized 149 women (GDM sufferers) to receive either a probiotic (*Lactobacillus salivarius*, 10^9 CFU per day) or a placebo, and the results showed no change between the two groups except for total cholesterol [107]. There was a considerable decrease in insulin resistance, which seemed to be primarily related to the species *Bifidobacterium* [108]. According to the findings, bigger, longer-term studies comparing various probiotic strains were required.

A modest number of RCTs have looked at probiotic supplementation's potential to stop GDM. In the Finnish "Probiotics and Pregnancy Outcome Study, " pregnant women were randomly assigned to receive dietary advice with probiotic supplementation (10^{10} CFU per day of *Lactobacillus rhamnosus* and *Bifidobacterium lactis*), dietary advice alone, or a placebo. In the probiotic group, the rate of GDM was much lower as compared to the other groups. There were no abnormalities in fetal development [109]. **Table 5** provides an overview of important studies demonstrating the effect of probiotics on human subjects with gestational diabetes. Recently, a probiotic intervention study for women at risk of GDM in New Zealand has been carried out. At 14–16 weeks of gestation, the scientists randomly assigned women to take either a probiotic (*Lactobacillus rhamnosus*, 6×10^9 CFU per day) or a placebo. They also noticed that the probiotic intervention dramatically reduced the occurrence of GDM [110]. Even though the results are encouraging, further research is required to decide if probiotic supplements should be widely utilized in early pregnancy to prevent GDM.

5. Conclusion

Our hypothesis is that the manipulation of the intestinal flora by probiotics may be useful for the prevention and treatment of diabetes. Experimental and clinical trials have shown the significant potential of probiotic strains in the management of diabetes. Probiotics may increase insulin signaling molecules and insulin sensitivity, reduce inflammation and inflammatory cytokines, suppress the nuclear factor-κB pathway, activate gut microbiota short-chain fatty acids (SCFAs)-hormone axis, and enhance the barrier property of the gastrointestinal mucosa by altering the intestinal flora. The studies discussed in this chapter provide insights into the impact of probiotics on diabetes, although further investigation is required to clarify the molecular processes involved in the regulation of intestinal flora by probiotic administration and their effects on the onset of diabetes.

Conflict of interest

The authors declare no conflict of interest.

Author details

Akash Kumar[1*], Jhilam Pramanik[2], Nandani Goyal[3], Bhupendra G. Prajapati[4] and Dimple Chauhan[5]

1 Department of Food Technology, SRM University, Sonepat, Haryana, India

2 Department of Food Technology, ITM University, Madhya Pradesh, India

3 Skill Department of Agriculture, Shri Vishwakarma Skill University, India

4 Shree S.K. Patel College of Pharmaceutical Education and Research, Ganpat University, Kherva, India

5 Shoolini University of Biotechnology and Management Sciences, Solan, Himachal Pradesh, India

*Address all correspondence to: akashksr@gmail.com

References

[1] Blair M. Diabetes mellitus review. Urologic Nursing. 2016;**36**:27-36

[2] Papatheodorou K, Banach M, Bekiari E, Rizzo M, Edmonds M. Complications of diabetes 2017. Journal Diabetes Research. 2018;**2018**:4. Article ID 3086167. DOI: 10.1155/2018/3086167

[3] Delahanty LM, Halford BN. The role of diet behaviors in achieving improved glycemic control in intensively treated patients in the diabetes control and complications trial. Diabetes Care. 1993;**16**:1453-1458. DOI: 10.2337/DIACARE.16.11.1453

[4] Papatheodorou K, Papanas N, Banach M, Papazoglou D, Edmonds M. Complications of diabetes 2016. Journal Diabetes Research. 2016;**2016**:4. Article ID 3086167. DOI: 10.1155/2016/6989453

[5] World Health Organization. World Malaria Report 2015. Geneva, Switzerland: World Health Organization; 2016

[6] Seuring T, Archangelidi O, Suhrcke M. The economic costs of type 2 diabetes: A global systematic review. PharmacoEconomics. 2015;**33**:811-831. DOI: 10.1007/S40273-015-0268-9

[7] Ramachandran A, Snehalatha C. Current scenario of diabetes in India. Journal of Diabetes. 2009;**1**:18-28. DOI: 10.1111/J.1753-0407.2008.00004.X

[8] Ramachandran A, Snehalatha C, Mary S, Mukesh B, Bhaskar AD, Vijay V. The Indian Diabetes Prevention Programme shows that lifestyle modification and metformin prevent type 2 diabetes in Asian Indian subjects with impaired glucose tolerance (IDPP-1). Diabetologia. 2006;**49**:289-297. DOI: 10.1007/S00125-005-0097-Z

[9] Association AD. Classification and diagnosis of diabetes. Diabetes Care. 2017;**40**:S11-S24. DOI: 10.2337/DC17-S005

[10] Association AD. Classification and diagnosis of diabetes. Diabetes Care. 2015;**38**:S8-S16. DOI: 10.2337/DC15-S005

[11] Association AD. Diagnosis and classification of diabetes mellitus. Diabetes Care. 2009;**32**:S62-S67. DOI: 10.2337/DC09-S062

[12] Bhat IA, Kabeer SW, Reza MI, Mir RH, Dar MO. AdipoRon: A novel insulin sensitizer in various complications and the underlying mechanisms: A review. Current Molecular Pharmacology. 2020; **13**:94-107. DOI: 10.2174/1874467212666191022102800

[13] Lamichhane S, Ahonen L, Dyrlund TS, Siljander H, Hyöty H, Ilonen J, et al. A longitudinal plasma lipidomics dataset from children who developed islet autoimmunity and type 1 diabetes. Scientific Data. 2018;**5**:1-9. DOI: 10.1038/sdata.2018.250

[14] Rewers M, Hyöty H, Lernmark Å, Hagopian W, She JX, Schatz D, et al. The environmental determinants of diabetes in the young (TEDDY) study: 2018 update. Current Diabetes Reports. 2018;**2018**:18. DOI: 10.1007/S11892-018-1113-2

[15] Battaglia M, Atkinson MA. The streetlight effect in type 1 diabetes. Diabetes. 2015;**64**:1081-1090. DOI: 10.2337/DB14-1208

[16] Cho NH, Shaw JE, Karuranga S, Huang Y, da Rocha Fernandes JD, Ohlrogge AW, et al. IDF Diabetes Atlas:

Global estimates of diabetes prevalence for 2017 and projections for 2045. Diabetes Research and Clinical Practice. 2018;**138**:271-281. DOI: 10.1016/J.DIABRES.2018.02.023

[17] Lyssenko V, Jonsson A, Almgren P, Pulizzi N, Isomaa B, Tuomi T, et al. Clinical risk factors, DNA variants, and the development of type 2 diabetes. New England Journal of Medicine. 2008;**359**:2220-2232. DOI: 10.1056/nejmoa0801869

[18] Bellamy L, Casas JP, Hingorani AD, Williams D. Type 2 diabetes mellitus after gestational diabetes: A systematic review and meta-analysis. Lancet. 2009;**373**:1773-1779. DOI: 10.1016/S0140-6736(09)60731-5

[19] Kubo A, Ferrara A, Windham GC, Greenspan LC, Deardorff J, Hiatt RA, et al. Maternal hyperglycemia during pregnancy predicts adiposity of the offspring. Diabetes Care. 2014;**37**:2996-3002. DOI: 10.2337/DC14-1438

[20] Asemi Z, Tabassi Z, Samimi M, Fahiminejad T, Esmaillzadeh A. Favourable effects of the dietary approaches to stop hypertension diet on glucose tolerance and lipid profiles in gestational diabetes: A randomised clinical trial. The British Journal of Nutrition. 2013;**109**:2024-2030. DOI: 10.1017/S0007114512004242

[21] Valdes AM, Walter J, Segal E, Spector TD. Role of the gut microbiota in nutrition and health. BMJ. 2018;**361**:36-44. DOI: 10.1136/BMJ.K2179

[22] Li W-Z, Stirling K, Yang J-J, Zhang L. Gut microbiota and diabetes: From correlation to causality and mechanism. 2020;**11**:293-308. DOI: 10.4239/WJD.V11.I7.293

[23] Larsen N, Vogensen FK, van den Berg FWJ, Nielsen DS, Andreasen AS, Pedersen BK, et al. Gut microbiota in human adults with type 2 diabetes differs from non-diabetic adults. PLoS One. 2010;**2010**:5. DOI: 10.1371/JOURNAL.PONE.0009085

[24] Lê KA, Li Y, Xu X, Yang W, Liu T, Zhao X, et al. Alterations in fecal *Lactobacillus* and *Bifidobacterium* species in type 2 diabetic patients in southern China population. Frontiers in Physiology. 2013;**2013**:3. DOI: 10.3389/FPHYS.2012.00496

[25] Derrien M, Vaughan EE, Plugge CM, de Vos WM. *Akkermansia muciniphila* gen. nov., sp. nov., a human intestinal mucin-degrading bacterium. International Journal of Systematic and Evolutionary Microbiology. 2004;**54**:1469-1476. DOI: 10.1099/IJS.0.02873-0

[26] Brown CT, Davis-Richardson AG, Giongo A, Gano KA, Crabb DB, Mukherjee N, et al. Gut microbiome metagenomics analysis suggests a functional model for the development of autoimmunity for type 1 diabetes. PLoS One. 2011;**2011**:6. DOI: 10.1371/JOURNAL.PONE.0025792

[27] Karlsson CLJ, Önnerfält J, Xu J, Molin G, Ahrné S, Thorngren-Jerneck K. The microbiota of the gut in preschool children with normal and excessive body weight. Obesity (Silver Spring). 2012;**20**:2257-2261. DOI: 10.1038/OBY.2012.110

[28] Wen L, Ley RE, Volchkov PY, Stranges PB, Avanesyan L, Stonebraker AC, et al. Innate immunity and intestinal microbiota in the development of type 1 diabetes. Nature. 2008;**455**:1109-1113. DOI: 10.1038/NATURE07336

[29] Cani PD, Amar J, Iglesias MA, Poggi M, Knauf C, Bastelica D, et al. Metabolic endotoxemia initiates obesity and insulin

resistance. Diabetes. 2007;**56**:1761-1772. DOI: 10.2337/DB06-1491

[30] Padwal R, Majumdar SR, Johnson JA, Varney J, McAlister FA. A systematic review of drug therapy to delay or prevent type 2 diabetes. Diabetes Care. 2005;**28**:736-744. DOI: 10.2337/DIACARE.28.3.736

[31] Kumar A, Prajapati B, Pramanik J. Prebiotics as adjunctive therapy in diabetes: A review prebiotics in diabetes. Current Nutraceuticals. 2022;**2022**:03. DOI: 10.2174/2665978603666220818085437

[32] Walker KZ, O'Dea K, Gomez M, Girgis S, Colagiuri R. Diet and exercise in the prevention of diabetes. Journal of Human Nutrition and Dietetics. 2010;**23**:344-352. DOI: 10.1111/J.1365-277X.2010.01061.X

[33] Norris SL, Zhang X, Avenell A, Gregg E, Bowman B, Schmid CH, et al. Long-term effectiveness of weight-loss interventions in adults with pre-diabetes: A review. American Journal of Preventive Medicine. 2005;**28**:126-139. DOI: 10.1016/J.AMEPRE.2004.08.006

[34] Norris SL, Zhang X, Avenell A, Gregg E, Brown T, Schmid CH, et al. Long-term non-pharmacological weight loss interventions for adults with type 2 diabetes mellitus. Cochrane Database of Systematic Reviews. 2005;**2010**(2):CD004095. DOI: 10.1002/14651858.CD004095.PUB2/INFORMATION/EN

[35] Diabetes Management. Community Health Workers | the Community Guide. n.d. https://www.thecommunityguide.org/findings/diabetes-management-interventions-engaging-community-health-workers.html [Accessed December 9, 2022]

[36] Gismondo MR, Drago L, Lombardi A. Review of probiotics available to modify gastrointestinal flora. International Journal of Antimicrobial Agents. 1999;**12**:287-292. DOI: 10.1016/S0924-8579(99)00050-3

[37] Lilly DM, Stillwell RH. Probiotics: Growth-promoting factors produced by microorganisms. Science. 1979;**1965**(147):747-748. DOI: 10.1126/SCIENCE.147.3659.747

[38] Parker RB. Probiotics, the other half of the antibiotic story. Animal Nutrition and Health. 1974;**29**:4-8

[39] Reid G, Sanders ME, Gaskins HR, Gibson GR, Mercenier A, Rastall R, et al. New scientific paradigms for probiotics and prebiotics. Journal of Clinical Gastroenterology. 2003;**37**:105-118. DOI: 10.1097/00004836-200308000-00004

[40] Hegar B, Waspada MI, Gunardi H, Vandenplas Y. A double blind randomized trial showing probiotics to be ineffective in acute Diarrhea in Indonesian children. Indian Journal of Pediatrics. 2015;**82**:410-414. DOI: 10.1007/S12098-014-1408-5

[41] Cammarota M, de Rosa M, Stellavato A, Lamberti M, Marzaioli I, Giuliano M. In vitro evaluation of *Lactobacillus plantarum* DSMZ 12028 as a probiotic: Emphasis on innate immunity. International Journal of Food Microbiology. 2009;**135**:90-98. DOI: 10.1016/J.IJFOODMICRO.2009.08.022

[42] Amara AA, Shibl A. Role of probiotics in health improvement, infection control and disease treatment and management. Saudi Pharmaceutical Journal: SPJ. 2015;**23**:107. DOI: 10.1016/J.JSPS.2013.07.001

[43] Bourdichon F, Casaregola S, Farrokh C, Frisvad JC, Gerds ML,

Hammes WP, et al. Food fermentations: Microorganisms with technological beneficial use. International Journal of Food Microbiology. 2012;**154**:87-97. DOI: 10.1016/J.IJFOODMICRO.2011.12.030

[44] Metchnikoff I. The Prolongation of Life: Optimistic Studies. United States: Springer Publishing Company; 2004

[45] Sanders ME, Merenstein D, Merrifield CA, Hutkins R. Probiotics for human use. Nutrition Bulletin. 2018;**43**:212-225. DOI: 10.1111/NBU.12334

[46] Pawar R, Zambare V, Nabar B. Comparative assessment of antibiotic resistance in lactic acid Bacteria isolated from healthy human adult and infant Feces. Nepal Journal of Biotechnology. 2020;**8**:69-75. DOI: 10.3126/NJB.V8I2.31893

[47] Choudhari G, Zambare V, Pawar R. Screening, isolation and characterization of probiotically safe lactic acid bacteria from human faeces for biofilm formation. International Journal of Research in BioSciences. 2018;**7**:10-18

[48] Topping DL, Clifton PM. Short-chain fatty acids and human colonic function: Roles of resistant starch and nonstarch polysaccharides. Physiological Reviews. 2001;**81**:1031-1064. DOI: 10.1152/PHYSREV.2001.81.3.1031

[49] Versalovic J. The human microbiome and probiotics: Implications for pediatrics. Annals of Nutrition & Metabolism. 2013;**63**(Suppl. 2):42-52. DOI: 10.1159/000354899

[50] Pawar R, Dhawal P, Nabar B, Barve S, Zambare V. Mechanisms and applications of probiotics in healthcare industry. Biotechnology in Healthcare. 2022;**2022**:225-257. DOI: 10.1016/B978-0-323-90042-3.00002-5

[51] Kristensen NB, Bryrup T, Allin KH, Nielsen T, Hansen TH, Pedersen O. Alterations in fecal microbiota composition by probiotic supplementation in healthy adults: A systematic review of randomized controlled trials. Genome Medicine. 2016;**2016**:8. DOI: 10.1186/S13073-016-0300-5

[52] Sanders ME, Heimbach JT, Pot B, Tancredi D, Lenoir-Wijnkoop I, Lähteenmäki-Uutela A, et al. Health claims substantiation for probiotic and prebiotic products. Gut Microbes. 2011;**2**:127-133. DOI: 10.4161/GMIC.2.3.16174

[53] Nagpal R, Wang S, Ahmadi S, Hayes J, Gagliano J, Subashchandrabose S, et al. Human-origin probiotic cocktail increases short-chain fatty acid production via modulation of mice and human gut microbiome. Scientific Reports. 2018;**2018**:8. DOI: 10.1038/S41598-018-30114-4

[54] Ang Z, Ding JL. GPR41 and GPR43 in obesity and inflammation - protective or causative? Frontiers in Immunology. 2016;**2016**:7. DOI: 10.3389/FIMMU.2016.00028

[55] Psichas A, Sleeth ML, Murphy KG, Brooks L, Bewick GA, Hanyaloglu AC, et al. The short chain fatty acid propionate stimulates GLP-1 and PYY secretion via free fatty acid receptor 2 in rodents. International Journal of Obesity. 2015;**39**:424-429. DOI: 10.1038/IJO.2014.153

[56] Christiansen CB, Gabe MBN, Svendsen B, Dragsted LO, Rosenkilde MM, Holst JJ. The impact of short-chain fatty acids on GLP-1 and PYY secretion from the isolated perfused rat colon. American Journal of Physiology. Gastrointestinal and Liver Physiology. 2018;**315**:G53-G65. DOI: 10.1152/AJPGI.00346.2017

[57] Abdelazez A, Abdelmotaal H, Evivie SE, Melak S, Jia FF, Khoso MH, et al. Screening potential probiotic characteristics of lactobacillus brevis strains in vitro and intervention effect on type I diabetes in vivo. Biomedical Research International. 2018;**2018**:20. Article ID 7356173. DOI: 10.1155/2018/7356173

[58] Dolpady J, Sorini C, di Pietro C, Cosorich I, Ferrarese R, Saita D, et al. Oral probiotic VSL#3 prevents autoimmune diabetes by modulating microbiota and promoting indoleamine 2,3-dioxygenase-enriched tolerogenic intestinal environment. Journal Diabetes Research. 2016;**2016**:12. Article ID 7569431. DOI: 10.1155/2016/7569431

[59] van Endert P, Mauvais FX, Diana J. Beta cell antigens in type 1 diabetes: Triggers in pathogenesis and therapeutic targets. F1000Res. 2016;**2016**:5. DOI: 10.12688/F1000RESEARCH.7411.1/DOI

[60] Takiishi T, Korf H, van Belle TL, Robert S, Grieco FA, Caluwaerts S, et al. Reversal of autoimmune diabetes by restoration of antigen-specific tolerance using genetically modified *Lactococcus lactis* in mice. The Journal of Clinical Investigation. 2012;**122**:1717-1725. DOI: 10.1172/JCI60530

[61] Calcinaro F, Dionisi S, Marinaro M, Candeloro P, Bonato V, Marzotti S, et al. Oral probiotic administration induces interleukin-10 production and prevents spontaneous autoimmune diabetes in the non-obese diabetic mouse. Diabetologia. 2005;**48**:1565-1575. DOI: 10.1007/S00125-005-1831-2

[62] Yadav R, Dey DK, Vij R, Meena S, Kapila R, Kapila S. Evaluation of anti-diabetic attributes of *Lactobacillus rhamnosus* MTCC: 5957, *Lactobacillus rhamnosus* MTCC: 5897 and *Lactobacillus fermentum* MTCC: 5898 in streptozotocin induced diabetic rats. Microbial Pathogenesis. 2018;**125**:454-462. DOI: 10.1016/J.MICPATH.2018.10.015

[63] Le TKC, Hosaka T, Nguyen TT, Kassu A, Dang TO, Tran HB, et al. *Bifidobacterium* species lower serum glucose, increase expressions of insulin signaling proteins, and improve adipokine profile in diabetic mice. Biomedical Research. 2015;**36**:63-70. DOI: 10.2220/BIOMEDRES.36.63

[64] Zhang J, Motyl KJ, Irwin R, MacDougald OA, Britton RA, McCabe LR. Loss of bone and Wnt10b expression in male type 1 diabetic mice is blocked by the probiotic *Lactobacillus reuteri*. Endocrinology. 2015;**156**:3169-3182. DOI: 10.1210/EN.2015-1308

[65] Wei SH, Chen YP, Chen MJ. Selecting probiotics with the abilities of enhancing GLP-1 to mitigate the progression of type 1 diabetes in vitro and in vivo. Journal of Functional Foods. 2015;**18**:473-486. DOI: 10.1016/J.JFF.2015.08.016

[66] Valladares R, Sankar D, Li N, Williams E, Lai KK, Abdelgeliel AS, et al. *Lactobacillus johnsonii* N6.2 mitigates the development of type 1 diabetes in BB-DP rats. PLoS One. 2010;**2010**:5. DOI: 10.1371/JOURNAL.PONE.0010507

[67] Lau K, Benitez P, Ardissone A, Wilson TD, Collins EL, Lorca G, et al. Inhibition of type 1 diabetes correlated to a *Lactobacillus johnsonii* N6.2-mediated Th17 bias. Journal of Immunology. 2011;**186**:3538-3546. DOI: 10.4049/JIMMUNOL.1001864

[68] Bejar W, Hamden K, Salah R, Chouayekh H. *Lactobacillus plantarum* TN627 significantly reduces complications of alloxan-induced diabetes in rats. Anaerobe. 2013;**24**:4-11. DOI: 10.1016/J.ANAEROBE.2013.08.006

[69] Vatanen T, Franzosa EA, Schwager R, Tripathi S, Arthur TD, Vehik K, et al. The human gut microbiome in early-onset type 1 diabetes from the TEDDY study. Nature. 2018;**562**:589-594. DOI: 10.1038/S41586-018-0620-2

[70] Uusitalo U, Liu X, Yang J, Aronsson CA, Hummel S, Butterworth M, et al. Association of Early Exposure of probiotics and islet autoimmunity in the TEDDY study. JAMA Pediatrics. 2016;**170**:20-28. DOI: 10.1001/JAMAPEDIATRICS.2015.2757

[71] Marcial GE, Ford AL, Haller MJ, Gezan SA, Harrison NA, Cai D, et al. *Lactobacillus johnsonii* N6.2 modulates the host immune responses: A double-blind, randomized trial in healthy adults. Frontiers in Immunology. 2017;**2017**:8. DOI: 10.3389/FIMMU.2017.00655

[72] Weir GC, Bonner-Weir S. Dreams for type 1 diabetes: Shutting off autoimmunity and stimulating beta-cell regeneration. Endocrinology. 2010;**151**:2971-2973. DOI: 10.1210/EN.2010-0538

[73] Yadav H, Lee JH, Lloyd J, Walter P, Rane SG. Beneficial metabolic effects of a probiotic via butyrate-induced GLP-1 hormone secretion. The Journal of Biological Chemistry. 2013;**288**:25088-25097. DOI: 10.1074/JBC.M113.452516

[74] Burrows MP, Volchkov P, Kobayashi KS, Chervonsky A, v., Medzhitov R. Microbiota regulates type 1 diabetes through toll-like receptors. Proceedings of the National Academy of Sciences of the United States of America. 2015;**112**:9973-9977. DOI: 10.1073/PNAS.1508740112

[75] Groele L, Szajewska H, Szypowska A. Effects of *Lactobacillus rhamnosus* GG and Bifidobacterium lactis Bb12 on beta-cell function in children with newly diagnosed type 1 diabetes: Protocol of a randomised controlled trial. BMJ Open. 2017;**2017**:7. DOI: 10.1136/BMJOPEN-2017-017178

[76] Ahola AJ, Harjutsalo V, Forsblom C, Freese R, Makimattila S, Groop P. The self-reported use of probiotics is associated with better glycaemic control and lower odds of metabolic syndrome and its components in type 1 diabetes. Journal of Probiotics Health. 2017;**2017**:05. DOI: 10.4172/2329-8901.1000188

[77] Yang J, Tamura RN, Uusitalo UM, Aronsson CA, Silvis K, Riikonen A, et al. Vitamin D and probiotics supplement use in young children with genetic risk for type 1 diabetes. European Journal of Clinical Nutrition. 2017;**71**:1449-1454. DOI: 10.1038/EJCN.2017.140

[78] Lee YK, Margolles A, Mayo B, Ruas-Madiedo P, Gueimonde M, de los Reyes-Gavilán C, et al. Probiotic Microorganisms. Handbook of Probiotics and Prebiotics. Second ed. New York, United States. 2008. pp. 1-176. DOI: 10.1002/9780470432624.CH1

[79] Li X, Wang N, Yin B, Fang D, Jiang T, Fang S, et al. Effects of *Lactobacillus plantarum* CCFM0236 on hyperglycaemia and insulin resistance in high-fat and streptozotocin-induced type 2 diabetic mice. Journal of Applied Microbiology. 2016;**121**:1727-1736. DOI: 10.1111/JAM.13276

[80] Lee E, Jung SR, Lee SY, Lee NK, Paik HD, Lim S. *Lactobacillus plantarum* strain Ln4 attenuates diet-induced obesity, insulin resistance, and changes in hepatic mRNA levels associated with glucose and lipid metabolism. Nutrients. 2018;**2018**:10. DOI: 10.3390/NU10050643

[81] Balakumar M, Prabhu D, Sathishkumar C, Prabu P, Rokana N,

Kumar R, et al. Improvement in glucose tolerance and insulin sensitivity by probiotic strains of Indian gut origin in high-fat diet-fed C57BL/6J mice. European Journal of Nutrition. 2018;**57**:279-295. DOI: 10.1007/S00394-016-1317-7

[82] Dang F, Jiang Y, Pan R, Zhou Y, Wu S, Wang R, et al. Administration of *Lactobacillus paracasei* ameliorates type 2 diabetes in mice. Food & Function. 2018;**9**:3630-3639. DOI: 10.1039/C8FO00081F

[83] Memarrast F, Ghafouri-Fard S, Kolivand S, Jafary-Nodooshan S, Neyazi N, Sadroddiny E, et al. Comparative evaluation of probiotics effects on plasma glucose, lipid, and insulin levels in streptozotocin-induced diabetic rats. Diabetes/Metabolism Research and Reviews. 2017;**2017**:33. DOI: 10.1002/DMRR.2912

[84] Lin Y, Ren Y, Zhang Y, Zhou J, Zhou F, Zhao Q, et al. Protective role of nano-selenium-enriched *Bifidobacterium longum* in delaying the onset of streptozotocin-induced diabetes. Royal Society Open Science. 2018;**2018**:5. DOI: 10.1098/RSOS.181156

[85] Sakai T, Taki T, Nakamoto A, Shuto E, Tsutsumi R, Toshimitsu T, et al. *Lactobacillus plantarum* OLL2712 regulates glucose metabolism in C57BL/6 mice fed a high-fat diet. Journal of Nutritional Science and Vitaminology (Tokyo). 2013;**59**:144-147. DOI: 10.3177/JNSV.59.144

[86] Wang G, Li X, Zhao J, Zhang H, Chen W. *Lactobacillus casei* CCFM419 attenuates type 2 diabetes via a gut microbiota dependent mechanism. Food & Function. 2017;**8**:3155-3164. DOI: 10.1039/C7FO00593H

[87] Zeng Z, Yuan Q, Yu R, Zhang J, Ma H, Chen S. Ameliorative effects of probiotic *Lactobacillus paracasei* NL41 on insulin sensitivity, oxidative stress, and Beta-cell function in a type 2 diabetes mellitus rat model. Molecular Nutrition & Food Research. 2019;**2019**:63. DOI: 10.1002/MNFR.201900457

[88] Jia L, Li D, Feng N, Shamoon M, Sun Z, Ding L, et al. Anti-diabetic effects of *Clostridium butyricum* CGMCC0313.1 through promoting the growth of gut butyrate-producing Bacteria in type 2 diabetic mice. Scientific Reports. 2017:7. DOI: 10.1038/S41598-017-07335-0

[89] Manaer T, Yu L, Nabi XH, Dilidaxi D, Liu L, Sailike J. The beneficial effects of the composite probiotics from camel milk on glucose and lipid metabolism, liver and renal function and gut microbiota in db/db mice. BMC Complementary Medicine Therapy. 2021;**21**:1-13. DOI: 10.1186/S12906-021-03303-4/FIGURES/6

[90] Zhao D, Zhu H, Gao F, Qian Z, Mao W, Yin Y, et al. Antidiabetic effects of selenium-enriched *Bifidobacterium longum* DD98 in type 2 diabetes model of mice. Food & Function. 2020;**11**:6528-6541. DOI: 10.1039/D0FO00180E

[91] Zhang J, Wang S, Zeng Z, Qin Y, Shen Q, Li P. Anti-diabetic effects of *Bifidobacterium animalis* 01 through improving hepatic insulin sensitivity in type 2 diabetic rat model. Journal of Functional Foods. 2020;**67**:103843. DOI: 10.1016/J.JFF.2020.103843

[92] Sabico S, Al-Mashharawi A, Al-Daghri NM, Yakout S, Alnaami AM, Alokail MS, et al. Effects of a multi-strain probiotic supplement for 12 weeks in circulating endotoxin levels and cardiometabolic profiles of medication naïve T2DM patients: A randomized clinical trial. Journal of Translational Medicine. 2017;**2017**:15. DOI: 10.1186/S12967-017-1354-X

[93] Sabico S, Al-Mashharawi A, Al-Daghri NM, Wani K, Amer OE, Hussain DS, et al. Effects of a 6-month multi-strain probiotics supplementation in endotoxemic, inflammatory and cardiometabolic status of T2DM patients: A randomized, double-blind, placebo-controlled trial. Clinical Nutrition. 2019;**38**:1561-1569. DOI: 10.1016/J.CLNU.2018.08.009

[94] Karczewski J, Troost FJ, Konings I, Dekker J, Kleerebezem M, Brummer RJM, et al. Regulation of human epithelial tight junction proteins by *Lactobacillus plantarum* in vivo and protective effects on the epithelial barrier. American Journal of Physiology. Gastrointestinal and Liver Physiology. 2010;**298**:851-859. DOI: 10.1152/AJPGI.00327.2009/ASSET/IMAGES/LARGE/ZH30051056450004.JPEG

[95] Hummel S, Veltman K, Cichon C, Sonnenborn U, Schmidt MA. Differential targeting of the E-cadherin/β-catenin complex by gram-positive probiotic *lactobacilli* improves epithelial barrier function. Applied and Environmental Microbiology. 2012;**78**:1140-1147. DOI: 10.1128/AEM.06983-11/ASSET/F277D377-DD28-48F7-8448-623CFA15F5AD/ASSETS/GRAPHIC/ZAM9991029470006.JPEG

[96] Hsieh MC, Tsai WH, Jheng YP, Su SL, Wang SY, Lin CC, et al. The beneficial effects of *Lactobacillus reuteri* ADR-1 or ADR-3 consumption on type 2 diabetes mellitus: A randomized, double-blinded, placebo-controlled trial. Scientific Reports. 2018;**8**:1-11. DOI: 10.1038/s41598-018-35014-1

[97] Mobini R, Tremaroli V, Ståhlman M, Karlsson F, Levin M, Ljungberg M, et al. Metabolic effects of *Lactobacillus reuteri* DSM 17938 in people with type 2 diabetes: A randomized controlled trial. Diabetes, Obesity & Metabolism. 2017;**19**:579-589. DOI: 10.1111/DOM.12861

[98] B F, M Z, L D, X Z, F R, S G. Probiotic camel milk powder improves glycemic control, dyslipidemia, adipose tissue and skeletal muscle function in T2DM patients: A randomized trial. 2020. 10.21203/RS.3.RS-34115/V1

[99] Raygan F, Rezavandi Z, Bahmani F, Ostadmohammadi V, Mansournia MA, Tajabadi-Ebrahimi M, et al. The effects of probiotic supplementation on metabolic status in type 2 diabetic patients with coronary heart disease IRCT2017082733941N5 IRCT. Diabetology and Metabolic Syndrome. 2018;**10**:1-7. DOI: 10.1186/S13098-018-0353-2/TABLES/3

[100] Kobyliak N, Falalyeyeva T, Mykhalchyshyn G, Kyriienko D, Komissarenko I. Effect of alive probiotic on insulin resistance in type 2 diabetes patients: Randomized clinical trial. Diabetes & Metabolic Syndrome: Clinical Research & Reviews. 2018;**12**:617-624. DOI: 10.1016/J.DSX.2018.04.015

[101] Firouzi S, Majid HA, Ismail A, Kamaruddin NA, Barakatun-Nisak MY. Effect of multi-strain probiotics (multi-strain microbial cell preparation) on glycemic control and other diabetes-related outcomes in people with type 2 diabetes: A randomized controlled trial. European Journal of Nutrition. 2016;**56**:1535-1550. DOI: 10.1007/S00394-016-1199-8

[102] Palacios T, Vitetta L, Coulson S, Madigan CD, Lam YY, Manuel R, et al. Targeting the intestinal microbiota to prevent Type 2 diabetes and enhance the effect of metformin on glycaemia: A Randomised Controlled Pilot Study. Nutrients. 2020;**12**:2041. DOI: 10.3390/NU12072041

[103] Khalili L, Alipour B, Jafar-Abadi MA, Faraji I, Hassanalilou T, Abbasi MM, et al. The effects of *Lactobacillus casei* on Glycemic response, serum Sirtuin1 and Fetuin-A levels in patients with type 2 diabetes mellitus: A randomized controlled trial. Iranian Biomedical Journal. 2019;**23**:68-77. DOI: 10.29252/.23.1.68

[104] Dolatkhah N, Hajifaraji M, Abbasalizadeh F, Aghamohammadzadeh N, Mehrabi Y, Abbasi MM. Is there a value for probiotic supplements in gestational diabetes mellitus? A randomized clinical trial. Journal of Health, Population, and Nutrition. 2015;**33**:1-8. DOI: 10.1186/S41043-015-0034-9/TABLES/3

[105] Karamali M, Dadkhah F, Sadrkhanlou M, Jamilian M, Ahmadi S, Tajabadi-Ebrahimi M, et al. Effects of probiotic supplementation on glycaemic control and lipid profiles in gestational diabetes: A randomized, double-blind, placebo-controlled trial. Diabetes & Metabolism. 2016;**42**:234-241. DOI: 10.1016/J.DIABET.2016.04.009

[106] Jafarnejad S, Saremi S, Jafarnejad F, Arab A. Effects of a multispecies probiotic mixture on Glycemic control and inflammatory status in women with gestational diabetes: A randomized controlled clinical trial. Journal of Nutrition Metabolism. 2016;**2016**. DOI: 10.1155/2016/5190846

[107] Lindsay KL, Kennelly M, Culliton M, Smith T, Maguire OC, Shanahan F, et al. Probiotics in obese pregnancy do not reduce maternal fasting glucose: A double-blind, placebo-controlled, randomized trial (probiotics in pregnancy study). The American Journal of Clinical Nutrition. 2014;**99**:1432-1439. DOI: 10.3945/AJCN.113.079723

[108] Taylor BL, Woodfall GE, Sheedy KE, O'Riley ML, Rainbow KA, Bramwell EL, et al. Effect of probiotics on metabolic outcomes in pregnant women with gestational diabetes: A systematic review and Meta-analysis of randomized controlled trials. Nutrients. 2017;**2017**:9. DOI: 10.3390/NU9050461

[109] Luoto R, Laitinen K, Nermes M, Isolauri E. Impact of maternal probiotic-supplemented dietary counselling on pregnancy outcome and prenatal and postnatal growth: A double-blind, placebo-controlled study. The British Journal of Nutrition. 2010;**103**:1792-1799. DOI: 10.1017/S0007114509993898

[110] Wickens KL, Barthow CA, Murphy R, Abels PR, Maude RM, Stone PR, et al. Early pregnancy probiotic supplementation with *Lactobacillus rhamnosus* HN001 may reduce the prevalence of gestational diabetes mellitus: A randomised controlled trial. British Journal of Nutrition. 2017;**117**:804-813. DOI: 10.1017/S0007114517000289

[111] Reyes-Muñoz E, Espino Y, Sosa S, Flores-Robles CM, Arce-Sánchez L, Martínez-Cruz N, et al. Uso de mioinositol más *Bifidobacterium lactis* y *Lactobacillus rhamnosus* para la prevención de diabetes mellitus gestacional en mujeres mexicanas. Gaceta Médica de México. 2020;**156**:S51-S57. DOI: 10.24875/GMM.M20000438

Chapter 9

Probiotics as a Beneficial Modulator of Gut Microbiota and Environmental Stress for Sustainable Mass-Reared *Ceratitis capitata*

Meriem Msaad Guerfali, Haytham Hamden, Kamel Charaabi, Salma Fadhl, Amor Mosbah and Amer Cherif

Abstract

The Mediterranean fruit fly *Ceratitis capitata* (medfly) is a major pest throughout the world and one of the most destructive. Several strategies for controlling this pest have been proposed, including the sterile insect technique (SIT). The SIT's effectiveness against the medfly is well documented. Sterile medflies, on the other hand, can perform poorly. Reduced mating compatibility and mating competitiveness in the field may be caused by genetic and symbiotic differences between natural and laboratory medfly populations. Probiotic gut symbionts have been shown to facilitate control strategies and improve male medfly fitness. They are equally effective in the live and inactivated forms when administered to medfly adults or larvae. They have been shown to modulate a large set of inducible effector molecules including antimicrobial peptides (AMP) and stress-responsive proteins. The selection procedures of probiotics for their use in the medfly rearing process are reviewed, and other pathways for selection are proposed based on recent in silico studies. This chapter summarizes the most relevant evidence from scientific literature regarding potential applications of probiotics in medfly as an innovative tool for biocontrol, while also shedding light on the spectrum of symbiotic relationships in medfly that may serve as a powerful symbiotic integrative control approach.

Keywords: *Ceratitis capitata*, probiotic, selection, *in vivo*, *in silico*, probiogenomics

1. Introduction

The development of insect farming is critical for achieving agricultural sustainability goals and dealing with rising food demand, ongoing natural resource depletion, and global climate change. Insects are now being mass-produced as entomophagous arthropods for pest management or for food and feed. During the 1950s and 1960s, the field of insect mass-rearing began with the mass production and release of sterile males for autocidal control of flies such as the screwworm and later with natural enemies during the 1970s, 1980s, and 1990s. By far the sterile insect technique (SIT) is the technique that makes the most use of mass-rearing. Pests are reared in large numbers before being sterilized with ionizing radiation and released into the wild as a viable alternative to chemical pesticides. Male sterile insects compete with male wild insects of the target pest. Females inseminated with sterile sperm are not fertilized and will not give birth. The worldwide directory of SIT facilities (DIR-SIT) indicates that there are more than 142 facilities breeding mainly Diptera, Lepidoptera, and Coleoptera.

The innovation of mass-rearing necessitates the development of artificial diets, as well as a controlled environment with clear and reproducible procedures to achieve the best yields at the lowest costs. For the Mediterranean fruit fly *Ceratitis capitata* (medfly), which is a major key pest that attacks more than 400 hosts, standard rearing procedures were developed by the USDA, IAEA, and the FAO in the 2000s [1]. This document represents the recommendations, reached by consensus of an international group of quality control experts, on the standard procedures for product quality control (QC) that are used now for sterile mass-reared and released tephritid flies. Indeed, despite years of improving the various breeding and release procedures, laboratory sterile males tend to have reduced performance compared to their wild counterparts. Recently microbiome disturbance or dysbiosis has been increasingly recognized as a significant contributor to the poor performance of sterile medfly males, which play a key role in shaping health and fitness. The presence of minor communities such as *Pseudomonas aeruginosa* in the medfly gut at the expense of major communities such as Enterobacteriaceae would result in a decrease in host nutrients and energy metabolic activity in sterile medfly males [2, 3]. Both culture-dependent and culture-independent techniques were used to identify potential dysbiosis after domestication, irradiation, mass-rearing, and handling, highlighting the potential risks to host immunity, development, nutrition, and health. The dominant presence of the enterobacterial community in the medfly's gut contributes to the fly's nitrogen and carbon metabolism, development, and copulatory success [2, 4], as well as its host fitness by acting as a barrier against deleterious bacteria [2]. The dominant species in wild and laboratory medfly populations were identified as *Klebsiella oxytoca* and *Enterobacter agglomerans*, respectively [5].

Even though prevention is preferable to cure, the development of health-enhancing additives such as probiotics began in the 1950s–1980s [6]. Because of their prophylactic efficacy against bacterial infections of the gut and immunomodulating activity, there is agreement on the efficacy of supplementing probiotics to human health conditions [7], poultry [8], and, more recently, aquaculture [9].

With the development of mass-rearing, concern for insects' health increased. Probiotics are already sold to beekeepers to restore the gut microbiota of honey bees following antibiotic treatment. First, anaerobic gut bacteria obtained from bees were studied, along with strains from several additional sources [10]. The most popular probiotic strains for bees are *Lactobacillus* and *Bacillus*, two strains that are associated with honey bees and/or have been chosen from the bee environment [11]. Over the past decade, experimental supplementation of probiotics to the medfly diet has provided key insights. Probiotics stimulate production and modulate the immune system. To what extent are these probiotics thought to be a preventative measure for medfly mass-rearing? This chapter describes ongoing research in this field and attempts to analyze how probiotics might aid sterile medflies in fighting diseases, dealing with pesticides, and dealing with the effects of climate change.

2. What causes dysbiosis in the medfly gut microbiome?

Gut symbionts are claimed to positively influence the development and ecological fitness of tephritidae. It could be through the provision of essential nutrients such as amino acids, vitamins, nitrogen, and carbon compounds [12–15], the suppression of pathogen establishment [2, 16, 17], the enhancement of host resistance to pesticides [18], or the mediation of mate selection [19]. As a result, dysbiosis of the gut microbiota has recently emerged as the cause of the sterile medfly males' low fitness. Indeed, these males face a variety of constraints during mass-rearing, treatment with ionizing radiation, and release conditions that favor minor bacterial genera such as *Providencia* and *Pseudomonas*, which are considered potential pathogens for the fly [16, 20]. The reduced fitness of released sterile males usually means that they are less competitive [21–23].

3. Probiotics used in mass-reared *Ceratitis capitata*: biological and functional properties

3.1 Current status and application of the probiotics to medfly sterile males production system

The term "probiotic" is derived from the Greek words pro and bios, which mean "life" [24]. It was coined in 1965 by Lilly and Stillwell [25] to contrast the term "antibiotic". The definition of probiotic' has evolved. The Food and Agricultural Organization and World Health Organization (FAO/WHO) define probiotics as "live microorganisms that, when administered in adequate amounts, confer a health benefit on the host" [26]. Many species have been designated as "Generally Recognized As Safe" (GRAS) with the origin of the strain, antibiotic resistance, and lack of pathogenicity determining the safety of probiotic strains [27]. Different Gram-positive bacteria belonging to the genus *Lactobacillus*, *Enterococcus*, *Bacillus*, and *Bifidobacterium* have been studied extensively for their role as probiotics.

Pioneering studies on the experimental use of probiotics were initiated following the interesting findings of Ben Ami et al. [16], working on medfly, that regenerating the original microbiota community could result in enhanced competitiveness of the sterile flies. We should also mention that this study, which partially replicated the work of Niyazi et al., [28], shed light on the composition of the intestinal microbiota in sterile males.

As demonstrated by Ben Ami et al., [16], the addition of Streptomycin-resistant *K. oxytoca* strain to the post-irradiation adult diet allowed this probiotic to colonize the guts of *C. capitata* sterile males. Currently, the most common method of medfly administration is oral administration via diet [17, 29, 30]. Indeed, probiotics could be given to medfly at two stages: larval and adult. If the addition occurs during the larval stage, there is only one option: add the probiotics as a suspension, usually 10^7, 10^8, 10^9 CFU/g mixed with the diet (carrot or wheat bran). If the addition occurs during the adult stage, there are two options: the first is to incorporate it into the adult diet as a bacteria-containing diet (granular sugar and yeast mixture or agar) [28], and the second is to introduce it through a cotton pad soaked with the bacterial suspension [2, 13, 16, 29, 31–35]. If multiple strain preparation is of interest in aquaculture, single administration for insects in general and medfly, in particular, is the option. As shown in **Table 1**, most of the studies exploited the probiotic strains as live; however, other

Strain	Orig	Stage	Diet	Stat	Single/ multi	C_i	Inoc T	Contact duration	Pf col	Ref
Enterobacter agglomerans *Klebtiella pneumoniae*		A	Granular sugar-yeast 3:1 ratio	Live	Single	50%		Ad libitum	yes	[28]
			Granular sugar-yeast diet 6:1 ratio							
			Prerelease sucrose-agar diet							
			Sucrose-agar diet containing a small amount of yeast							
Pectobacterium cypripedi *Citrobacter freundii* *Enterobacter* spp. *Klebtiella oxytoca* *Pantoea* spp.	Wild caught flies	A	Bacterial suspension in 20% sucrose solution		Multi	10^8 CFU/ml	Daily until death			[2]
Klebtiella oxytoca SmKo	Wild caught flies	A		Live/ inactive		10^6 CFU/ml			Yes	[16]
Klebsiella oxytoca N8-S	Wild caught flies	A	Cotton wool soaked with bacterial culture	Live		10^9 CFU/ml	Daily	5 days	Yes	[34]
Enterobacetr spp. *Klebtiella pneumoniae* *Citrobacter freundii*	Other	L	Wheat bran diet	Live	Multi	5.6 μg/g	Daily	10 days	No	[13]
Enterobacter spp.	Vienna 8 GSS	L	Carrot diet	Live/ Inactive		10^6, 10^7, 10^8 CFU/g			No	[29]
Klebtiella oxytoca	Vienna 8 $^{D53+}$	L	Carrot diet	Live/ Inactive		10^6, 10^7, 10^8 CFU/g				[30]

DOI: http://dx.doi.org/10.5772/intechopen.110126

Strain	Orig	Stage	Diet	Stat	Single/ multi	C_i	Inoc T	Contact duration	Pf col	Ref
Enterobacter AA26 *Klebtiella oxytoca*	Wild caught flies Vienna 8 $^{D53+}$,	A	Cotton pad soaked with 5 ml of bacterial suspension	Live	Single	10^8 bacteria/ ml	Daily	5–6 days		[30]
Enterobacter AA26		L	Carrot diet with full yeast replacement with *EAA26* biomass	Dry biomass		7%, 3.5% and 0%				[32]
			Carrot diet with partial yeast replacement with *EAA26* biomass							
Morganella morganii *Enterobacter* spp. *Klebtiella oxytoca* *Rahnella aquatilis* *Lactococcus lactis* *Pluralibacter gergoviae* *Enterobacter asburiae*	Wild caught flies	L	Wheat bran	Live	Single	10^9 CFU/g			No	[35]
Enterobacter spp.	Wild caught flies	L	Wheat bran	Live/ inactive		10^5, 10^7, 10^9 CFU/g			No	[31]

Abbreviations: Origin (Orig), Stat (Status), Ci (species concentration), Inoc t (inoculation times), Pf col. (Proof of colonization), Ref (references), A (Adult), L (larvae).

Table 1.
Summary of probiotics use in medfly SIT application.

	Adult						Larvae										
	E. agglomernas *K. pneumoniae*	*P. cyppripedi* *C. freundii* *Enterobacter* spp. *K .oxytoca* *Pantoea* spp.	*K. oxytoca N8-S*	*K. oxytoca SmKo*	*Enterobacter AA26*	*Enterobacter* spp. *C. freundii* *K. pneumoniae*		*Enterobacter* spp.		*Enterobacter AA26*		*K. oxytoca*	*M. morganii*	*R. aquatilis*	*L. lactis*	*P. gergoviae*	*E. asburiae*
References	[28]	[2]	[34]	[16]	[30]	[17]	[29]	[35]	[31]	[30]	[32]	[30]			[35]		
Parameters									#		*	#					
Egg to pupae recovery							+				+	—					
Egg to adult recovery							—	+			+	—	+	+	+	+	+
Sex ratio							—	—			—	—					
Egg to pupae development time							+	+			+						
Egg to adult development time							+	—				+					
Larvae development time										+		+					
Pupa stage duration (♀)							+					—					
Pupa stage duration (♂)												+					
Fecundity											—						
Pupal weight						+	—	+	+		+		+	+	+	+	+
Emergence						+			+				+	+	+	+	+
Flight ability						+	—	+	+		—	+	+	+	+	+	+
Morphometric traits						+											
Pheromone calling	—																
Latency time				+													
Remating			+														

	Adult						Larvae									
	E. agglomernas ***K. pneumoniae***	***P. cypripedi*** ***C. freundii*** ***Enterobacter* spp.** ***K .oxytoca*** ***Pantoea* spp.**	***K. oxytoca N8-S***	***K. oxytoca SmKo***	***Enterobacter AA26***	***Enterobacter* spp.** ***C. freundii*** ***K. pneumoniae***		***Enterobacter* spp.**		***Enterobacter AA26***	***K. oxytoca***	***M. morganii***	***R. aquatilis***	***L. lactis***	***P. gergoviae***	***E. asburiae***
Longevity	+/−	+	—				—	+		—	—	+	+	+	+	+
Sexual competitiveness	+/−		+		—		—	+	—	—	—	—	+	+	+	+
Sperm transfer						+										

Abbreviations: (*) inactivated, (#) live and inactivated (+) positive effect, (−) no effect, (+/−) inconsistent findings between diet substrates, field and laboratory.

Table 2.
Summary of the affected parameters after probiotic supplementation to the reared sterile medfly males.

forms such as inactivated (autoclaved suspension) [16, 29–31] or biomass as a replacement for yeast in the diet can be used [32]. Until now, the use has been limited to non-spore-forming bacteria, with the exception of Hamden et al. 2013's work, which used *Citrobacter* sp. of non-host origin. Spores are chemically resistant forms that could be a good candidate as a probiotic, particularly in the medfly larvae diet, which contains acidulants and antimicrobials [33].

Furthermore, Hamden et al. [17] tested the administration of a probiotic mixture, and as previously stated, the strains were of non-host origin, which is one of the agreed-upon selection criteria for a good probiotic candidate. The intervals of administration were also variable across experiments, with adult diet supplementation being frequent [2, 28, 34], whereas larval diet administration is limited to diet preparation, except for Hamden et al. [17].

3.2 Ameliorative effects on medfly colonies productivity and biological quality of sterile males

The initial interest in probiotics for medfly was focused on their use to improve colony productivity and the biological quality of released sterile males, such as longevity, flight ability, and mating competitiveness; however, new areas have been found, such as their effect on stress tolerance, although this requires more scientific development. The following section discusses some functional properties of gut bacteria supplemented as probiotics in medfly feeding. **Table 2** provides an overview of the main results obtained in several studies. There have been several studies in which potential bacterial strains such as *K. oxytoca* and *Enterobacter* sp. have been used to improve the egg to the adult recovery of medfly colonies [29, 32, 35] as well as the biological quality of released sterile males in the laboratory and/or field cages [16, 17, 28, 31, 32, 34, 35]. These studies revealed that the incorporation of gut bacteria in larval or adult artificial diets can positively affect pupal weight [17, 31, 35], adult size [17], survival ability [2, 17, 28, 32, 35], flight ability [17, 30, 35], mating competitiveness [17, 28, 34, 35], and sperm transfer [17].

However, **Table 2** also demonstrates that inconsistencies between results for the same bacterial strain can be found for some parameters, including pupal weight and sexual competitiveness [28, 29, 35]. This might be explained by the methodological setup used in each study. Since experiments are conducted with different medfly strains, isolated bacterial taxa, feeding stages, and lab or field-based applications, the different effects of the bacteria additives on medfly fitness may be explained. Probiotic bacteria have the potential to establish themselves, modify the existing gut microbial community, and play a more discrete role in nutrition and development. Follow-up experiments regarding the localization/quantification of these bacteria after incorporation in larval or adult artificial diets in the medfly's gut during development can provide more insight into how probiotic diets work. More research could enhance mass-rearing even further by upscaling the experimental design, using more replicates and generations, and potentially combining these beneficial isolates (consortium) or testing new bacteria isolated either from the medfly or other insect species. In general, increased pupal and adult productivity, decreased developmental time of the immature stages, and improved fly longevity would result in increased production of insects in shorter periods. This would facilitate mass-rearing of this insect pest species for SIT applications as well as small-scale laboratory rearing required for research.

3.3 Colonization of the probiotics and host origin importance

An effective probiotic should be able to adhere to and colonize the mucus layer of the insect gut [36]. According to **Table 1**, some studies chose to supplement the probiotic daily [17], whereas others only did so once. The initial step in establishing a symbiotic relationship between a microorganism and its host is colonization. Since the ingested food moves from the oral to the anal opening, the digestive tract is exposed to the environment. The term "colonization" can therefore be used for a wide range of associations, ranging from the simple transition of environmental bacteria to the replication, proliferation, and persistence of specific symbionts in the insect gut [37, 38]. The research on *Drosophila* revealed that each strain had a different capacity to reside in the gut following initial colonization [39]. The first day after consuming probiotics, the gut's probiotic levels grew quickly. After ceasing the probiotics, their number in the *Drosophila* intestine dropped and remained at a low level [39]. On the contrary, Lee et al., [40] did not find any differences in the extent of colonization and proliferation in the *Drosophila* gut among the tested bacteria. Successful colonization of the probiotics was demonstrated for medfly by [16, 28, 34]. However, to confirm the presence of *E. agglomerans* and *K. pneumoniae* in the guts of the probiotically treated insects, Niyazi et al., [28] only stated that the later strains were retrieved from the treated males, whereas control flies were found to be largely free of these bacteria (90% of the cases) (**Table 1**). There was no information provided about the isolates' identification procedure. Similarly, Gavriel et al., [34] confirmed that they recovered probiotics (*K. oxytoca* N8-S stereptomycine-resistant strain) from enriched sterile flies even after more than 7 days with no bacteria replacement by comparing bacterial counts on an antibiotic (Sm) treated LB agar and LB agar without antibiotics. However, Ben Ami et al., [16] went further in their explanation of the colonization by comparing the total bacterial count (SmKo strain) from adult guts on chromogenic medium and LB medium containing antibiotics for five consecutive days for the enriched diet and two additional days with a diet devoid of bacteria. Colonization is a fairly complex phenomenon that would also depend on stochastic factors and preexisting populations. The latter reduces the chances of subsequent colonization as was suggested for irradiated males of *B. dorsalis* fed with *K. oxytoca* BD177 [3], thus increasing the stability of the highly-diverse guts [41]. The direct and indirect colonization resistance from the commensal gut microbiota will limit the long-term effect of the probiotic. Indeed, Akami et al., [42], working on *Bactrocera dorsalis*, discovered that axenic flies preferred probiotic diets over symbiotic flies, confirming colonization resistance due to resident microbiota. They hypothesize that the native probiotic isolates were able to recolonize their natural habitat in the axenic flies' guts and revive appetitive behaviors that had been slowed due to bacterial suppression.

The provenance of the strain studied, however, is something we want to highlight here since it is crucial. All of the aforementioned studies used the *Drosophila* model to examine the probiotic human strains. Isolating putative probiotics from the host or environment where the bacteria are intended to exert their beneficial effect, on the other hand, makes more sense. The origin of the host should be considered even if for human purposes this requirement was negated since some strains showed to be effective even if they were of not human origin [43]. Recently, a study used a mixture of non-native and native bacteria for honey bees [44], however, without any proof of persistence in bee guts.

3.4 Isolation and characterization strategies of probiotics for mass-reared *Ceratitis capitata*

The majority of probiotics have thus far been isolated from medfly using the classical methods. Culture-dependent approaches have been used and adjusted to isolate and identify most of the probiotics. In the culture-dependent approach, the culture is using solid media allowing growth of bacteria such as Luria Bertani (LB), tryptic soy agar (TSA) [28], or a chromogenic medium such as CHROMagar orientation [16]. However, the morphological characterization by itself is unresponsive because bacteria's morphological characteristics, such as their color and shape, are not always constant. Further accurate identification approaches have been used such as the 16SrRNA gene amplification and sequencing. To reassemble bacterial colonies in haplotypes while minimizing sequencing, Hamden et al., [35] used the universal primers S-D-Bact-1494-a-20 and L-D-Bact-0035-a-15 to perform DNA amplification of the 16S–23S rRNA internal transcribed spacers region (ITS-PCR) (**Table 3**). While Augustinos et al., [29] combined morphological examination of colonies and RFLP assays, Ben Ami et al., [16] chose amplified rDNA restriction analysis (ARDRA), both techniques are based on restriction enzymes that provide the same digestion pattern.

Probiotics	Isolation	Identification	Reference
Enterobacter agglomerans *Klebsiella oxytoca*	Tryptic soy agar	—	[28]
Pectobacterium cypripedi *Citrobacter freundii* *Enterobacter* spp. *Klebsiella oxytoca* *Pantoea* spp.	—	16S rRNA eubacterial GC-clamp 968F-1401	[2]
Klebsiella oxytoca SmKo	Antibiotic LB medium CHROMagar medium	16S rRNA eubacterial 63F-907R 784F-1401R	[16]
	LB medium	16S rRNA	[17]
Klebsiella oxytoca	LB medium	16S rRNA ubacterial 63F-907R 784F-1401R	[34]
		16S rRNA	[30]
Lactococcus lactis *Rahnella aquatilis* *Pluralibacter gergoviae Klebsiella oxytoca* *Enterobacter* spp. *Enterobacter asburiae*	LB medium	16S–23S rRNA S-D-Bact-1494-a-20 L-D-Bact-0035-a-1	[35]
Enterobacter spp.	LB medium	16S rRNA 27F/1492R	[29]

Table 3.
Isolation and selection approaches of probiotics for medfly mass-rearing.

4. Mechanism of action and selection process of probiotics

Probiotics' mechanisms of action are not fully understood [45]. These mechanisms have been reviewed for humans through *in vitro* and *in vivo* animal models such as *Drosophila* [46, 47]. The effects of probiotics on medfly were studied, but the mechanisms underlying this were not explored. In general, probiotics affect microorganisms through antimicrobial secretion, competitive adhesion to epithelium and mucosa, intestinal epithelial barrier reinforcement, and immune system regulatory impact [48].

The probiotics used in the initial studies were selected from the prevailing population. The effectiveness of the aforementioned probiotic was then confirmed using the quality control criteria, which can be referred to as *in vivo* analyses, that were used to rate the quality of sterile males [1]. None of the studies adopted the basic selection approaches developed for human or aquaculture. The recent study by Hamden et al., [35] was the first to select strains based on specific criteria established in accordance with probiotics selection criteria and SIT requirements. Stress tolerance (tolerance to irradiation), adhesion ability (hydrophobicity, autoaggregation and coaggregation assays (biofilm formation), and antipathogenic activity (Exopolysaccharides production (EPS)) at specific diet incubation temperatures were the minimum criteria for a probiotic strain prior to integration into medfly food for SIT application. It consists of a series of *in vitro* tests that allowed all of the isolated strains to be screened as a first step before being proven *in vivo*. **Table 1** also shows that *Enterobacter* AA26, isolated from the gut of the Vienna 8D53+ genetic sexing strain (GSS), is a promising probiotic for medfly. When this strain was added to the larval diet, it increased the strain's productivity. Azis et al., [49] thoroughly investigated this strain *in vitro* for its biokinetic properties and nutritional values. Indeed, as demonstrated by this strain, a probiotic can be chosen for its functional molecules' secretory abilities, which could provide amino acids, vitamins, and increased α- and β-glucosidase activities.

From a scientific standpoint, the selection criteria for medfly probiotics could be expanded to include immunostimulatory activity, anti-inflammatory activity, and safety assessment [50]. Combined "omics" approaches including genomics, proteomics, transcriptomics, and metabolomics analyses in a novel scientific discipline called "Probiogenomics" [51] could provide a better comprehension and new insights about the selection of the "best" probiotic strain (see Section 5).

5. In silico approaches for probiotics selection

The conventional approaches of validating and selecting new probiotics using *in vitro* and *in vivo* assays are still not yielding robust results. Indeed, the molecular mechanisms through which probiotic microorganisms benefit insect health are, in fact, largely unknown. Thus, in order to fully benefit from probiotics, methodological evolution is required to discover a new potential probiotic. The advancement of sequencing technologies and related bioinformatic techniques enables the development of predictive models tailored to insect rearing conditions for the rational selection of new probiotics. In this context, the complete genome sequencing data of potential probiotic candidates have enabled the development of new effective approaches that serve as the basis for "in silico" screening of metabolic capability prediction and microbial interactions that operate in a microbial community following probiotic treatment [52, 53]. Furthermore, the reproducibility of metagenomics results can enter interpretative variations at many steps of the SIT protocol, including long-term mass-rearing conditions, pupae irradiation, insect diet variability, etc., all of which may map variations in *C. capitata* intestinal microbiota. Such data could be combined with bioinformatics tools to modulate microbial composition within insects on a personalized beneficial population basis. Currently, the taxonomic microbiome characterization as well as the relative abundance of each taxonomic level is increasingly being combined with metagenomics sequencing of 16S rRNA V3-V4 hypervariable regions data through various existing NGS platforms sequencing technologies (pyrosequencing (www.454.com); sequencing-by-synthesis (www.illumina.com); sequencing-by-ligation (www.solid.appliedbiosystems.com); semiconductor sequencing (www.lifetechnologies.com); and nanoball sequencing (www.genomics.cn)). As a result, the taxonomic classification of metagenomic sequencing data of intestinal microbiota as well as diversity studies after probiotic treatment can reveal the probiotic potential parameters of bacteria candidates such as viability after mass-rearing, persistence or transience post-irradiation, capacity for intestinal colonization in the host, and effect on gut community structure [54]. Moreover, the integration of metagenomic data in various software programs (e.g., Prodigal, PICRUST, etc.) and Web-based bioinformatic pipelines (e.g., MicFunPred, available at: http://micfunpred.microdm.net.in/ [55]; Microbiome Analyst, available at: https://www.microbiomeanalyst.ca [56]; Galaxy/Hutlab, available at: https://huttenhower.sph.harvard.edu/galaxy [57]) can be used as a metagenome genes prediction approach to identify the likely functions of the intestinal microbiota before and after probiotic treatment for interpretive variations. Various functional databases, such as the Kyoto Encyclopedia of Genes and Genomes (KEGG) level 1 to 3, Gene Ontology Resource (GO), Clusters of Orthologous Genes (COG), and Carbohydrate Active Enzymes (CAZY), can be used for the identification and functional analysis of genes related to metabolic pathways. For instance, using NGS and bioinformatics platforms to examine changes in the composition and metabolic processes of medfly intestinal microorganisms after probiotic supplementation in the diet of the larval and adult stages serves as a reference for further studies and application of probiotics for SIT improvement.

This approach can be associated to the novel scientific discipline known as "Probiogenomics", which is a combination of "omics" methods using genomics, transcriptomics, metabolomics, and proteomics assays, that has been successfully applied in human health and aquaculture [51–53]. The "omics" assays provide in-depth details of the molecular features related to physiology, functionality, and mechanisms of action of the microorganism [58]. Based on the available whole genome sequence (WGS), "Probiogenomics" approach can be used to gene prediction of probiotic metabolic function [59]. However, there are a number of stressors that the probiotics must deal with during insect mass-rearing, including the composition of the larval and adult diets, irradiation, etc., which can affect their viability and abundance in the insect's digestive system. Consequently, the functional prediction would not be sufficient. Such models can be used not only for discovery and prediction, but also for elucidating the mechanisms of action of potential probiotic microbes on insect health, as well as for accurately identifying probiotics in multistrain mixes and the presence of potential contaminants [60]. Nonetheless, none will replace the need for *in vivo* assessments, which remain the gold standard for probiotic efficacy in the SIT mass-rearing process (**Figure 1**).

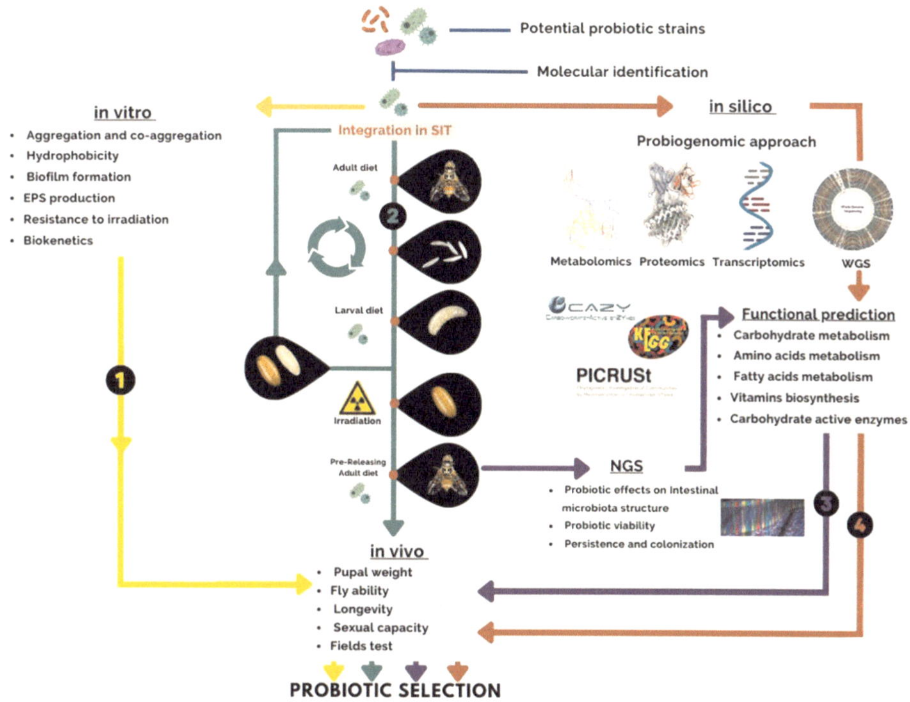

Figure 1.
Probiotics selection strategy for mass-reared Ceratitis capitata *for SIT application. Pathway1: Classical approach using "*in vitro*" and "*in vivo*" assays; Pathway2: Integration of potential probiotic strain into SIT procedures; Pathway3: Probiogenomic approach using different "omics" methods and functional prediction; Pathway4: Probiotic selection using metagenomics analysis and functional prediction of genes related to metabolic pathways.*

6. Probiotics' role in stress mitigation

6.1 Stress related to long-term mass-rearing and irradiation procedures

The biological quality of sterile males can be affected by a variety of significant stressors, including handling, artificial conditions for rearing, and radiation exposure. The ability of male medflies' to fly, attract females, compete for mates, and maintain longevity are all negatively impacted by sterilizing irradiation techniques used for SIT, which are also a significant source of microbiome perturbation [16, 61]. As a result, more focus has been placed on evaluating the impact of irradiation on the survival and mating abilities of the medfly sterile males in order to identify and pinpoint the primary drawbacks of these treatments. The changes in the diversity of the gut microbiota and the decline in the physical quality of sterile males are related. According to Ben-Ami et al. [16], industrial strains exhibit an increase in potentially pathogenic species like *Pseudomonas* and *Providencia*, which are known to harm insects, while levels of dominant gut bacteria (such as *Klebsiella* spp.) decrease after sterilization. It is interesting to note that adding *K. oxytoca* to the post-irradiation diet promotes colonization of these bacteria in the gut while lowering *Pseudomonas* spp. levels. The same authors, Ben Ami et al. [16], indicate that copulatory success tests show that the addition of these bacteria to male diets significantly improved sterile male performance. Similarly, a probiotic adult diet enriched with *E. agglomerans* and

K. pneumonia significantly improved the gut environment of medflies whose alimentary canal had been damaged by the radiation used in the sterilization process of medfly [61]. A more recent study on the effect of irradiation on medfly immunity discovered that molecular changes occur at different time points via regulation of stress and immunity genes such as *Hsp* 70, *Hsp* 83, *cecropin*, *attacin*, and *PGPR*. The expression of *attacin* and *PGPR-LC* was increased, whereas *cecropin* was decreased. *Hsp* genes, on the other hand, showed decreased levels between 0 and 18 h, peaking at 72 h. Only the *attacin* was induced after supplementation with the probiotic *Enterobacter* sp. [35].

6.2 Environmental stress

Along with the increase in agrochemicals, climate change and modifications in land use can all lead to unfavorable stress conditions for sterile males in agroecosystems. Sterile males are regularly exposed to unfavorable environments, including cold, heat, ultraviolet stress, lack of food resources, insecticide exposure, parasites, and infectious diseases or pathogens. Stress conditions can impair sterile males, physiology, biochemistry, and gene regulation, as well as the interaction between medfly and microorganisms, which lowers male performances. Given the range of beneficial functions provided by microbiota, it may also shape the ability of hosts to tolerate environmental stress [62]. Beneficial bacteria can help sterile males maintain their inherent resistance to these challenges; thus, adding these bacteria to the medfly diet can help reduce the negative impact of environmental stress conditions on sterile males. However, novel approaches are needed to explore medfly–bacteria and bacteria–bacteria interactions under abiotic and biotic stress conditions to identify potential stress-tolerant or -resistant bacteria to improve medfly performance.

6.2.1 Temperature tolerance

Among multiple stress factors, the temperature has profound effects on the physiology, behavior, and performance of insects [63]. There is evidence supporting that the ongoing climate change is expected to impose strong selection pressures on the heat tolerance of insects [64], and that gut microbiota can contribute to host thermal tolerance [65–67]. Alteration of energy reserves, metabolism, or gene expression by microbiota may indirectly affect thermal tolerance, which strongly depends on these traits [68]. Since the global surface annual temperature has increased at an average rate of 0.1°C, almost double compared to 20 years ago, and increases of 1.5°C and 2–4°C are expected by 2050 and 2100, respectively [69], rising temperatures can severely affect an AW-IPM program because temperature changes can influence the longevity, flight ability, and mating performance of sterile males. An elevated temperature could lead to the death of sterile males released during SIT [70]. Numerous studies have recently suggested that the gut microbiota is sensitive to environmental temperature, which induces changes in its composition and diversity, and may have significant consequences on host phenotype and fitness [71–73]. For instance, it has been shown that *K. michiganensis* was implicated in promoting insect resistance to long-term low-temperature stress in the tephritid fly *B. dorsalis*. The mechanisms by which gut symbionts modulate host physiologies and the molecules involved in these changes have been reported as follows: Gut symbionts, particularly *K. michiganensis*, help the host *B. dorsalis* upregulate the levels of "cryoprotectant" transcripts and metabolites, which increases its resistance to long-term low-temperature stress by stimulating the host arginine and proline metabolism pathway [74]. It has also been noted in *Drosophila melanogaster*, the disruption of its gut microbiota leads to decreased cold tolerance [75] that can be rescued by supplementing a single member of its natural microbiota, the yeast *Lachancea kluyveri*. Similarly, increases in temperature have been associated with increased relative abundances of *Proteobacteria*. Developmental temperature has been shown to impact the composition of the gut microbiota of fruit flies, with higher temperatures (31°C) leading to increased abundances of *Acetobacter*, a genus of *Proteobacteria*, relative to lower temperatures (13°C) [76]. Additionally, in aphid, obligatory endosymbionts contribute to host performance at high temperatures [77, 78], whereas facultative endosymbionts also confer tolerance to high temperature in aphids [79, 80] and *Drosophila* [81]. Although *C. capitata's* acute tolerance of extreme temperatures, under ecologically relevant conditions, and the relative costs and benefits of acclimation have attracted significant attention [82–87], little is known about how microbial symbionts affect medfly sensitivity to toxins, desiccation resistance, and thermal tolerance.

Medflies are exposed to a variety of environmental stresses in the wild. The wild flies seem to be remarkably temperature-variation resistant [83, 84]. Even if this is true, it does not follow that laboratory sterile medfly males will be the same once released. The performance of released sterile males could be improved by enhancing their phenotypic characteristics with probiotic bacteria that confer thermal tolerance. This might be a simple and affordable way to improve the effectiveness of an SIT program. The role of the gut microbiota in the adaptive response to climate change is a new area of study, and future research must balance mechanistic approaches to understand host-microbiota interactions with holistic approaches to understanding the role of the gut microbiota in insect ecology and evolution.

6.2.2 Pesticides tolerance

The management of *C. capitata* is currently based on the implementation of an integrated pest management (IPM) program that employs a variety of techniques, including insecticides [88, 89], mass trapping [90], the sterile insect technique [91, 92], and also biological control using parasitoids [93]. However, the area under IPM includes a large number of cultivated plant species that are attacked by other pests [94]. Pesticides are usually used when these pests exceed their economic thresholds. The compatibility of the existing programs will be determined by the interaction between SIT and other pest management strategies when SIT is used [95]. The impact of pesticides and their residues on sterile Vienna-8 males has been investigated in citrus-integrated pest management. San Andrés et al., [96] observed high mortality of sterile Vienna-8 males on proteinaceous malathion and spinosad baits under laboratory conditions. Additionally, Juan-Blasco et al., [97] showed that both chlorpyrifos and spinosad formulations at authorized concentrations against other citrus pests were toxic by contact with Vienna-8 males, resulting in significant mortality. Pesticides have deleterious effects on Vienna-8 males. Thus, a solution is needed to limit these off-target effects. Naturally, reducing pesticide use would expose Vienna-8 males to fewer pesticides, but this solution may reduce crop yield and burden the food supply. The use of alternative, non-chemical control methods, particularly against serious pests, is another suggestion. However, these approaches are subject to the legislative process and competing interests and do not give growers the ability to address the pesticide issue on their own.

According to recent findings, the insect-associated microbial community, that is exposed to pesticides, as a source of selection pressure, may help the host metabolize these substances by enhancing enzyme activity through a wide range of metabolic pathways able to break down and/or modify xenobiotics [98–100]. It might also act as a source of variation, which would make the host less vulnerable to pesticides [101]. In some model organisms, it has been demonstrated that administering bacteria as probiotics lowers toxicity and has protective effects on the host. Future studies can use this foundation to explore the possibility of enhancing SIT to control medfly [102–104]. It might be a novel idea to include probiotics in the diet of sterile medfly males to lessen the effects of pesticides. Recently, some authors have drawn attention to the capacity of bacteria, such as lactic acid bacteria, to be developed into probiotic products capable of reducing the oxidative damage brought on by pesticides *in vivo* [105, 106]. These authors also emphasized how bacterial strains differ in their resistance to organophosphorus pesticides and their capacity to degrade them [107].

Pesticide-degrading bacteria are common in nature and have been found in a variety of insect orders, including Lepidoptera [108, 109], Hemiptera [110], Diptera [18, 111], and Coleoptera [101]. The surface communities of the Tephritid fruit fly *Rhagoletis pomonella* contained the first bacteria with this characteristic to be identified [112] (**Table 4**). It has been demonstrated that this bacterial symbiont degrades up to six different insecticides from three major groups (chlorinated hydrocarbons, organophosphates, and carbamates). Since then, evidence has shown that various other bacterial microbiota, such as those in the guts of herbivores, are capable of degrading insecticides [113]. For instance, it was found that in *Bactrocera tau*, bacteria were involved in the degradation of the toxic substances the host insect ingested, leading to insecticide resistance [111]. *Bactrocera dorsalis*, an oriental fruit fly, detoxifies trichloroethylene as another fascinating example of symbiont-mediated detoxification in Tephritid fruit flies [18]. The findings of this study showed that a bacterium

Pesticides families	Pesticides name	Gut microbiota	Tephritidae pests	References
Carbamate	Carbaryl	*Pseudomonas melophthora*	*Rhagoletis pomonella*	[12]
Organochloride	Dieldrin	*Pseudomonas melophthora*	*Rhagoletis pomonella*	[12]
	Endosulfan	*Klebsiella oxytoca, Pantoea agglomerans, and Staphylococcus* sp.	*Bactrocera tau*	[111]
Organophosphate	Dichlorovos, Diazinon, Parathion, Diisopropyl phosphorofluoridate	*Pseudomonas melophthora*	*Rhagoletis pomonella*	[12]
	Malathion	*Klebsiella oxytoca, Pantoea agglomerans, and Staphylococcus* sp	*Bactrocera tau*	[111]
	Trichlorphon	*Citrobacter freundii*	*Bactrocera dorsalis*	[17]
Neonicotinoid	*Imidacloprid*	*Pantoea agglomerans, Staphylococcus* sp	*Bactrocera tau*	[111]

Table 4.
List of tephritidae gut microbiota involved in pesticide degradation.

called *Citrobacter freundii*, isolated from the gut of the *B. dorsalis*, can break down the toxin trichlorphon into less toxic compounds called chloral hydrate and dimethyl phosphite, possibly by activating genes called organophosphorus hydrolase (OPH-like) genes and conferring host resistance in the oriental fruit fly [18]. Higher trichlorphon resistance was seen when isolated *Citrobacter* species were inoculated with *B. dorsalis*, whereas flies treated with antibiotics exhibited lower resistance. Based on this evidence, it is possible to reduce pesticide uptake and increase pathogen resistance by supplementing the diet of larval and adult sterile medfly males with suitable bacteria that degrade insecticide (multiple strains or single strain). This would reduce the sublethal effects of pesticides. The ability to supplement sterile medfly males with probiotics could aid the insects in combating the unintended pernicious effects and improving the SIT application while chemical agents are still being used in agriculture.

7. Safety and efficacy of probiotics

7.1 Safety considerations

Probiotics formulated for use in mass-rearing facilities have been shown to be beneficial due to their ability to improve a multitude of parameters and contribute to the restoration of dysbiosis in the medfly digestive tract. The probiotics selected so far are exclusively from the family of Enterobacteriaceae, and they are the cause of enteric human diseases that can lead to illness and death [114]. The use of Enterobacteriaceae in medfly mass-rearing procedures is still under experimentation; researchers have not yet addressed the issue of handler safety and environmental risk in general. The use of the probiotic in the larval rearing medium at the rearing facility and the administration of the probiotic to the adult sterile males intended for release are the two processes to be considered for safety issues. In the first case, it has long been recognized that facility workers can become infected by the agents they manipulate, thus making the nature of their work an occupational hazard. In the second case, introducing pathogenic bacteria into the adult diet allows bacteria to be transmitted horizontally to the environment. Implementing biosecurity procedures in rearing units, such as daily decontamination of all surfaces and equipment with specific disinfectants and limiting ventilation inside production modules, is difficult and will incur additional costs. However, it is clear that an increasing number of experiments are based on the use of the inactivated form of the probiotic, which is prebiotic, which appears to be less complicated to handle and yields comparable results [29, 31, 35].

7.2 Microencapsulation of probiotics for medfly mass-rearing

Acidulants are present in the mass-rearing medfly larval diet and play an important role in preventing microorganism growth, buffering diets, decreasing diet rancidity, and modifying the viscosity and consistency of the diet [115]. The pH of the larval diet is adjusted to 3.5–4.5 in insectaries. Acid stress inhibits bacterial proliferation and changes the phenotypes and morphology of bacterial cells in the medfly diet as a result [116, 117]. This is not in the probiotic's favor because it will be subjected to pre-ingestion stress, reducing its stability and effectiveness. Encapsulation will stabilize the probiotics during processing, storage, and the site of action to safeguard them in the medfly diets. Given that edible polymers can be used as coating materials to provide a protective environment for the long-term viability of microorganisms, encapsulation is a successful food industry technique [118]. The polymer systems used to encapsulate probiotics are alginate, carrageenan, gelatin, chitosan, cellulose acetate phthalate, locust bean gum, modified starch, chitosan, gellan, xanthan, gum arabic, and animal proteins [119].

Probiotic encapsulation in mass-rearing is a new and unexplored area. Remarkably, some research has suggested that entomopathogenic bacteria be microencapsulated for pest control. Due to its low residual activity in the field, the most notable example is the microencapsulation of *Bacillus thuringiensis* (B.t.) with arabic gum, gelatin, and chitosan against some Coleoptera, Lepidoptera, and Hemiptera at larval and adult stages. Laboratory tests on *Trichoplusia ni* larvae (Lepidoptera: Noctuidae) revealed that the microencapsulation process had no effect on B. t. bioactivity. After 12 days, the mean number of larvae in microencapsulated formulations in colloidosomal microparticles (50 mm) was significantly lower than in a commercial B. t. formulation, and the effect of microencapsulated formulations was comparable to that of a chemical pesticide (lambda-cyhalothrin) [120]. The spray dryer produced a particle size of 32 nm against *Helicoverpa armigera* (Lepidoptera: Noctuidae) larvae damaging cotton, and the results show that even low doses of this encapsulation significantly reduced the larval population [121]. These and other experiments show promise for the use of microencapsulation to ensure the stability of probiotics throughout the medfly rearing process while paying attention to functionality, which is impaired in some experiments [122].

8. Waste conversion in mass-rearing facilities

The most common insect for which the sterile insect technique has been used is *Ceratitis*. Following that, a large number of mass-rearing facilities were established around the world. Mexico and Guatemala have facilities that rear over 1.5 billion medflies per week. The most important factor in mass-rearing is diet. Each mass-rearing facility generates a large amount of waste on a daily basis, the majority of which comes from the remaining rearing diet that does not respond to increasing requirements for economic efficiency and environmental standards [123], combined with global warming. At the El Piño biofactory in Guatemala, 31 tons of larval diet per day are produced [124]. Waste recycling initiatives are not published even if they exist. It is obvious that this waste is autoclaved before being used in order to eliminate any stage of the pest. Mastrangelo et al., (2009) [124] stated after conducting analyses on medfly diet that it has the potential as an alternative ruminant feedstuff. Likewise, Sayed et al., [125] showed that this diet is a potential feed ingredient for the production of BSF pre-pupae and could be applied to valorize this rearing waste into high-value feed.

The conversion of waste, such as agricultural by-products and food preparation wastes, into novel animal feeds, has received a lot of attention. The addition of exogenous probiotics is a promising strategy that enhances the biotransformation of food wastes [126], water treatment [127], and compost production [128]. The probiotics were shown to exert a positive effect through the extracellular enzyme secretions to break down carbohydrates, proteins, and fats into micronutrients in the waste that is transformed into feed [126]. Consequently, the probiotics added to the medfly larvae diet in the rearing facilities could improve the degradation of the diet and its use as feed for livestock after the larvae have left the medium. Probiotics may also reduce antinutritional compounds and lignocellulose from the finisher diet bran, which is used as a substrate [129], and inhibit endogenous pathogens [130]. Therefore, WHO specifies that converted products for the animal feed chain should not be degraded or contaminated while maintaining an acceptable nutritional value [131].

9. Conclusion

The introduction of probiotics into the insect industry and their mass-rearing could be game changers. Insect farming is useful for biocontrol, such as the sterile insect technique, but it is also useful for edible insects. Probiotics used in mass-rearing can provide enormous benefits by increasing production quality and quantity. However, when using them, certain security aspects must be considered. We believe that the proposed schemes for probiotic selection in medfly rearing are well suited to all insects mass-reared for SIT application and can be adapted for other types of rearing and modified according to the specificity of the insect in question. However, the global approach incorporating new OMICs techniques is applicable to all types of insect farming and can provide answers to all of the interactions that the selected probiotic will have with the host microbiota.

Funding information

This study was supported by Grant 1: PRF2019-D6P2 and Grant 2 PRIMA2019/INTOMED under the Ministry of higher education and scientific research, Tunisia.

Conflict of interest

"The authors declare no conflict of interest."

Author details

Meriem Msaad Guerfali[1*], Haytham Hamden[1], Kamel Charaabi[1], Salma Fadhl[1], Amor Mosbah[2] and Amer Cherif[2]

1 Laboratory of Biotechnology and Nuclear Techniques LRCNSTN01, National Centre of Nuclear Sciences and Technologies, Ariana, Tunisia

2 Laboratory of Biology and Bio-Geo Resources LR11ES31, Higher Institute of Biotechnology of Sidi Thabet, University of Manouba, Ariana, Tunisia

*Address all correspondence to: msaad_tn@yahoo.fr

References

[1] FAO/IAEA/USDA. Product Quality Control for Sterile Mass-Reared and Released Tephritid Fruit Flies. Vienna, Austria: International Atomic Energy Agency; 2019. p. 148

[2] Behar A, Yuval B, Jurkevitch E. Gut bacterial communities in the Mediterranean fruit fly (*Ceratitis capitata*) and their impact on host longevity. Journal of Insect Physiology. 2008;**54**:1377-1383. DOI: 10.1016/j.jinsphys.2008. 07.011

[3] Cai P, Hong J, Wang C, Yang Y, Yi C, Chen J, et al. Effects of Co-60 radiation on the activities of three main antioxidant enzymes in *Bactrocera dorsalis* (Hendel) (Diptera: Tephritidae). Journal of Asia-Pacific Entomology. 2018;**21**(1):345-351. DOI: 10.1016/j.aspen.2018.01.006

[4] Ben-Yosef M, Jurkevitch E, Yuval B. Effect of bacteria on nutritional status and reproductive success of the Mediterranean fruit fly *Ceratitis capitata*. Physiological Entomology. 2008;**33**: 145-154. DOI: 10.1111/j.1365-3032.2008.00617.x

[5] Marchini D, Rosetto M, Dallai R, Marri L. Bacteria associated with the oesophageal bulb of the medfly *Ceratitis capitata* (Diptera:Tephritidae). Current Microbiology. 2002;**44**:120-1240. DOI: 10.1007/s00284-001-0061-1

[6] McFarland LV. From yaks to yogurt: The history, development, and current use of probiotics. Clinical Infectious Diseases. 2015;**60**(2):85-90. DOI: 10.1093/cid/civ054

[7] Dunne C, Murphy L, Flynn S, O'Mahony L, O'Halloran S, Feeney M, et al. Probiotics: From myth to reality. Demonstration of functionality in animal models of disease and in human clinical trials. Antonie Van Leeuwenhoek. 1999; **76**(1–4):279-292. DOI: 10.1093/ajcn/73.2.386s

[8] Kozasa M. Toyocerin (*Bacillus toyoi*) as growth promoter for animal feeding. Microbiologie, Aliments, Nutrition. 1986;**4**:121-135

[9] Lakshmi B, Viswanath B, Sai Gopal DV. Probiotics as antiviral agents in shrimp aquaculture. Journal of Pathogens. 2013;**2013**:424123

[10] Máchová M, Rada V, Huk J, Smékal F. Development of probiotics for bees. Apiacta. 1997;**4**:99-111

[11] Audisio MC. Gram-positive Bacteria with probiotic potential for the *Apis mellifera* L. honey bee: The experience in the northwest of Argentina. Probiotics and antimicrobial. Proteins. 2017;**9**: 22-31. DOI: 10.1007/s12602-016-9231-0

[12] Lauzon CR, Sjogren RE, Prokopy RJ. Enzymatic capabilities of bacteria associated with apple maggot flies: A postulated role in attraction. Journal of Chemical Ecology. 2000;**26**:953-967. DOI: 10.1023/A:1005460225664

[13] Kuzina LV, Peloquin JJ, Vacek DC, Miller TA. Isolation and identification of bacteria associated with adult laboratory Mexican fruit flies, *Anastrepha ludens* (Diptera: Tephritidae). Current Microbiology. 2001;**42**:290-294. DOI: 10.1007/s002840110219

[14] Behar A, Ben-Yosef M, Lauzon CR, Yuval B, Jurkevich E. Structure and function of the bacterial community associated with the Mediterranean fruit fly. In: Bourtzis K, Miller T, editors. Insect Symbiosis. Vol. 3. Boca Raton: CRC Press; 2009. pp. 251-271

[15] Saha P, Ray RR. Production of polysaccharide degrading enzymes by the gut microbiota of *Leucinodes Orbonalis* and *Bactrocera dorsalis*. Journal of Entomology and Zoology Studies. 2015;**3**:122-125

[16] Ben Ami E, Yuval B, Jurkevitch E. Manipulation of the microbiota of mass-reared Mediterranean fruit flies Ceratitis capitata (Diptera: Tephritidae) improves sterile male sexual performance. The ISME Journal. 2010;**4**:28-37. DOI: 10.1038/ismej.2009.82

[17] Hamden H, M'saad Guerfali M, Fadhl S, Saidi M, Chevrier C. Fitness improvement of mass-reared sterile males of *Ceratitis capitata* (Vienna 8 strain) (Diptera: Tephritidae) after gut enrichment with probiotics. Journal of Economic Entomology. 2013;**106**: 641-647. DOI: 10.1603/EC12362

[18] Cheng DF, Guo ZJ, Riegler M, Xi ZY, Liang GW, Xu YJ. Gut symbiont enhances insecticide resistance in a significant pest, the oriental fruit fly *Bactrocera dorsalis* (Hendel). Microbiome. 2017;**5**(1):13. DOI: 10.1186/s40168-017-0236-z

[19] Sacchetti P, Ghiardi B, Granchietti A, Stefanini F, Belcari A. Development of probiotic diets for the olive fly: Evaluation of their effects on fly longevity and fecundity. Annals of Applied Biology. 2017;**164**:138-150. DOI: 10.1111/aab.12088

[20] Bel Mokhtar N, Catalá-Oltra M, Stathopoulou P, Asimakis E, Remmal I, Remmas N, et al. Dynamics of the gut Bacteriome during a laboratory adaptation process of the Mediterranean fruit Fly, *Ceratitis capitata*. Frontiers in Microbiology. 2022;**13**:919760. DOI: 10.3389/fmicb.2022.919760

[21] McInnis D, Lance D, Jackson C. Behavioral resistance to the sterile insect technique by Mediterranean fruit fly (Diptera: Tephritidae) in Hawaii. Annals of the Entomological Society of America. 1996;**89**:739-744

[22] Rendon P, McInnis D, Lance D, Stewart J. Medfly (Diptera: Tephritidae) genetic sexing: Large-scale field comparison of males-only and bisexual sterile fly releases in Guatemala. Journal of Economic Entomology. 2004;**97**: 1547-1553. DOI: 10.1603/0022-0493-97.5.1547

[23] Virginio JF, Gòmez M, Pinto AM, Aniely GG, Paranhois BJ, Gava CAT, et al. Male sexual competitiveness of two *Ceratitis capitata* strains, tsl Vienna 8 and OX3864A transgenics, in field cage conditions. Entomologia Experimentalis Et Applicata. 2017;**164**(3):318-326. DOI: 10.1111/cea.12615

[24] Schrezenmeir J, de Vrese M. Probiotics, prebiotics, and synbiotics-approaching a definition. The American Journal of Clinical Nutrition. 2001;**73**(2): 361-364. DOI: 10.1093/ajcn/73.2.361s

[25] Lilly DM, Stillwell RH. Probiotics. Growth-promoting factors produced by microorganisms. Science. 1965;**147**: 747-748. DOI: 10.1093/ajcn/73.2.361s

[26] World Health Organization. Food and Agriculture Organization of the United Nations Probiotics in Food, Health Nutritional Proprieties and Guidelines for Evaluation. Geneva, Switzerland: FAO/WHO; 2016

[27] Markowiak P, Śliżewska K. Effects of probiotics, prebiotics, and Synbiotics on human health. Nutrients. 2017;**9**(9): 1021. DOI: 10.3390/nu9091021

[28] Niyazi N, Lauzon CR, Shelly TE. The effect of probiotic adult diet on fitness

components of sterile male Mediterranean fruit flies (Diptera: Tephritidae) under laboratory and field conditions. Journal of Economic Entomology. 2004;**97**:1581-1586. DOI: 10.1371/journal.pone.0136459

[29] Augustinos AA, Kyritsis GA, Papadopoulos NT, Abd-Alla AMM, Cáceres C, Bourtzis K. Exploitation of the medfly gut microbiota for the enhancement of sterile insect technique: Use of *Enterobacter* sp. Larval Diet-Based Probiotic Applications. PLoS ONE. 2015; **10**(9):e0136459. DOI: 10.1371/journal.pone.0136459

[30] Kyritsis GA, Augustinos AA, Cáceres C, Bourtzis K. Medfly gut microbiota and enhancement of the sterile insect technique: Similarities and differences of *Klebsiella oxytoca* and *Enterobacter sp*. AA26 probiotics during the larval and adult stages of the VIENNA 8D53+ genetic sexing strain. Frontiers in Microbiology. 2017;**8**:2064. DOI: 10.3389/fmicb.2017.02064

[31] Msaad Guerfali M, Charaabi K, Hamden H, Djobbi W, Fadhl S, Mosbah A, et al. Probiotic based-diet effect on the immune response and induced stress in irradiated mass reared *Ceratitis capitata* males (Diptera: Tephritidae) destined for the release in the sterile insect technique programs. Plos One. 2012;**16**(9):e0257097. DOI: 10.1371/journal.pone.0257097

[32] Kyritsis GA, Augustinos AA, Ntougias S, Papadopoulos N, Bourtzis K, Caceres C, et al. AA26 gut symbiont as a protein source for Mediterranean fruit fly mass-rearing and sterile insect technique applications. BMC Microbiology. 2019;**19**(1):288. DOI: 10.1186/s12866-019-1651-z

[33] Tanaka N, Steiner LF, Ohinata K, Okamoto R. Low-cost larval rearing medium for mass production of oriental and Mediterranean fruit flies. Journal of Economic Entomology. 1969;**62**(4): 967-968. DOI: 10.1093/jee/62.4.967

[34] Gavriel S, Jurkevitch E, Gazit Y, Yuval B. Bacterially enriched diet improves sexual performance of sterile male Mediterranean fruit flies. Journal of Applied Entomology. 2011;**135**:564-573. DOI: 10.1111/j.14390418.2010.01605.x

[35] Hamden H, Guerfali MM, Charaabi K, Djobbi W, Fadhl S, Mahjoubi M, et al. Screening and selection of potential probiotic strains from the Mediterranean fruit fly (*Ceratitis capitata*) guts origin based on SIT application. Journal of Radiation Research and Applied Science. 2020; **13**(1):776-791. DOI: 10.1080/16878507.2020.1848010

[36] Vine NG, Leukes WD, Kaiser H. Probiotics in marine larviculture. FEMS Microbiology Reviews. 2006;**30**(3): 404-427. DOI: 10.1111/j.1574-6976.2006.00017.x

[37] Leftwich Philip T, Edgington Matthew P. Chapman Tracey. Transmission efficiency drives host-microbe associations. Proceedings of the Royal Society B: Biological Sciences. 2020;**287**:20200820. DOI: 10.1098/rspb.2020.0820

[38] Schmidt K, Engel P. Mechanisms underlying gut microbiota-host interactions in insects. Journal of Experimental Biology. 2021;**224**: jeb207696. DOI: 10.1242/jeb.207696

[39] Laomongkholchaisri P, Teanpaisan R, Wonglapsuwan M, Piwat S. Impact of potential probiotic *Lactobacillus* strains on host growth and development in a *Drosophila melanogaster* model. Probiotics

Antimicrobial Proteins. 2021;**13**:390-397. DOI: 10.1007/s12602-020-09705-z

[40] Lee HY, Lee SH, Lee JH, Lee WJ, Min KJ. The role of commensal microbes in the lifespan of *Drosophila melanogaster*. Aging (Albany NY). 2019; **11**(13):4611-4640. DOI: 10.18632/aging.102073

[41] Benjamin Obadia ZT, Güvener VZ, Ceja-Navarro JA, Brodie EL, Ja WW, Ludington WB. Current Biology. 2017; **27**(13):1999-2006. DOI: 10.1016/j.cub.2017.05.034

[42] Akami M, Ren X, Wang Y, Mansour A, Cao S, Qi X, et al. Host fruits shape the changes in the gut microbiota and development of *Bactrocera dorsalis* (Diptera: Tephritidae) larvae. International journal of tropical insect. Science. 2022:1-15. DOI: 10.1007/s42690-022-00733-66

[43] Sanders ME, Merenstein D, Merrifield CA, Hutkins R. Probiotics for human use. Nutrition Bulletin. 2018;**43**: 212-225. DOI: 10.1111/nbu.12334

[44] Chmiel JA, Pitek AP, Burton JP, Thompson GJ, Reid G. Meta-analysis on the effect of bacterial interventions on honey bee productivity and the treatment of infection. Apidologie. 2021; **52**:960-972. DOI: 10.1007/s13592-021-00879-1

[45] Vieira AT, Fukumori C, Ferreira CM. New insights into therapeutic strategies for gut microbiota modulation in inflammatory diseases. Clinical and Translational Immunology. 2016;**5**:e87. DOI: 10.1038/cti.2016.38

[46] Westfall S, Lomis N, Prakash S. Longevity extension in *Drosophila* through gut-brain communication. Scientific Reports. 2018;**8**:8362. DOI: 10.1038/s41598-018-25382-z

[47] Milner E, Stevens B, An M, Lam V, Ainsworth M, Dihle P, et al. Utilizing probiotics for the prevention and treatment of gastrointestinal diseases. Frontiers in Microbiology. 2021;**9**(12): 689958. DOI: 10.3389/fmicb.2021.689958

[48] Bermudez-Brito M, Plaza-Díaz J, Muñoz-Quezada S, Gómez-Llorente C, Gil A. Probiotic mechanisms of action. Annals of Nutrition & Metabolism. 2012; **61**:160-174. DOI: 10.1159/000342079

[49] Azis K, Zerva I, Melidis P, Caceres C, Bourtzis K, Ntougias S. Biochemical and nutritional characterization of the medfly gut symbiont *Enterobacter* sp. AA26 for its use as probiotics in sterile insect technique applications. BMC Biotechnology. 2019;**18**(19):90. DOI: 10.1186/s12896-019-0584-9

[50] De Melo Pereira GV, de Oliveira CB, Magalhães Júnior AI, Thomaz-Soccol V, Soccol CR. How to select a probiotic? A review and update of methods and criteria. Biotechnology Advances. 2018; **36**(8):2060-2076. DOI: 10.1016/j.biotechadv.2018.09.003

[51] Castro-Lopez C, Garcia HS, Martinez-Avila GCG, Gonzalez-Cordova AF, Vallejo-Cordoba B, Hernandez-Mendoza A. Genomics-based approaches to identify and predict the health-promoting and safety activities of promising probiotic strains–a probiogenomics review. Trends in Food Science and Technology. 2021;**108**: 148-163. DOI: 10.1016/j.tifs.2020.12.017

[52] Fang Z, Lu W, Zhao J, Zhang H, Qian L, Wang Q, et al. Probiotics modulate the gut microbiota composition and immune responses in patients with atopic dermatitis: A pilot study. European Journal of Nutrition.

2020;**59**(5):2119-2130. DOI: 10.1007/s00394-019-02061-x

[53] Devika NT, Jangam AK, Katneni VK, Patil PK, Nathamuni S, Shekhar MS. In silico prediction of novel probiotic species limiting pathogenic vibrio growth using constraint-based genome scale metabolic modeling. Frontiers in Cellular and Infection Microbiology. 2021;**2021**:11. DOI: 10.3389/fcimb.2021.752477

[54] Zhang Q, Wang S, Zhang X, Zhang K, Li Y, Yin Y, et al. Beneficial Bacteria in the intestines of housefly larvae promote larval development and humoral Phenoloxidase activity. While Harmful Bacteria do the Opposite. Frontiers in Immunology. 2022;**13**: 938972. DOI: 10.3389/fimmu.2022.938972

[55] Mongad DS, Chavan NS, Narwade NP, Dixit K, Shouche YS, Dhotre DP. MicFunPred: A conserved approach to predict functional profiles from 16S rRNA gene sequence data. Genomics. 2021;**113**(6):3635-3643. DOI: 10.1016/j.ygeno.2021.08.016

[56] Chong J, Liu P, Zhou G, Xia J. Using MicrobiomeAnalyst for comprehensive statistical, functional, and meta-analysis of microbiome data. Nature Protocols. 2020;**15**(3):799-821. DOI: 10.1038/s41596-019-0264-1

[57] Afgan E, Baker D, Batut B, Van den Beek M, Bouvier D, Čech M, et al. The galaxy platform for accessible, reproducible and collaborative biomedical analyses: 2018 update. Nucleic Acids Research. 2018;**46**(W1): 537-544. DOI: 10.1093/nar/gky379

[58] Yadav R, Kumar V, Baweja M, Shukla P. Gene editing and genetic engineering approaches for advanced probiotics: A review. Critical Reviews in Food Science and Nutrition. 2018;**58**(10):1735-1746. DOI: 10.1080/10408398.2016.1274877

[59] Lugli GA, Longhi G, Alessandri G, Mancabelli L, Tarracchini C, Fontana F, et al. The Probiotic Identity Card: A Novel "Probiogenomics" Approach to Investigate Probiotic Supplements. Frontiers in Microbiology. 2021;**2021**:12. DOI: 10.3389/fmicb.2021.790881

[60] Patro JN, Ramachandran P, Barnaba T, Mammel MK, Lewis JL, Elkins CA. Culture independent metagenomic surveillance of commercially available probiotics with high throughput next-generation sequencing. mSphere. 2016;**1**(2):e00057-e00016. DOI: 10.1128/mSphere.00057-16

[61] Lauzon CR, Potter S. Description of the irradiated and nonirradiated midgut of *Ceratitis capitata* Wiedemann (Diptera: Tephritidae) and *Anastrepha ludens* Loew (Diptera: Tephritidae) used for sterile insect technique. Journal of Pesticide Science. 2012;**85**(2):217-226. DOI: 10.1007/s10340-011-0410-1

[62] Soen Y. Environmental disruption of host–microbe co-adaptation as a potential driving force in evolution. Frontiers in Genetics. 2014;**5**:168. DOI: 10.3389/fgene.2014.00168

[63] Angilletta MJ Jr. Looking for answers to questions about heat stress: Researchers are getting warmer. Functional Ecology. 2009;**23**(2):231-232. DOI: 10.1111/j.1365-2435.2009.01548.x

[64] Hoffmann AA, Sgrò CM. Climate change and evolutionary adaptation. Nature. 2011;**470**(7335):479-485. DOI: 10.1038/nature09670

[65] Kokou F, Sasson G, Nitzan T, Doron-Faigenboim A, Harpaz S, Cnaani A, et al. Host genetic selection for

cold tolerance shapes microbiome composition and modulates its response to temperature. eLife. 2018;**7**:e36398

[66] Renoz F, Pons I, Hance T. Evolutionary responses of mutualistic insect–bacterial symbioses in a world of fluctuating temperatures. Current Opinion in Insect Science. 2019;**35**:20-26. DOI: 10.1016/j.cois.2019.06.006

[67] Sepulveda J, Moeller AH. The effects of temperature on animal gut microbiomes. Frontiers in Microbiology. 2020;**11**:384. DOI: 10.3389/fmicb.2020.00384

[68] Teets NM, Denlinger DL. Physiological mechanisms of seasonal and rapid cold-hardening in insects. Physiological Entomology. 2013;**38**(2):105-116. DOI: 10.1111/phen.12019

[69] Pörtner HO, Roberts DC, Adams H, Adler C, Aldunce P, Ali E, et al. Climate Change 2022: Impacts, Adaptation and Vulnerability. Netherlands: IPCC; 2022. p. 3675

[70] Sollazzo G, Gouvi G, Nikolouli K, Martinez EIC, Schetelig MF, Bourtzis K. Temperature sensitivity of wild-type, mutant and genetic sexing strains of *Ceratitis capitata*. Insects. 2022;**13**(10):943. DOI: 10.3390/insects13100943

[71] Wernegreen JJ. Mutualism meltdown in insects: Bacteria constrain thermal adaptation. Current Opinion in Microbiology. 2012;**15**(3):255-262. DOI: 10.1016/j.mib.2012.02.001

[72] Alberdi A, Aizpurua O, Bohmann K, Zepeda-Mendoza ML, Gilbert MTP. Do vertebrate gut metagenomes confer rapid ecological adaptation? Trends in Ecology & Evolution. 2016;**31**(9):689-699. DOI: 10.1016/j.tree.2016.06.008

[73] Mesas A, Jaramillo A, Castañeda LE. Experimental evolution on heat tolerance and thermal performance curves under contrasting thermal selection in *Drosophila subobscura*. Journal of Evolutionary Biology. 2021;**34**(5):767-778. DOI: 10.1111/jeb.13777

[74] Raza MF, Wang Y, Cai Z, Bai S, Yao Z, Awan UA, et al. Gut microbiota promotes host resistance to low-temperature stress by stimulating its arginine and proline metabolism pathway in adult *Bactrocera dorsalis*. PLoS Pathogens. 2020;**16**(4):e1008441. DOI: 10.1371/journal.ppat.1008441

[75] Henry Y, Colinet H. Microbiota disruption leads to reduced cold tolerance in Drosophila flies. The Science of Nature. 2018;**105**(9):1-5. DOI: 10.1007/s00114-018-1584-7

[76] Moghadam NN, Thorshauge PM, Kristensen TN, de Jonge N, Bahrndorff S, Kjeldal H, et al. Strong responses of *Drosophila melanogaster* microbiota to developmental temperature. Fly. 2018;**12**(1):1-12. DOI: 10.1080/19336934.2017.1394558

[77] Dunbar HE, Wilson ACC, Ferguson NR, Moran NA. Aphid thermal tolerance is governed by a point mutation in bacterial symbionts. PLoS Biology. 2007;**5**(5):e96. DOI: 10.1371/journal.pbio.0050096

[78] Zhang B, Leonard SP, Li Y, Moran NA. Obligate bacterial endosymbionts limit thermal tolerance of insect host species. Proceedings of the National Academy of Sciences. 2019;**116**(49):24712-24718. DOI: 10.1073/pnas.1915307116

[79] Montllor CB, Maxmen A, Purcell AH. Facultative bacterial endosymbionts benefit pea aphids *Acyrthosiphon pisum* under heat stress.

Ecological Entomology. 2002;**27**(2): 189-195. DOI: 10.1046/j.1365-2311.2002.00393.x

[80] Russell JA, Moran NA. Costs and benefits of symbiont infection in aphids: Variation among symbionts and across temperatures. Proceedings of the Royal Society B: Biological Sciences. 2006; **273**(1586):603-610. DOI: 10.1098/rspb.2005.3348

[81] Gruntenko NE, Ilinsky YY, Adonyeva NV, Burdina EV, Bykov RA, Menshanov PN, et al. Various *Wolbachia* genotypes differently influence host *Drosophila* dopamine metabolism and survival under heat stress conditions. BMC Evolutionary Biology. 2017;**17**(2): 15-22. DOI: 10.1186/s12862-017-1104-y

[82] Nyamukondiwa C, Terblanche JS. Thermal tolerance in adult Mediterranean and Natal fruit flies (*Ceratitis capitata* and *Ceratitis rosa*): Effects of age, gender and feeding status. Journal of Thermal Biology. 2009;**34**(8): 406-414. DOI: 10.1016/j.jtherbio.2009.09.002

[83] Nyamukondiwa C, Terblanche JS. Within-generation variation of critical thermal limits in adult Mediterranean fruit flies *Ceratitis capitata* and *Ceratitis rosa*: Thermal history affects short-term responses to temperature. Physiological Entomology. 2010;**35**:255-264. DOI: 10.1111/j.1365-3032.2010.00736.x

[84] Terblanche JS, Nyamukondiwa C, Kleynhans E. Thermal variability alters climatic stress resistance and plastic responses in a globally invasive pest, the Mediterranean fruit fly (*Ceratitis capitata*). Entomologia Experimentalis et Applicata. 2010;**137**(3):304-315. DOI: 10.1111/j.1570-7458.2010.01067.x

[85] Esterhuizen N, Clusella-Trullas S, Van Daalen CE, Schoombie RE, Boardman L, Terblanche JS. Effects of within-generation thermal history on the flight performance of *Ceratitis capitata*: Colder is better. The Journal of Experimental Biology. 2014;**217**(19): 3545-3556. DOI: 10.1242/jeb.106526

[86] Steyn VM, Mitchell KA, Nyamukondiwa C, Terblanche JS. Understanding costs and benefits of thermal plasticity for pest management: Insights from the integration of laboratory, semi-field and field assessments of *Ceratitis capitata* (Diptera: Tephritidae). Bulletin of Entomological Research. 2022:1-11. DOI: 10.1017/S0007485321000389

[87] Huisamen EJ, Karsten M, Terblanche JS. Consequences of thermal variation during development and transport on flight and low-temperature performance in false codling moth (*Thaumatotibia leucotreta*): Fine-tuning protocols for improved field performance in a sterile insect programme. Insects. 2022;**13**(4):315. DOI: 10.3390/insects13040315

[88] Primo Millo E, Argilés Herrero R, Alfaro-Lassala F. Plan de actuación c ontra la mosca de las frutas (*Ceratitis ca pitata*) en la Comunidad Valenciana Ph ytoma España. La revista profesional de sanidad vegetal. 2003;**153**:127-130

[89] Magaña C, Hernández-Crespo P, Ortego F, Castañera P. Resistance to malathion in field populations of *Ceratitis capitata*. Journal of Economic Entomology. 2007;**100**(6):1836-1843. DOI: 10.1603/0022-0493(2007)100[1836:RTMIFP]2.0.CO;2

[90] Katsoyannos BI, Heath RR, Papadopoulos NT, Epsky ND, Hendrichs J. Field evaluation of Mediterranean fruit fly (Diptera: Tephritidae) female selective attractants for use in monitoring programs. Journal

of Economic Entomology. 1999;**92**(3):583-589

[91] Navarro-Llopis V, Alfaro F, Domínguez J, Sanchis J, Primo J. Evaluation of traps and lures for mass trapping of Mediterranean fruit fly in citrus groves. Journal of Economic Entomology. 2008;**101**(1):126-131. DOI: 10.1093/jee/101.1.126

[92] Hendrichs J, Robinson AS, Cayol JP, Enkerlin W. Medfly areawide sterile insect technique programmes for prevention, suppression or eradication: The importance of mating behavior studies. Florida Entomologist. 2022;**85**(1):1-13. DOI: 10.1653/0015-4040(2002)085[0001:MASITP]2.0.CO;2

[93] Montoya P, Cancino J, Zenil M, Gómez E, Villaseñor A. Parasitoid releases in the control of *Ceratitis capitata* (Diptera: Tephritidae) outbreaks, in coffee growing zones of Chiapas, Mexico. Vedalia. 2005;**12**(1):85-89

[94] Jacas JA, Karamaouna F, Vercher R, Zappalà L. Citrus pest management in the northern Mediterranean basin (Spain, Italy and Greece). In: Integrated Management of Arthropod Pests and Insect Borne Diseases. Dordrecht: Springer; 2010. pp. 3-27

[95] Gurr GM, Kvedaras OL. Synergizing biological control: Scope for sterile insect technique, induced plant defences and cultural techniques to enhance natural enemy impact. Biological Control. 2010;**52**(3):198-207. DOI: 10.1016/j.biocontrol.2009.02.013

[96] Andrés VS, Pérez-Panadés J, Carbonell EA, Castañera P, Urbaneja A. Effects of post-teneral nutrition and ginger root oil exposure on longevity and mortality in bait treatments of sterile male *Ceratitis capitata*. Entomologia Experimentalis et Applicata. 2009;**132**:256-263. DOI: 10.1111/j.1570-7458.2009.00893.x

[97] Juan-Blasco M, Sabater-Muñoz B, Argilés R, Jacas JA, Ortego F, Urbaneja A. Effects of pesticides used on citrus grown in Spain on the mortality of *Ceratitis capitata* (Diptera: Tephritidae) Vienna-8 strain sterile males. Journal of Economic Entomology. 2013;**106**(3):1226-1233. DOI: 10.1603/EC12464

[98] Itoh H, Hori T, Sato Y, Nagayama A, Tago K, Hayatsu M, et al. Infection dynamics of insecticide-degrading symbionts from soil to insects in response to insecticide spraying. The ISME Journal. 2018;**12**:909-920. DOI: 10.1038/s41396-017-0021-9

[99] Itoh H, Tago K, Hayatsu M, Kikuchi Y. Detoxifying symbiosis: Microbe-mediated detoxification of phytotoxins and pesticides in insects. Natural Product Reports. 2018b;**35**:434-454. DOI: 10.1039/c7np00051k

[100] Gangola S, Bhatt P, Kumar AJ, Bhandari G, Joshi S, Punetha A, et al. Biotechnological tools to elucidate the mechanism of pesticide degradation in the environment. Chemosphere. 2022;**8**:133916. DOI: 10.1016/j.chemosphere.2022.133916

[101] Akami M, Njintang NY, Gbaye OA, Andongma AA, Rashid MA, Niu CY, et al. Gut bacteria of the cowpea beetle mediate its resistance to dichlorvos and susceptibility to *Lippia adoensis* essential oil. Scientific Reports. 2019;**9**:6435. DOI: 10.1038/s41598-019-42843-1

[102] Bouhafs L, Moudilou EN, Exbrayat JM, Lahouel M, Idoui T. Protective effects of probiotic *Lactobacillus plantarum* BJ0021 on liver and kidney oxidative stress and apoptosis induced by endosulfan in

pregnant rats. Renal Failure. 2015;**37**: 1370-1378. DOI: 10.3109/0886022X.2015.1073543

[103] Daisley BA, Trinder M, McDowell TW, Welle H, Dube JS, Ali SN, et al. Neonicotinoid-induced pathogen susceptibility is mitigated by Lactobacillus plantarum immune stimulation in a *Drosophila melanogaster* model. Scientific Reports. 2017;**7**(1):1-13. DOI: 10.1038/s41598-017-02806-w

[104] Lili Z, Junyan W, Hongfei Z, Baoqing Z, Bolin Z. Detoxification of cancerogenic compounds by lactic acid bacteria strains. Critical Reviews in Food Science and Nutrition. 2018;**58**: 2727-2274. DOI: 10.1080/10408398.2017.1339665

[105] Pinto GDA, Castro IM, Miguel MAL, Koblitz MGB. Lactic acid bacteria-promising technology for organophosphate degradation in food: A pilot study. Lwt. 2019;**110**:353-359. DOI: 10.1016/j.lwt.2019.02.037

[106] Zhang YH, Xu D, Liu JQ, Zhao XH. Enhanced degradation of five organophosphorus pesticides in skimmed milk by lactic acid bacteria and its potential relationship with phosphatase production. Food Chemistry. 2014;**164**:173-178

[107] Yuan S, Li C, Yu H, Xie Y, Guo Y, Yao W. Screening of lactic acid bacteria for degrading organophosphorus pesticides and their potential protective effects against pesticide toxicity. Lwt. 2021;**147**:111672. DOI: 10.1016/j.lwt.2021.111672

[108] Ramya SL, Venkatesan T, Murthy KS, Jalali SK, Varghese A. Degradation of acephate by *Enterobacter asburiae*, *Bacillus cereus* and *Pantoea agglomerans* isolated from diamondback moth Plutella xylostella (L), a pest of cruciferous crops. Journal of Environmental Biology. 2016;**37**(4):611 PMID: 27498509

[109] Almeida LGD, Moraes LABD, Trigo JR, Omoto C, Consoli FL. The gut microbiota of insecticide-resistant insects houses insecticide-degrading bacteria: A potential source for biotechnological exploitation. PLoS One. 2017;**12**(3):e0174754. DOI: 10.1371/journal.pone.0174754

[110] Kikuchi Y, Hayatsu M, Hosokawa T, Nagayama A, Tago K, Fukatsu T. Symbiont-mediated insecticide resistance. Proceedings of the National Academy of Sciences. 2012; **109**(22):8618-8622. DOI: 10.1073/pnas.120023110

[111] Prabhakar CS, Sood P, Mehta PK. Protein hydrolyzation and pesticide tolerance by gut bacteria of *Bactrocera tau* (Walker). Pest Management and Economic Zoology. 2008;**16**:123-129

[112] Boush MG, Matsumura F. Insecticidal degradation by *Pseudomonas melophthora*, the bacterial symbiote of the apple maggot. Journal of Economic Entomology. 1967;**60**(4):918-920

[113] Miller A, Dearing D. The metabolic and ecological interactions of oxalate-degrading bacteria in the mammalian gut. Pathogens. 2013;**2**:636-652. DOI: 10.3390/pathogens2040636

[114] Bublitz DC, Wright PC, Bodager JR, Rasambainarivo FT, Bliska JB, Gillespie TR. Epidemiology of pathogenic enterobacteria in humans, livestock, and peridomestic rodents in rural Madagascar. PLoS One. 2014;**9**, **9**(7):e101456. DOI: 10.1371/journal.pone.0101456

[115] Vargas RI, Williamson DL, Chang H, Komura M. Effects of

larval-diet pH on worker comfort and insect quality during mass production of mediterranean fruit fly (Diptera: Tephritidae) in Hawaii. Journal of Environmental Science and Health Part A: Environmental Science and Engineering. 1984;**19**(5):621-630. DOI: 10.1080/10934528409375181

[116] De Angelis M, Gobbetti M. Environmental stress responses in *Lactobacillus*: A review. Proteomics. 2004;**4**(1):106-122. DOI: 10.1002/pmic.200300497

[117] Lee Yuan K, Salminen S. Handbook of Probiotics and Prebiotics. 2nd ed. New Jersey: Johns Wiley & Sons; 2009. p. 596. DOI: 10.1002/9780470432624

[118] Eslami P, Davarpanah L, Vahabzadeh F. Encapsulating role of β-cyclodextrin in formation of Pickering water-in-oil-in-water (W1/O/W2) double emulsions containing *Lactobacillus dellbrueckii*. Food Hydrocolloids. 2017;**64**:133-148. DOI: 10.1016/j.foodhyd.2016.10.035

[119] Iravani S, Korbekandi H, Mirmohammadi SV. Technology and potential applications of probiotic encapsulation in fermented milk products. Journal of Food Science and Technology. 2015;**52**(8):4679-4696. DOI: 10.1007/s13197-014-1516-2

[120] Bashir O, Claverie JP, Lemoyne P, Vincent C. Controlled-release of *Bacillus thurigiensis* formulations encapsulated in light-resistant colloidosomal microcapsules for the management of lepidopteran pests of *Brassica* crops. PeerJ. 2016;**11**(4):e2524. DOI: 10.7717/peerj.2524

[121] Murthy KS, Vineela V, Devi PSV. Generation of nanoparticles from technical powder of the insecticidal bacterium *Bacillus thuringiensis* Var. Kurstaki for improving efficacy. International Journal of Biomedical Nanoscience and Nanotechnology. 2014;**3**(3):236-2014. DOI: 10.1504/IJBNN.2014.065470

[122] Yoha KS, Nida S, Dutta S, Moses JA, Anandharamakrishnan C. Targeted delivery of probiotics: Perspectives on research and commercialization. Probiotics & Antimicrobial Proteins. 2022;**14**:15-48. DOI: 10.1007/s12602-021-09791-7

[123] Parker AG. Mass-rearing for sterile insect release. In: Dyck VA, Hendrichs J, Robinson AS, editors. Sterile Insect Technique. Principles and Practice in Area-Wide Integrated Pest Management. Dordrecht, The Netherlands: Springer; 2005. pp. 209-232

[124] Mastrangelo T, Silva J, Abdalla AL, Peçanha MR, Melges Walder JM. Potential use of larval diet disposal from medfly mass-rearing as alternative livestock feed. Livestock Research for Rural Development. 2010;**22**(3):Article #58 Retrieved November 21, 2022, from http://www.lrrd.org/lrrd22/3/mast22058.htm

[125] Sayed WAA, Alm-Eldin MMS, Hassan RS, Sileem TH, Rumpold BA. Recycling of Mediterranean fruit Fly rearing waste by black soldier Fly, *Hermetia illucens*. Waste Biomass Valor. 2022;**14**:93-104. DOI: 10.1007/s12649-022-01847-1

[126] Du G, Shi J, Zhang J, Ma Z, Liu X, Yuan C, et al. Exogenous probiotics improve fermentation quality, microflora phenotypes, and trophic modes of fermented vegetable waste for animal feed. Microorganisms. 2021;**9**(3):644. DOI: 10.3390/microorganisms9030644

[127] Liu J, Liu Y, Li G, Shen J, Tao Z, Tian Y, et al. Dynamic comparison on

the usage of probiotics in organic wastewater treatment under aerobic conditions in a diurnal environment. Journal of the Air & Waste Management Association. 2016;**66**(12):1183-1190. DOI: 10.1080/10962247.2016.1158131

[128] Tortosa G, Fernández-González AJ, Lasa AV, Aranda E, Torralbo F, González-Murua C, et al. Involvement of the metabolically active bacteria in the organic matter degradation during olive mill waste composting. Science of The Total Environment. 2021;**789**:147975. DOI: 10.1016/j.scitotenv.2021.147975

[129] Shi CY, Zhang Y, Lu ZQ, Wang YZ. Solid-state fermentation of cornsoybean meal mixed feed with *Bacillus subtilis* and *Enterococcus faecium* for degrading antinutritional factors and enhancing nutritional value. Journal of Animal Science and Biotechnology. 2017;**8**:50. DOI: 10.1186/s40104-017-0184-2

[130] Wang C, Su W, Zhang Y, Hao L, Wang F, Lu Z, et al. Solid-state fermentation of distilled dried grain with solubles with probiotics for degrading lignocellulose and upgrading nutrient utilization. AMB Express. 2018;**8**(1):188. DOI: 10.1186/s13568-018-0715-z

[131] W.H. Organization. Hazards Associated with Animal Feed: Report of the Joint FAO/WHO Expert Meeting, 12–15 May 2015. Rome, Italy: FAO headquarters. Food & Agriculture Org; 2019

Chapter 10

Intestinal Microbiomics in Physiological and Pathological Conditions

Ruxandra Florentina Ionescu, Elena Codruta Cozma, Robert Mihai Enache, Sanda Maria Cretoiu, Maria Iancu, Matei Mandea, Monica Profir, Oana Alexandra Roşu and Bogdan Severus Gaspar

Abstract

Microbiomics represents a new science studying the microbiome, consisting of all the microorganisms of a given community. This new science collects data about all the members of the microbial community and quantifies the molecules responsible for the structure, function, and dynamics of the microbiome. The human microbiome plays a very important role in the healthy state and in a variety of disease states. The human microbiome knowledge has evolved during the last decades and nowadays one can consider that, in particular, the gut microbiota is seen as a significant organ holding 150 times more genes compared to the human genome. This chapter will focus on discussing the normal and modified phyla and species of the gut microbiome in a variety of conditions, providing a better understanding of host-microbiome interactions. We will highlight some new associations between intestinal dysbiosis and acute or chronic inflammatory and metabolic diseases.

Keywords: microbiomics, gut microbiome, microbiota, dysbiosis, eubiosis

1. Introduction

Microbiomics is the science that distinguishes the structure, role, and passage of molecules involved in the microbial group [1]. In the "omics" era, it became more and more clear that gut microbiota is probably impacting the entire metabolism of the host. The study of the microbial community in their own habitat allows us to understand the complex interactions between microorganisms and the molecules responsible for their maintenance and correct functioning [1]. The microbiome, considered the metagenome of the microbiota, consists of the genetic material of bacteria, fungi, protozoa, and viruses, which can be found on the skin or hair surfaces, on mucosal surfaces (oral, intestinal, airways [2], vaginal [3]); uterus [4], eyes [5], and lungs [6]) [7].

Humans and microorganisms have coexisted for millennia under symbiotic relationships [7]. Any alteration in the human microbiome can lead to an imbalance stated, called dysbiosis, which influences the evolution of different conditions [8]. Dysbiosis can occur due to a series of factors like environment conditions (cold temperatures, poor economic status), treatment with antibiotics, probiotics intake, acute or chronic infections, or even the immune status of the host [9].

The gut microbiota is responsible for generating biologically active metabolites, with important roles in homeostasis, but also in pathophysiological processes [7].

Gut microbiota is involved in maintaining the immunological barrier, providing nutrients, and generating energy [10].

2. Structure and dynamics of the healthy adult microbiota

Oral microbiota was described to be dominated by *Streptococcus*, followed by *Haemophilus* (buccal mucosa), *Actinomyces* (supragingival plaque), and *Prevotella* (near the subgingival plaque) [11, 12]. *Porphyromonas gingivalis (P. gingivalis)*, a bacterium that colonizes the oral mucosa, was found through immunohistochemical techniques in 61% of the cancerous esophageal tissue examined. Thus, experts suggest it is a potential biomarker for assessing cancer progression. Originally located in the mouth, *Fusobacterium nucleatum* is linked with colonic adenocarcinoma development, strong evidence of its tumor protective role against the immune system cells arises from recent research [13].

Skin microbiota differs between different topographical regions, being under the influence of lifestyle conditions, hygiene, and antibiotic use. The microorganisms present on the skin are involved in the pathophysiology of different dermatological conditions, such as atopic dermatitis, psoriasis, acne, and seborrheic dermatitis. In a study conducted by Grice et al., although based on a limited number of subjects, the most frequent phyla identified were *Actinobacteria, Firmicutes, Proteobacteria* and *Bacteroidetes* and the most common genera were *Corynebacteria (Actinobacteria), Propionibacteria (Actinobacteria)*, and *Staphylococci (Firmicutes)*. Propionibacterium species preponderate in sebaceous locations, *Corynebacteria* in moist locations, while *Staphylococci* species were present in significant amounts in both sebaceous and moist sites [14]. Regarding dry areas, high levels of *beta-Proteobacteri*a and *Flavobacteriales* were observed [14]. Although human skin microbiota consists mostly of bacteria, several types of fungi are also present. A combination of the genera: *Malassezia, Aspergillus, Cryptococcus Rhodotorula*, and *Epicoccum* was found located mostly in the foot skin area [15].

The vaginal microbiome is dominated by bacteria that can produce lactic acid, mostly *Lactobacillus* species (*Lactobacillus iners*, *Lactobacillus crispatus*, *Lactobacillus gasseri, Lactobacillus jensenii*), coexisting with other types of bacteria, such as *Gardnerella, Atopobium, Megasphaera, Eggerthella, Aerococcus, Alloiococcus, Streptococcus, Leptotrichia/Sneathia, Prevotella, Papillibacter* and anaerobic microorganisms [16]. They lower the local pH due to lactic acid production and have bacteriostatic and bactericidal properties [17, 18]. The uterine microbiome is similar in composition to the vaginal population with a predominance of *Lactobacillus* colonies together with *Bifidobacterium, Gardnerella, Prevotella,* and *Streptococcus* types of microorganisms. Uterine dysbiosis due to contraceptive medication usage, untreated or chronic bacterial vaginosis, or other physiological factors can lead to fertility issues (loss of fetal implantation ability, bacterial overpopulation, and uro-genital infections) [4]. The uterine microbiome and the interactions between the microbiome and the human reproductive system are currently being studied for enhancing the current approach to assist reproductive techniques, by targeting specific phyla and the results are promising [19].

The predominant bacterial genera found in the eyes conjunctiva and ocular surface are gram-positive pathogens like *Staphylococcus, Streptococcus, Propionibacterium, Diphtheroid* bacteria, and *Micrococcus*. While gram-negative genus is mostly found in the gut, anaerobes or fungi are rarely observed in this particular site. It is unclear how the intraocular immune environment and microbiome interact to control inflammatory eye disorders like uveitis [20].

Airways are largely populated by *Actinobacterium (Corynebacterium, Aureobacterium,* and *Rhodococcus)*, but there is a significant microbiome diversity difference between nasopharynx microbiota and pharynx commensal bacterial population. *Corynebacterium, Aureobacterium, Rhodococcus*, and *Staphylococcus*, including *S. epidermis, Staphylococcus capitis, Staphylococcus hominis, Staphylococcus haemolyticus, Staphylococcus lugdunensis,* and *Staphylococcus warneri,* compose the majority of the nasal microbiota [2].

Although previously believed that the lungs are sterile, and the first evidence of commensal bacterial population in the lungs where initially attributed to contamination from upper airways through bronchoscopy, it is now clear that the majority of lung microbiota consists of *Firmicutes, Bacteroidetes, Proteobacteria, Fusobacteria,* and *Actinobacteria* and alterations at this level can be linked to lung diseases (asthma, chronic obstructive pulmonary disease, and chronic suppurative lung disease) occurrence [6].

The human gut hosts thousands of microbial species [21], which have a gene pool larger than the human genome, which determined its name as a metagenome [22, 23]. There are two major phyla, *Bacteroidetes* and *Firmicutes*, representing 90% of the total bacterial species found in the human gut, the remaining 10% consisting of *Actinobacteria, Cyanobacteria, Fusobacteria, Proteobacteria,* and *Verrucomicrobia* [7, 23].

Several factors can alter the composition and evolution of gut microbiota over the years. Firstly, differences between newborns are noted: babies delivered vaginally have gut microbiota consisting of *Lactobacillus, Prevotella, and Atopobium*, while, in comparison, the gut of babies delivered by caesarian section has maternal epidermal microflora, mostly represented by *Staphylococcus* [18, 23]. With age, anaerobic microorganisms become more abundant, with significant concentrations of *Bifidobacteria* and *Clostridia* in teenagers when compared to adults and higher levels of facultative anaerobes in the elderly [10]. The microbiota of infants was observed to be rich in *Clostridium coccoides* and *Clostridium leptum*, while elevated levels of *Escherichia Coli* and *Bacteroidetes* were observed in older people [10, 23].

Changes in the gut microbiota composition are in correlation with the physiological age-related processes. A systematic review conducted by Badal and colleagues presented some of the microbiota variations throughout the years. In older subjects, alpha diversity of the microbial taxa, functional pathways, and metabolites were enhanced, while beta diversity fluctuated significantly through different age groups. *Akkermansia* was described to be relatively plentiful with aging, while *Faecalibacterium, Bacteroidaceae,* and *Lachnospiraceae* were relatively diminished [24]. Elders possess different properties and functions of the microbiota: decreased activity of carbohydrate metabolism pathways and amino acid synthesis, higher production of short-chain fatty acids (SCFA) and butyrate derivatives (gamma-aminobutyric acid - GABA and DL-3-amino isobutyric acid) [24, 25].

For older people with ages ranging from 66 to 80 years old, lower levels of *Bifidobacterium, Faecalibacterium, Bacteroides*, and *Clostridium* cluster XIVa were noted. However, elevated aggregations of the *Akkermansia* and *Lactobacillus* group were detected in the cluster of people over 80 years old, compared with adults. Moreover, lower fecal SCFA concentrations were associated with aging, with statistical significance [26].

Diet plays a major role in the diversity of the human gut microorganisms and David et al. [27] compared plant-based diet microbiome with animal produce consumption microbiome and concluded that a shift in diet from mostly fibers to high fats and proteins can lead to only 24 hours to an increased population of *Alistipes, Bilophila* and *Bacteroides* and decreased levels of *Firmicutes (Roseburia, Eubacterium rectale,* and *Ruminococcus bromii)* known for their ability to metabolize dietary plant polysaccharides [27]. Several studies comparing the African diet with European food underline the same conclusion: different food components can alter the human gut microbiota very quickly and in different ways, leading to variability in the microorganism population found in the digestive tract [28, 29].

3. The role of the microbiota in specific diseases and conditions

3.1 Inflammatory bowel disease

Inflammatory Bowel Disease (IBD) defines a group of chronic disorders that includes Crohn's disease (CD) and Ulcerative colitis (UC). Though they are two different diseases, they both affect the intestinal tract and are characterized by intestinal inflammation with periods of remission and relapse [30]. The incidence of IBD is consistently growing in the recent few decades, having a peak onset age between 15 and 35 years that was initially described in the western populations, and now is also more frequent in other countries, as processed food and animal-based diets are overtaking the plant-based diet [31].

The etiology of IBD is an important subject of discussion as it is not fully understood. The key ways proposed as mechanisms for developing inflammation in IBD are the genetic susceptibility and environmental factors that interact with the immune system. Thus, the host gives an inappropriate immune response to changes of the gut microbiome and modulates inflammation and disease involvement and activity [32, 33].

The interaction between the host and different environmental factors, such as infections, smoking, dietary habits, psychological stress, medications, and alcohol consumption leads to alterations in the balance between gut microbiota and the genetically predisposed host. This imbalance changes the complex interactions of the immune system and products of the commensal microbiota that trigger immune responses using inflammatory mediators and signaling pathways. Hence, prolonged imbalance of the gut microbiota (including the microbiome, mycobiome, virome, and protozoa) with changes of the composition with a decrease of the commensal phyla and increase of potential pathological microorganisms, defined as dysbiosis, induce the alterations and dysregulations of mucosal barrier [34–36].

The dysfunction of the mucosal immune barrier has been shown in mouse studies that can regulate the development of T regulatory (T reg) cells and T helper 17 (Th17) cells with important differentiation in healthy and sick subjects. The activation of Th17 cells is important in bacterial and fungal infections, releasing pro-inflammatory interleukine (IL) 17 cytokines, important in the pathogenesis of colitis. T reg cells play an important role in the suppression of inflammation through transforming-growth factor B (TGF-B), interleukine (IL) 35, and IL10. The deficiency of T reg cells leads to inflammation and IBD [33, 37–39]. Their role is important against *Citrobacter rodentium* and *Salmonella enterica* and was shown to be decreased in *Bacteroides* increased microbiome. Also, *Clostridium* clusters showed the ability to act on the differentiation of T reg cells [34, 37, 40, 41].

The dysbiosis occurring in IBD affecting bacterial microbiota is the most studied section of the gut microbiota. The most frequent phyla that are seen in healthy subjects are *Bacteroides, Bifidobacterium spp, Fecalibacterium spp, Firmicutes spp, Roseburia spp, Actinobacteria, and Verrucomicrobia* are regarded as over 90% of the gut microbial families [30, 32, 34]. Patients affected by IBD, in general show a decreased presence of mentioned phyla and an increase in *Proteobacteria spp, Escherichia coli spp*, *Fusobacterium spp, Ruminococcus spp, Pasteurellaceae spp, Veillonellaceae, Campylobacter spp,* and *Clostridioides spp*. There have been shown differences in composition and diversity regarding UC and CD, regarding also the extension of disease, aggressivity, and activity, thus being able to use the microbiome changes as a biomarker for disease activity and response to treatment [30, 34].

Regarding composition and diversity, there is a common agreement that in CD patients is a greater degree of dysbiosis compared to UC. Studies using 16 s rRNA sequencing characterized the gut microbiome in IBDs, showing a decrease of *Anaerostipes, Methanobrevibacter, Fecalibacterium* (especially *F.prausnitzii*), *Peptostreptococcaceae, Collinsella, Bifidobacteria* (especially *Bifidobacterium adolescentis*), *Dialister invisus, Clostridioides* cluster XIVa, *Bacteroides fragilis, Roseburia, Firmicutes* and *Erysipelotrichales* in CD and an increase of *Proteobacteria (Campylobacter), Yersinia enterocolitica, Bacteroides (vulgatus, fragilis), Helicobacterhepaticus, Mycobacteria spp, Enterobacteriaceae* (pathogenic *E.coli, Shigella*), *Ruminococcus gnavus, Veillonellaceae, Fusobacteriaceae,* and *Pasteurellaceae*, in human and animal models [30, 34].

These bacterial taxa are different from those expressed in UC, where a decrease of *Roseburia, Eubacterium, Faecalibacterium, Akkermansia, Bifidobacterium* and an increase *Helicobacteraceae, Mucispirillum, Desulfovibrio, Clostridioides ramnosum,* and *Porphyromonas* differentiate from common alterations of the microbiome seen in both CD and UC [34, 35, 42, 43].

Regarding disease phenotype, there have been a few studies about a range of specific gut bacteria changes associated with different patterns in CD. Li et al. [44] showed that individuals with ileal CD showed an increase in *Actinobacteria spp* and *Firmicutes/Bacillus* and a decrease in *Ruminococcus spp* [44]. Also, this phenotype was associated with an absence of *Roseburia* and *F. prausnitzii*, and an increase of *E. coli* [45]. In addition, decreased presence of *F. prausnitzii* in patients with ileal resection in CD, showed an increase in recurrence [46].

The regulation of gut mucosal immunity and host immune response is made through bacterial physiology and interaction on cell growth and interaction with metabolites produced by the microbiome. The stability of mucosal inflammation is disrupted in IBDs with the alteration of immunomodulatory metabolites such as SCFAs (acetate, propionate, and butyrate), bile acids, and tryptophan metabolites. SCFAs are mostly represented by acetate and are produced by *Bacteroidetes* and *Firmicutes*, and there has been demonstrated an important reduction in IBDs while associated also with reduced SCFA-producing bacteria such as *F. prausnitzii, R.intestinalis*. Another study also demonstrated decreased specific taxa for CD as *Phascolarctobacterium* and *Roseburia* and for UC *Leuconostocaceae spp* [32, 38, 47].

Given the alterations of gut microbiota and metabolites in IBD, there have been developed and proposed several management strategies for controlling the microbiome. Probably the most studied approach is using probiotics, which are bacterial species that may promote the maintenance of the immunological balance [48]. The effectiveness of probiotics in improving IBD evolution has been exhibited using different strains of *Lactobacillus, Bifidobacterium, Streptococcus,* and *Saccharomyces*. Their efficacy was seen in maintaining remission in UC patients by reducing pro-inflammatory cytokines and restoring normal gut microbiota. Nevertheless, the use of probiotics in CD showed little or no implication [31, 48, 49]. Often administered with oral probiotics, are the substrates, such as fructooligosaccharides, pectins, starch, and fibers, targeting microbiome composition by aiding the development of normal gut microbiota [50].

The use of antibiotics for their role in the modulation of microbiota is controversial. They function by decreasing the concentrations of different bacteria in the gut and reducing tissue invasion and translocation, acting also on metabolism with a decrease of pro-inflammatory metabolites and an increase of SCFAs. However, the non or very little selectivity character of antibiotics alter also the composition of some beneficial bacterial strains and their use is kept for septic and infectious complications, such as *Clostridioides difficile* infection [32, 48, 51, 52].

An important method of influencing the microbiome is Fecal Microbiota Transplantation (FMT), a very attractive method with significant rates of success, that is known from as early as fourth century [53]. As well as probiotics, FMT was better studied and showed important results in UC, and less in CD [34, 54, 55]. In UC, in mild-to-moderate cases, usage is still modest as it managed to induce response and remission in 20–55% of cases being comparable with active treatment as reflected in decreasing Mayo score and reducing symptoms [54, 56]. An important use of FMT is also recommended in recent guidelines for recurrent infection [57]. It remains a subject of future studies' better selection of FMT donors as currently being no possibility of predicting the success of a given donor to an IBD patient, thus defining an "ideal" donor [53].

The changes in lifestyle and diet represent the most common intervention on the microbiome, and of paramount interest being the first recommendation and the easiest to accept the measure. Diets rich in vegetables, fermented foods probiotic-rich (kimchi, kefir, yogurt, and pickled vegetables), fibers, and prebiotics have a positive impact on intestinal barrier health and microbiome balance [35, 50]. Currently, there are some diet recommendations for IBD and the most studied diets are Low Fermentable Oligosaccharides, Disaccharides, Monosaccharides and Polyols (FODMAP), Crohn's disease exclusion diet, and Mediterranean diet (MD). A low FODMAP diet was found to have a good improvement in disease clinical scores in mild cases of IBD that are associated with IBS (Irritable Bowel Syndrome). MD characterized by low saturated fat, high monounsaturated fat, fiber, high vitamin B, C, E, and moderate ethanol intake showed in a few studies on CD patients' improvements of the quality of life and mild reducing fecal calprotectin an serum CRP [35, 58–61]. Another diet studied is a plant-based diet that exerts anti-inflammatory effects, composed of whole grains, cereals, fruits, vegetables, and nuts showed good improvements regarding symptoms, lowering serum CRP, overall WBC, but with the price of requiring supplementation of micronutrients [31, 62].

3.2 Acute and chronic pancreatitis

Acute pancreatitis (AP) is defined as an inflammatory condition of the pancreas following the injury of the pancreatic serous acini, leading to premature activation of digestive enzymes (trypsin, chymotrypsin, lipase, and elastase) [63]. The clinical severity of AP cases depends on their complications, which can be localized (sterile or infected peri/pancreatic necrosis) or systemic (transient or persistent organ failure) into mild, moderate, severe, and critical AP [64]. The evolution of AP can be summarized in three stages: (1) local inflammation of the pancreas; (2) systemic inflammatory response syndrome; and (3) multiple organ dysfunction syndrome [65–67].

The revised Atlanta classification identifies two main stages of AP: (a) interstitial edematous pancreatitis and (b) necrotizing pancreatitis (NP) [68].

Although often overlooked, the gut microbial community and the gut barrier integrity disruption were described as aggravating factors responsible for the amplification of the initial inflammatory process accompanying AP [69]. Apparently, according to Liu et al. 2008 in AP patients, with mild and severe forms, there is an early gut mucosal dysfunction, leading to the development of multiple organ dysfunction [70]. The mucus layer integrity in the gut lining is lost after the onset of AP as shown by Fishman et al. 2014, leading to the failure of the gut barrier, apparently due to mechanisms independent of the activity of the pancreatic proteases in the intestinal lumen [71]. Pancreatic necrosis is accompanied by a lot of inflammatory cytokines and determines multiple changes in the gut such as a decrease in intestinal motility, favoring bacterial overgrowth and malnutrition and followed by gut barrier failure and increased permeability [72]. The intestinal permeability is highly increased in severe forms of AP and favors a poor prognosis.

The gut mucosal secretions also contain important quantities of secretory IgA, a key immunoglobulin that prevents the adhesion of pathogens and is responsible for the maintenance of immune homeostasis [73]. Usually, the amount of sIgA found in the small intestine is directly correlated with bacterial eubiosis and diversity. A decrease in sIgA is often correlated with low bacterial diversity in the small intestine and increased permeability and bacterial translocation leading to severe AP and infection [74].

The study by Yu et al. 2020 performed the 16S rRNA sequencing of gut microbiota species from fecal samples obtained through rectal swabs from 80 patients and described a correlation between gut microbiota and the severity of AP [75].

The microbiota profile was different, depending on the severity grade. In mild AP the main two phyla *Bacteroidetes* and *Firmicutes* were identified. *Bacteroides, Escherichia-Shigella,* and *Enterococcus* species were dominant while *Blautia* was highly decreased. *Finegoldia, Eubacterium hallii*, and *Lachnospiraceae* were considered to be potential diagnostic biomarkers for this stage of AP. In moderately severe AP, *Anaerococcus* was the most significantly increased and *E. hallii* the most decreased species, while in severe AP, *Enterococcus* was the most significantly increased and *E. hallii* the most decreased species. *Proteobacteria* phylum was the most increased in both, moderately severe and severe AP [75]. This study is impaired by several limitations such as possible contamination due to rectal swab samples and secondly by the impossibility to determine if microbiota dysbiosis is due to the presence of AP or is the main factor determining the AP severity. These findings are in correlation to those of the multihospital prospective clinical study performed by Tan et al. 2015 who describe dramatic alterations of the microbiota, determined by real-time quantitative polymerase chain reaction, in mild and severe forms of AP [76]. *Enterobacteriaceae* and *Enterococcus* were found to be increased by 3.2 and 9.3%, respectively, while the beneficial strains like *Bifidobacterium* were decreased by 9.2% in the severe forms of AP compared to mild forms [76]. The drawbacks of this study consist in the small sample size of patients with AP included and the lack of modern techniques like high-throughput sequencing. Another study performed by Zhu et al. 2019 describes the reduction of other beneficial strains like *Blautia* in patients with severe AP [77].

The gut mucosal lining is affected by dysbiosis mainly through the metabolites produced by certain bacterial species. *Firmicutes* and *Bacteroidetes* are mainly responsible for the production of short-chain fatty acids (SCFAs), mainly acetate, propionate, and butyrate, the main energy source of enterocytes, colonocytes, and hepatocytes [78]. SCFAs are very important for the maintenance of tight junctions between the intestinal epithelial cells and also for the mucosal immune barrier [79]. In AP patients, there is a decrease in SCFAs promoted by dysbiosis and moreover, because of the decreased pH, it creates the condition for potential pathogenic and pathogenic bacteria, such as *E. coli* and *Shigella,* to grow and aggravate the evolution [80].

Experimental studies performed on mice suggested that microbiota regulation by fecal transplantation might reduce the damage at the intestinal barrier level and create a more stable evolution, preventing severe forms [80, 81]. Ding et al. 2021 showed in a randomized, controlled study registered at https://clinicaltrials.gov (NCT02318134) that the fecal microbiota transplantation had no beneficial effects in the evolution of severe forms of AP and moreover, the intestinal permeability might have been adversely affected [82].

Chronic pancreatitis (CP) is defined as a progressive and irreversible inflammation of the pancreas that leads to pancreatic exocrine insufficiency (PEI) and diabetes mellitus [83]. A normal pancreatic function provides antimicrobial peptides, bicarbonate, and digestive enzymes that are necessary for digestive function but also for the maintenance of healthy microbiota [84, 85].

The evidence accumulated in recent years regarding pancreatic exocrine deficiency advocates for small intestinal bacterial overgrowth (SIBO) and gut dysbiosis-reduced diversity, and increased abundance of opportunistic pathogens [86, 87]. Capurso et al. 2016 also demonstrated in a meta-analysis that one-third of patients with CP have SIBO [88]. A study by Ní Chonchubhair et al. 2018 evaluated the relationship between SIBO and clinical symptoms in CP and found that SIBO was present in 15% of chronic pancreatitis patients [89]. Frost et al. 2020 recently determined the intestinal microbiota composition by bacterial 16S ribosomal RNA gene sequencing and found reduced alfa and beta microbial diversity index and an increased abundance of opportunistic pathogens in patients with CP. They found in CP cases an increase in abundance of *Enterococcus* and *Bacteroides* and an absolute reduction of *Faecalibacterium* and *Prevotella* [86]. Talukdar et al. 2017 also described in their study a reduction of *Fecalibacterium prausnitzii* and *R. bromii* in CP without and with diabetes. Apparently, the gut barrier integrity is disrupted due to low *Fecalibacterium* levels and this favors the passage of bacterial endotoxins in circulation followed by subsequent alterations in the functionality of beta pancreatic cells [90].

As the studies indicated, there are some significant alterations in the composition and function of the gut microbiota in patients with AP and CP, leading to severe forms of disease and in correlation with a poor prognosis. The disturbance of the gut microflora equilibrium needs to be further explored in close correlation with the gut mucosal integrity and systemic inflammatory status.

3.3 Colorectal cancer

Colorectal cancer (CRC) is the third most frequent cancer worldwide with more than 1.9 million new cases and 930.000 deaths reported in 2020. It is predicted that by 2040, the burden of the disease will be increased to 3.2 million cases per year and 1.6 million deaths per year [91]. Approximately 90% of CRC cases are sporadic [92], and various environmental and genetic factors contribute to CRC tumorgenesis [93]. Studies show that only a small percentage of CRC cases are genetically predisposed [93, 94], underlining the importance of environmental factors in the development of CRC. Diets rich in red and grilled meat, tobacco, high alcohol intake, disruption of circadian rhythm, and preexisting conditions, such as obesity, inflammatory bowel disease, and diabetes, have been associated with CRC [95]. In addition, the intestinal microbiota is getting more and more recognition among environmental factors implicated in the development of CRC, evidence dating as early as the 1960s. One study published in the late 1960s demonstrated that glucoside cycasin failed to produce its carcinogenic effect in germ-free mice and was only able to induce cancer in conventional rats [96]. In 1975 Reddy et al. showed that a large dose of 1,2-dimethylhydrazine induced multiple colonic tumors in 93% of the conventional rats included in the study, whereas 1,2-dimethylhydrazine-induced colonic tumors were observed in only 20% of the germ-free mice [97]. Moreover, subcutaneous administration of azoxymethane led to an increased incidence of colonic tumors in germ-free rats, indicating that intestinal bacterial populations can alter the carcinogenic effects of certain compounds in the colon [98].

Studies on humans, that have analyzed both mucosal and fecal samples, demonstrate that the gut microbiota of CRC patients differs significantly from that of healthy subjects, CRC patients presenting diminished richness and bacterial diversity [99–101]. Also, Chen et al. 2012 observed that the microbial composition in cancerous tissue is significantly different from that found in the intestinal lumen [102]. Numerous bacteria have been correlated with CRC in spite of variations in intestinal microbiota [99, 100].

B. fragilis, a bacteria that colonizes most humans [103] *F. nucleatum, Prevotella intermedia, Parvimonas micra, Porphyromonas asaccharolytica, Alistipes finegoldii,* and *Thermanaerovibrio* are bacteria identified by one meta-analysis to be enriched in CRC [104]. In 2019 two more meta-analyses investigating the fecal metagenome in CRC have been published, expanding the list of CRC-enriched bacteria [105, 106].

Not only has an increase in the population of *F. nucleatum* been associated with CRC, but also it is thought to promote disease progression [107]) and its presence in CRC tissues might be indicative of a worsen prognosis [108, 109]. A recent study found increased levels of *P. intermedia* and *F. nucleatum* in adenocarcinomas compared with paired adenomatous polyps. The presence of this bacteria was shown to exert an additive effect on the migration and invasion of CRC cells and was also associated with lymph node involvement and distant metastasis [110].

Increased levels of *Enterococcus faecalis, E. coli,* and *Peptostreptococcus anaerobiusi* in CRC patients in comparison with healthy controls was also reported by several authors, but the exact mechanisms by which these bacteria promote cancer development is still to be determined [100].

The enriched bacteria are also associated with reduced levels of benefic bacteria, such as *Clostridium butyicum and Streptococcus thermophilus*, [104] bacteria belonging to the genus *Roseburia* and other butyrate-producing bacteria [111]. *Wang et al. 2012* highlight that the decrease in butyrate-producing bacteria and the opportunistic pathogen multiplication might be responsible for the structural imbalance of gut microbiota in patients suffering from CRC [111]. Short-chain fatty acids (SCFAs) are fermentation end products produced by bacteria, with butyrate being the most intensively studied SCFA. Apart from being considered the energy source for colonocytes, they also promote the apoptosis of cancer cells [112]. The amount of SCFAs produced by the microbiota is however insufficient to inhibit CRC development and probiotic supplementation might result in increased SCFAs. One *in vitro* study showed that *Lactobacillus fermentum* NCIMB 5221 was able to increase SCFAs production, thus exerting antiproliferative effects against Caco-2 cancer cells and promoting normal epithelial cell growth [113]. Resistant starch (RS) is part of starch that is fermented into SCFAs in the cecum and this process leads to pH decrease. Prebiotic supplementation with RS has been demonstrated to reduce the proliferation of epithelial cells in the colon and rectum [114, 115]. Moreover, the administration of synbiotics, meaning the combinations of prebiotics and probiotics has also been investigated. In one RCT patients with a history of CCR received a synbiotic preparation composed of oligofructose-enriched inulin and two probiotics *Lactobacillus rhamnosus* GG and *Bifidobacterium lactis* Bb12. The synbiotic intervention resulted in significantly reduced colorectal proliferation, an increase in the number of beneficial bacteria, cytokine production modulation (decreased interleukin (IL) 2 and increased IFN-gamma production), and a decreased genotoxins exposure, which translates into a reduction in DNA alterations [116].

The role of the intestinal microbiota in CRC tumor progression is also supported by the differences in bacterial composition between patients with early-stage adenomas and those in advanced stages with definitive CRC [92].

Nevertheless, the CRC microbiome is also characterized by an imbalance in the composition of the viral and fungal species [92, 99]. A higher viral load has been observed in tumors compared to normal tissue of CRC patients [92]. Although some studies have identified cytomegalovirus, John Cunnningham virus, and human papilloma virus in CRC tumor samples, the data are however inconsistent [99]. Shotgun metagenomic analyses of viromes of fecal samples identified 22 viral taxa that differentiate the CRC virome from one of healthy controls [117]. Trans kingdom crosstalk between bacteria and viruses may play an important role in CRC tumorigenesis, as some studies indicate [118]. Although less studied, differences in terms of fungal composition were also observed [119, 120].

Existing studies suggest that several carcinogenesis mechanisms involved in the development of CRC are intimately linked to the gut microbiota. Among studies, authors have insisted on the mechanisms of inflammation, oxidative stress, pathogenic bacteria, genotoxins, and biofilm [100]. Studies have demonstrated that some bacterial species, such as *F. nucleatum* [121] and *P. anaerobius* [122], can induce a pro-inflammatory immune microenvironment, which leads to the progression of colorectal neoplasia. The immunomodulatory capacity of probiotics has led scientists to investigate probiotics in the management of CRC. Oral administration of a mixture of six viable strains of *Lactobacillus* and *Bifidobacterium* in patients with CRC 4 weeks after surgery resulted in a significant pro-inflammatory cytokine reduction compared to placebo administration. The levels of tumor necrosis factor (TNF-α), IL-6, IL-10, IL-12, IL-17A, IL-17C, and IL-22 were significantly reduced, and no severe adverse reactions were reported [123]. After comparing the intestinal microbiota of CRC patients with that of healthy patients, one study analyzed the possibility of preventing colorectal carcinogenesis by modulating the composition of the intestinal bacterial population using *L. gasseri*. Probiotic administration resulted in an increase in the *Lactobacillus* population and a decrease in the amount of *Clostridium perfringens* as well as a shift in fecal pH toward acidosis along with an increase in IL-1 and natural killer (NK) cell activity values starting with week 4 [124].

Additionally, through their adhesion capacities, pathogens and their virulence factors adhere to the intestinal epithelial cells (IECs) and promote tumor formation [122, 125–127]. Also, the gut microbiota can modulate the immune system response by stimulating the production of chemokine in tumoral cells with the purpose of recruiting T lymphocytes [128]. Moreover, bacterially produced genotoxins, exert DNA damage in IECs, which can further initiate carcinogenesis. For example, *E. coli* produces the genotoxin colibactin [129, 130] which is reported to induce transient DNA damage in epithelial cells [130]. Similarly, *Salmonella* damages the DNA in IECs by producing typhoid toxin [131]. Inflammation can lead to increased levels of ROS (reactive oxygen species) and RNS (reactive nitrogen species), its negative impact translating into DNA damage and the development of mutations. *E. faecalis* [132], *P. anaerobius* [133], *E. coli,* and enterotoxigenic *B. fragilis* [134, 135] promote ROS production by colonic cells. Enterotoxigenic *B. fragilis,* through its metalloprotease toxin and its effect on IL-17 pathway, is believed to promote carcinogenesis in colonic cell population [136, 137]. Microbiota, also found as a biofilm at the surface of the colon mucosa, can promote colonic tumor cell proliferation through modulating interleukin 6 and STAT3 signaling pathways [138, 139].

3.4 Cardiovascular disease

The abnormal interactions between the microbiota and the host compromise homeostatic mechanisms. Most cardiovascular risk factors, such as age, obesity, diet, and lifestyle, can generate gut dysbiosis, which is associated with intestinal inflammation and poor integrity of the intestinal barrier [7, 23].

Diets rich in fat lead to the stimulation of mast cells from the intestinal mucosa, generating inflammatory mediators, such as histamine, which can amplify intestinal permeability [140]. However, high carbohydrate diets can also raise intestinal permeability and endotoxins [141].

Cardiovascular diseases (CVD), the number one cause of death worldwide, are influenced by smoking, dyslipidemia, diabetes mellitus, and arterial hypertension [23].

Dysbiosis is involved in numerous pathophysiological chains of events, leading to different conditions, and cardiovascular afflictions making no exception. The perturbation of the gut microbiota can favor a pro-inflammatory state in the human body, therefore promoting the atherosclerotic process [7, 23, 142].

Atherosclerosis is, unfortunately, a frequent chronic inflammatory process, which comprises endothelial dysfunction, dysfunction of vascular smooth muscle cells differentiation, infiltration with inflammatory cells, and subendothelial lipid accumulation [143].

Microorganisms, such as *Chlamydophila* pneumoniae, *P. gingivalis, Helicobacter pylori*, Influenza A virus, Hepatitis C virus, cytomegalovirus, and human immunodeficiency virus, were associated with a high risk for developing CVD [23, 144]. Infections can influence atherosclerosis through arterial wall inflammation, favoring plaque formation, or through the production of pro-inflammatory mediators, which are the result of infections of various sites in the body [23, 145].

High blood levels of lipopolysaccharides (LPS) have been linked to adverse cardiac events in patients with CVD such as atrial fibrillation [146]. LPS are endotoxins, byproducts of gut microbiota that can reach systemic circulation through the intestinal mucosa [147]. A decrease in gut bacteria, such as *Bacteroides spp*, has been negatively correlated with atherosclerotic plaque progression and endothelial dysfunction, thus promoting inflammation [148].

Atherosclerosis is associated with trimethylamine-N-oxide (TMAO), a vasculotoxic metabolite resulting from L-carnitine, choline, and phosphatidylcholine. TMAO was indicated to promote the development of aortic lesions in apolipoprotein E (apoE) in mice by modifying bile acid profiles. TMAO inhibits the production of bile acids through the farnesoid X nuclear receptor (FXR) and small heterodimer partner (SHP) [149].

Elevated serum levels of TMAO have been shown to predict CVD outcomes in heart failure. Individual TMAO formation is dependent on microbial gut composition. A red meat diet consumption rich in choline and an omnivorous diet with high carnitine may account for TMAO levels elevation [150]. In an observational study of 155 patients with heart failure, elevated plasma levels of TMAO were found in chronic HF patients with higher levels in NYHA class III and IV and were associated with worse prognoses [151].

Microbiota in the colon metabolizes secondary bile acids (BA) from un-recycled bile acids through bile-salt hydrolase (BSH). BA synthesis is an important pathway for cholesterol elimination, thus having an athero-protective function. Composition of bile acids is altered in heart failure patients with a decrease in the primary to secondary bile acids ratio. A decrease in BSH levels subsequently causes cholesterol buildup and progression of CVD. Microbial BSH modulates stimulation of hepatic FXR, which acts as a bile acid signaling receptor and a potential target for bile acid therapy in reducing cardiovascular complications [152, 153].

Moreover, probiotic supplements may improve intestinal balance and select probiotics could have a cardioprotective role. Altered bacterial diversity was observed in two heart failure with reduced ejection fraction (HFrEF) cohorts with an increase in *Prevotella* genus and a decrease in genera belonging to *Lachnospiraceae* family and *Rumminococcaceae Faecalibacterium* and *Bifidobactericeae Bifidobacterium* [154]. Similar cohorts had increases in pathogenic bacteria, such as *Campylobacter, Shigella, Yersinia enterolytica*, and *Candida* species, associated with an increase in gut permeability [155]. The *Firmicutes/Bacteroidetes* ratio (F/B) in hypertensive patients is higher than in the normotensive individuals, by lower levels of *Bacteroidetes* [156]. *Roseburia*, one of the main producers of butyrate, is diminished in hypertensive patients. However, *Roseburia* can also produce linoleic acid, which has anti-inflammatory properties and a possible role in lowering blood pressure values, together with linolenic acid [156–159]. According to CARDIA study, *Robinsoniella* and *Catabacter* were positively associated with hypertension [160].

Animal studies suggest that gut dysbiosis is associated with arterial hypertension both directly and indirectly. Change in microbial diversity such as the ratio of *Firmicutes* to *Bacteroidetes* in the intestine yields a potential mechanism in hypertension formation and a pathway for future treatment. By fermentation of fibers, these bacteria produce short-chain fatty acids (SCFAs) such as propionate and butyrate [161].

SCFAs play an important role in homeostasis, including blood pressure variations, through their interaction with certain receptors: G-protein-coupled receptors (GPCRs), such as Gpr41 or Olfr78. Studies on mice null for Olfr78 led to the conclusion that those animals were hypotensive, while mice null for Gpr41 were hypertensive [162].

In a metabolomic analysis of prehypertensive and hypertensive patients, it was shown that overgrowth of opportunistic bacteria, such as *Klebsiella* and *Prevotella copri,* was present in prehypertensive (pHTN) patients compared to healthy individuals, where higher levels of *Faecalibacterium, Bifidobacterium, Roseburia* and *Butyrivibrio* were found. This suggests alteration of the microbial profile occurs well before clinical findings. Probiotics and antibiotics could be proven as potential therapies for BP. Furthermore, small-scale fecal transplant from hypertensive patients to germ-free mice has led to higher blood pressure levels compared to controls [163].

Atrial fibrillation (AF) is another important CVD that has been linked in recent studies with dysbiosis. Patients with persistent AF manifest an increase in *Ruminococcus, Streptococcus,* and *Enterococcus,* and bacteria, such as *Faecali bacterium, Oscillobacter,* and *Biliophilus,* were decreased [164]. An imbalance of microbiota leads to damage in the intestinal barrier function that in turn can promote atrial electrical remodeling by increasing the activity of NLRP3 inflammasome [165, 166].

A metagenomic analysis by Zhang et al. 2021 in a cohort of patients with AF showed that species with SCFA-synthesis enzymes such as *Coprococcus catus* and *Firmicutes bacterium* were decreased in the gut of AF patients compared to controls. Furthermore, homeostasis of gut microbiota metabolites such as bile acids can modulate the risk of AF [167].

3.5 Obesity and diabetes mellitus

The microbiota of obese individuals significantly differs in composition and function from that of healthy individuals [168]. Thus, the microbiota of obese people is characterized by an increased ratio of *Firmicutes* vs. *Bacteroidetes*, mainly *Ruminiococcus, Candida*, and *Lactobacillus* [169, 170], increased amount of *Actinobacteria*, which produce SCFA and *Proteobacteria* [171]. Human studies have shown that obese people had more *Firmicutes* and approximately 90% fewer *Bacteroidetes* and a low-fat or low-carbohydrate diet can restore the *Firmicutes* to *Bacteroidetes* ratio but never be the same as the people that were lean from the beginning [169]. Some other studies demonstrated that a higher caloric intake increased *Firmicutes* by 20% and reduced *Bacteroidetes* by 20%, leading to a gain in body weight [172]. Studies on infants observed that obese children have a lower level of *Bifidobacterial* and a higher level of *Staphylococcus aureus* [173].

As it is already known, the diet has an important role in modulating microbiota composition, in both healthy and obese people. Some types of diets, like the Western diet, can modify microbiota, especially by increasing *Firmicutes* levels, leading to dysbiosis, metabolic stress, and obesity [174, 175]. Compared to the Western diet, a diet based on dietary fiber, plant polysaccharides, and lower fat and animal protein is characterized by a lower level of *Firmicutes* and a higher level of *Bacteroidetes* [28, 176]. Importantly, some mice and human studies underlined that a high-fat/high-sugar Western diet can modify the microbiota in just 1 day [177, 178]. Chen J et al. 2019 have shown that dietary intake has more impact on microbiota changes in mice than genetic etiology [179]. Moreover, Pols et al. 2011 have demonstrated that an improper diet has significantly negative consequences leading to the disappearance of species and strains of microbiota [180].

The obesity-microbiota relationship and its mechanisms have been studied for a long time [168] Many studies have shown that alterations in the microbiota community modify the process of energy extraction from food and consequently the adiposity of the body [176]. The gut microbiota of obese people has a larger capacity for absorbing energy from meals, thus their gut bacteria lead to weight growth [170]. Some studies have shown that gut microbiota can influence adiposity by modulating host gene expression, metabolic and inflammatory pathways, and gut-brain axis [181]. Inflammation mediated by gut microbiota can increase circulating lipopolysaccharide (LPS) levels and gut permeability and thus adipose tissue inflammation, commonly seen in obesity [182]. Microbiota metabolites like SCFA are increased in obese people, being involved in glucose homeostasis (improving glucose sensitivity) and lipid metabolism through free-fatty acid receptors, leading to activation of hepatic gluconeogenesis and lipogenesis [183] and inhibition of fatty acid oxidation in muscles [184]. Nondigestible carbohydrates can increase SCFA levels, which can modify the level of enteric hormones [185]. Alterations of the microbiota can reduce organisms that temper CD36 expression, such as products produced by *Clostridia*, which can increase lipid absorption, leading to obesity and metabolic syndrome [186]. Microbiota dysbiosis can reduce fasting-induced adipose factor expression, being involved in lipoprotein lipase (LPL) activation with lipid accumulation in adipose tissue [187]. Gut bacteria influence two key signaling pathways, glycemic reaction component binding domain, and cholesterol control component related proteins causing fat accumulation in the liver, where lipids can be then absorbed via visceral fat, thanks to LPL [170]. A lack of dietary fiber and poorly digestible carbohydrates reduce the diversity of bacterial flora [188]. Some studies have shown that lower microbiota diversity is associated with increased abdominal adiposity [189], but can be reversible in humans with cardiorespiratory fitness [190]. Human studies underlined that obese humans have a low fecal bacterial diversity, promoting adiposity, dyslipidemia, impaired glucose homeostasis, and higher low-grade inflammation [191]. Hormonal, neurological, and immunological pathways connect the brain with the microbiota [170]. Microbiota can modulate the synthesis of neuropeptides like dopamine, which regulate gastrointestinal function and thus can influence cognitive activity and increase hunger [192]. Among the metabolites secreted by the microbiota, serotonin, and γ-aminobutyric acid (GABA) control appetite and body weight regulation [193]. Alterations of the intestinal microbiota can modify the secretion of gastrointestinal hormones, such as glucagon-like-peptide-1 (GLP-1), which is involved in food intake control [194]. The dysbiosis of the microbiota in obese people can increase the level of acetate, enhancing the secretion of glucose-stimulated insulin and ghrelin, consequently increasing obesity [195]. Some studies underlined that the risk of obesity is associated with prenatal and perinatal antibiotic use by influencing microbial colonization and maturation [196].

Obesity-microbiota relationship and especially dysbiosis is associated with the risk of developing some other health problems, like diabetes mellitus (DM) [168, 197].

Schwartz et al. 2016 included for the first time gut microbiota modification as a mechanism implicated in DM [198]. The gut microbiota has an important role in influencing the immunologic system and developing type 1 DM (T1DM), as also as in developing metabolic disorders such as type 2 DM (T2DM) [197]. DM is considered an inflammatory clinical entity, characterized by inflammatory mechanisms that involve lipid accumulation, cytokines synthesized by a dysfunctional adipose tissue, a dysregulated immune system, as also as increased levels of inflammatory markers, such as C-reactive protein, Tumor Necrosis Factor-α, interleukins 6, 17 and 23, and Transforming Growth Factor β [199–201].

Studies have underlined that SCFAs, bile acid, branched-chain amino acids, imidazole propionate, and LPS have an important role in DM, among these the release of LPS with pro-inflammatory effects and decrease in SCFA production is the phenomena discussed in DM patients [197, 202].

In the case of dysbiosis, the LPS secreted by gram-negative bacteria from the gut generates a low-grade inflammatory state by interacting with type 4 toll-like receptors, increasing the risk of insulin resistance [203]. Physiological, the intestinal wall prevents the passage of LPS into the systemic circulation. High-fat diets increase the permeability of the intestinal wall and LPS circulation, by influencing the distribution of binding protein complexes and excessive and chronic production of biliary acids [197]. LPS binds then with the lipopolysaccharide-binding proteins and interacts with a membrane protein of differentiation 4, allowing the activation of TLR. A signaling cascade is then stimulated and focal adhesion kinase is phosphorylated and activated. In systemic circulations, LPS binds the TLR-4 in the membranes of immune and adipose cells, including pancreatic betta-cells, releasing TNF-α, IL-1, and IL-6, which can induce insulin resistance [204, 205].

Increased levels of *Firmicutes* in obese individuals, as was already mentioned, generate energy harvest, positive energy balance, and higher caloric bioavailability, leading to weight gain [197]. Modifications of *Firmicutes* to *Bacteroidetes* ratio have also been present in DM patients, being characterized by increased levels of *Bacteroidetes* [206], which are associated with decreased levels of *Akkermansia municiphila* [207]. Studies have observed an increased level of *Clostridium* and *Veillonella* genre in kids with T1DM, which ferment glucose and form propionate, succinate, and acetate from lactate and increase gut permeability [208]. Patients with DM and chronic pancreatitis have a low level of *Fecalibacterium prausnitzii*, which has anti-inflammatory properties and stimulate the synthesis of binding proteins [209]. Low levels of *R. bromii* have been observed in patients with DM, leading to the production of butyrate and energy [210]. T2DM is characterized especially by increased levels of *Bifidobacterium* and *Bacteroides* and to a lesser extent by *Faecalibacterium, Akkermansia, Roseburia, Ruminococcus, Fusobacterium,* and *Blautia* [211]. In patients with gestational diabetes mellitus, it was observed an increase in *Firmicutes* levels and a decrease in *Bacteroidetes* and *Actinobacteria* levels [212].

SCFAs are involved in T2DM by their immunomodulatory functions, but also stimulate the secretion of peptides that regulate the appetite and satiety, like GLP-1, the YY peptide, and ghrelin [213, 214]. In dysbiosis induced by a high-fat diet, it has been observed a decreased level of *Lactobacillus* and an increased level of *Bacteroides, Bukholderia*, and *Clostridium*, leading to an increased level of GLP-1 [215] and SCFA acetate, which affects insulin secretion, leading to obesity, hyperlipidemia, and insulin resistance [197, 216]. Studies have shown that increased levels of *Eubacterium* and *Roseburia* intestinalis in association with abnormal production and absorption of propionate, as also as postprandial insulin secretion and propionate generation in feces stimulated by butyrate, can increase the risk of T2DM [202].

Gut microbiota plays an important role in obesity and DM, especially in the case of dysbiosis, which influences the inflammatory and immune response, but also their pathophysiology. Throughout life gut microbiota is influenced by a lot of factors and has an important role in energy balance, being connected to obesity. Greater levels of LPS and lower levels of SCFA are the main characteristics of DM patients. Many mechanisms implicated in an obesity-microbiota-DM relationship were discussed in studies, a lot of them being still unwell known, so future research needs to investigate the function of the intestinal flora and its link to obesity and DM [170, 217].

3.6 Dermatological conditions

The skin, together with the intestinal epithelium, represent the largest interfaces between the body and the external environment, being the place where the most important processes of immune tolerance take place, allowing their colonization with essential commensal microorganisms that form the skin and gut microbiota [218, 219]. Thus, their alterations are associated with the appearance or progression of numerous inflammatory dermatological diseases, such as psoriasis, atopic dermatitis (AD), hidradenitis suppurativa (HS), acne, rosacea, alopecia areata, skin cancers, and seborrheic dermatitis [218]. Although most research groups have focused on the changes in the skin microbiota associated with dermatological diseases, recent studies have also observed alterations also in intestinal microbiota, probably through the systemic modulations determined by secreted molecules with the hormonal role and through the cells of the immune system [219, 220].

One of the most studied dermatological conditions associated with changes in the intestinal microbiota is psoriasis, a chronic inflammatory dermatosis, characterized by numerous pruritic, erythematous-scaly patches and plaques, distributed especially on the extension areas, associated or not with articular involvement [221]. Thus, a study conducted on a group of 30 patients with psoriasis and 30 healthy volunteers that evaluated the composition of the intestinal microbiota, observed that, although there is no difference statistically significant in terms of the type of bacteria in the analyzed samples (alpha diversity), their proportion is statistically significantly different between the two groups. Thus, the group with psoriasis showed an increase in the proportion of the families *Veillonellaceae* and *Ruminococcaceae* ($p < 0.05$) and of the genera *Faecalibacterium* and *Megamonas* ($p < 0.05$) compared to the healthy group [222]. The number of some of the microorganisms (*Bacteroides, Escherichia*, respectively *Dialister*) also seems to correlate negatively with different paraclinical markers like complement 3 (C3) ($p < 0.01$) respectively Interleukin 2 Receptor (IL2R) ($p < 0.001$). Moreover, *Prevotella*, respectively *Phascolarctobacterium* positively correlates positively with the level of C3 ($p < 0.01$), respectively IL2R ($p < 0.001$) [222]. Tan et al. 2015, observed a decrease in the classes of microorganisms *Mollicutes* and *Verrucomicrobiae* and the genus *Akkermansia* (species *Akkermansia muciniphila*), as well as an increase in the genera *Enterococcus* and *Bacteroides* in a study conducted on a group of 14 patients with psoriasis and 14 healthy volunteers [223].

Another study conducted by Hidalgo-Cantabrana et al. 2019 on a group of 19 patients with psoriasis and 20 healthy patients also highlighted the presence of the same phyla as in a healthy population, similar to the studies above. However, unlike Tan et al. [76], the populations of *Bacteroidetes* and *Proteobacteria* were lower than in the control group ($p < 0.001$), and *Actinobacteria* and *Firmicutes* were in a larger number ($p < 0.001$). This study also highlighted a decrease in *Verrucomicrobacteria* [224]. Scher et al. 2015 evaluated the variability of the microbiota in patients with early psoriatic arthritis, compared to patients with psoriasis and healthy patients, and found a decrease in *Akkermansia* and *Ruminoccocus* in those with psoriatic arthritis compared to patients with psoriasis. In the latter, a decrease in *Bacteroidetes* and *Coprobacillus* was observed. Also, lower levels of medium-chain fatty acids (involved in cell signaling) were found in patients with psoriatic arthritis ($p < 0.05$) and in those with psoriasis ($p < 0.01$) compared to the control group [225].

Regarding atopic dermatitis (AD), numerous studies evaluate both the changes in the microbiota, as well as the impact of the administration of probiotics on the evolution and severity of the disease. Thus, it was found that 1-week-old newborns who were later diagnosed with IgE-mediated eczema showed a decrease in *Enterobacteriaceae, Escherichia-Shigella* (statistically insignificant), and *Ruminococcaceae* ($p = 0.0047$). It was also found that the mothers of these children had an increased level of microorganisms from the *Bacilli* class and the *Streptoccocus* genus [226, 227]. AD was also associated in patients under 20 years, with a decrease in *Clostridium, Streptococcus, Enterobacteriaceae,* and *Bifidobacterium* ($p = 0.006$). Moreover, more severe forms of the disease were associated with a lower number of

Bifidobacterium ($p = 0.046$) and a higher number of *Bacteroides* ($p = 0.0443$) compared to children with average manifestations of AD [228]. Another study carried out on a pediatric population (28 children aged 6 months old with AD) demonstrates the existence of a statistically significant correlation between the severity of the disease and the decrease in the number of bacterial species in the microbiota ($r = -0.54$, $p = 0.002$). Moreover, the administration of hydrolyzed casein in these patients led to an improvement in the clinical score and the composition of the microbiota [229].

Another dermatological condition with a significant impact on the quality of life, in which the microbiota seems to play an important role is hidradenitis suppurativa (HS). Thus, in those patients, a decrease in the diversity of the intestinal bacterial flora was also found, but with an increase in *Ruminoccocus gnavus*, which also appears to increase in other inflammatory digestive or articular diseases [230]. Kam et al. also observed a decrease in the phylum *Firmicutes* compared to the healthy population ($p = 0.03$), with changes in the genera *Lachobacterium* and *Veillonella* in the same direction ($p = 0.019$, respectively $p = 0.005$). The genera *Biophila* and *Holdemania* were found in a higher proportion of these patients, although the small number of patients on which the study was conducted (3) makes it difficult to interpret the data [231]. Another difference between the microbiota of HS patients compared to healthy ones was highlighted by Lam et al. 2021 in a study carried out on 17 patients with HS. He observed colonization with *Robinsoniella* only in patients with HS, not in the healthy group, but also a greater number of microorganisms from the *Sellimonas* genus in these patients. The latter was also associated with the presence of several inflammatory joint diseases [232].

The immunological, neurological, and biochemical interrelations between skin and gut, explained by the existence of the skin-gut axis are also reflected in the way in which microbiota alterations are present in various dermatological inflammatory pathologies. Although the current studies show changes in the proportions of bacteria from the intestinal microbiota, the small groups of patients, as well as the contradictory data from some studies prevent us from drawing clear conclusions and associating changes in specific genera or species with certain diseases.

4. Conclusion and future perspectives

Although the complex mechanisms between gut dysbiosis and the etiology and progression of numerous systemic diseases are not fully understood and there are clear indications that gut homeostasis is very important. Future research is needed addressing also animal models and clinical trials to restore the microflora normal balance and gut mucosal barrier integrity in order to maintain health. As microbiomics develops as an equivalent of human genomics and the microbiome is seen as a second genome in the human body considered nowadays as a holobiont (the host organism and its microbiome), one can consider this as a very promising future step toward precision medicine. The continuous development of next-generation sequencing (NGS) technologies will allow us to gain new insights and perspectives about how to influence and modulate the microbiome through noninvasive procedures, such as prebiotics, probiotics, and dietary lifestyle changes.

Conflict of interest

The authors declare no conflict of interest.

Acronyms and abbreviations

AF	atrial fibrillation
AD	atopic dermatitis
apoE	apolipoprotein E
SCFAs	short-chain fatty acids
RS	resistant starch
TNF	tumor necrosis factor
IL	interleukin
NK	natural killer
IECs	intestinal epithelial cells
ROS	reactive oxidative species
RNS	reactive nitrogen species
CVD	cardiovascular disease
LPS	lipopolysaccharides
TMAO	trimethylamine-N-oxide
FXR	farnesoid X nuclear receptor
SHP	small heterodimer partner
BA	bile acids
BSH	bile-salt hydrolase
F/B	*Firmicutes/Bacteroidetes* ratio
GPCRs	G-protein-coupled receptors
GABA	aminobutyric acid
LPS	lipopolysaccharide
GLP-1	glucagon-like-peptide-1
DM	diabetes mellitus
T1DM	type 1 DM
T2DM	type 2 DM
HS	hidradenitis suppurativa
C3	complement 3
NGS	next-generation sequencing
pHTN	prehypertensive
HFrEF	heart failure with reduced ejection fraction

Author details

Ruxandra Florentina Ionescu[1,2], Elena Codruta Cozma[3,4], Robert Mihai Enache[5], Sanda Maria Cretoiu[2*], Maria Iancu[6], Matei Mandea[7,8], Monica Profir[9], Oana Alexandra Roşu[9] and Bogdan Severus Gaspar[10,11*]

1 Department of Cardiology I, "Dr. Carol Davila" Central Military Emergency Hospital, Bucharest, Romania

2 Department of Morphological Sciences, Cell and Molecular Biology and Histology, "Carol Davila" University of Medicine and Pharmacy, Bucharest, Romania

3 Department of Pathophysiology, University of Medicine and Pharmacy of Craiova, Craiova, Romania

4 Department of Dermatology, Elias Emergency University Hospital, Bucharest, Romania

5 Department of Radiology and Medical Imaging, Fundeni Clinical Institute, Bucharest, Romania

6 "Prof. Dr. C.C.Iliescu" Emergency Institute for Cardiovascular Diseases, Romania

7 Fundeni Clincal Institute, Bucharest, Romania

8 "Carol Davila" University of Medicine and Pharmacy, Bucharest, Romania

9 Department of Oncology, Elias University Emergency Hospital, Bucharest, Romania

10 Department of Surgery, "Carol Davila" University of Medicine and Pharmacy, Bucharest, Romania

11 Surgery Clinic, Bucharest Emergency Clinical Hospital, Bucharest, Romania

*Address all correspondence to: sanda@cretoiu.ro and bogdan.gaspar@umfcd.ro

References

[1] Kumar PS. Microbiomics: Were we all wrong before? Periodontology 2000. 2021;**85**(1):8-11. DOI: 10.1111/prd.12373

[2] Rasmussen TT, Kirkeby LP, Poulsen K, Reinholdt J, Kilian M. Resident aerobic microbiota of the adult human nasal cavity. APMIS. 2000;**108**(10):663-675. DOI: 10.1034/j.1600-0463.2000.d01-13.x

[3] Diop K, Dufour J-C, Levasseur A, Fenollar F. Exhaustive repertoire of human vaginal microbiota. Human Microbiome Journal. 2019;**11**:100051. DOI: 10.1016/j.humic.2018.11.002

[4] Toson B, Simon C, Moreno I. The endometrial microbiome and its impact on human conception. International Journal of Molecular Sciences. 2022;**23**(1):485. DOI: 10.3390/ijms23010485

[5] Dong Q, Brulc JM, Iovieno A, Bates B, Garoutte A, Miller D, et al. Diversity of bacteria at healthy human conjunctiva. Investigative Ophthalmology & Visual Science. 2011;**52**(8):5408-5413. DOI: 10.1167/iovs.10-6939

[6] Moffatt MF, Cookson WO. The lung microbiome in health and disease. Clinical Medicine (London, England). 2017;**17**(6):525-529. DOI: 10.7861/clinmedicine.17-6-525

[7] Ionescu RF, Enache RM, Cretoiu SM, Cretoiu D. The interplay between gut microbiota and miRNAs in cardiovascular diseases. Frontiers in Cardiovascular Medicine. 2022;**9**:856901. DOI: 10.3389/fcvm.2022.856901

[8] Parello CSL. 6 - Microbiomics. In: Sonis ST, Villa A, editors. Translational Systems Medicine and Oral Disease. United Kingdom: Academic Press, Elsevier Inc.; 2020. pp. 137-162. DOI: 10.1016/B978-0-12-813762-8.00006-2

[9] Feng Q, Chen W-D, Wang Y-D. Gut microbiota: An integral moderator in health and disease. Frontiers in Microbiology. 2018;**9**:151. DOI: 10.3389/fmicb.2018.00151

[10] Mariat D, Firmesse O, Levenez F, Guimarães V, Sokol H, Doré J, et al. The firmicutes/bacteroidetes ratio of the human microbiota changes with age. BMC Microbiology. 2009;**9**:123. DOI: 10.1186/1471-2180-9-123

[11] The Human Microbiome Project Consortium. Structure, function and diversity of the healthy human microbiome. Nature. 2012;**486**(7402):207-214. DOI: 10.1038/nature11234

[12] Segata N, Haake SK, Mannon P, Lemon KP, Waldron L, Gevers D, et al. Composition of the adult digestive tract bacterial microbiome based on seven mouth surfaces, tonsils, throat and stool samples. Genome Biology. 2012;**13**(6):R42. DOI: 10.1186/gb-2012-13-6-r42

[13] Jia G, Zhi A, Lai PFH, Wang G, Xia Y, Xiong Z, et al. The oral microbiota - a mechanistic role for systemic diseases. British Dental Journal. 2018;**224**(6):447-455. DOI: 10.1038/sj.bdj.2018.217

[14] Grice EA, Kong HH, Conlan S, Deming CB, Davis J, Young AC, et al. Topographical and temporal diversity of the human skin microbiome. Science. 2009;**324**(5931):1190-1192. DOI: 10.1126/science.1171700

[15] Byrd AL, Belkaid Y, Segre JA. The human skin microbiome. Nature Reviews

Microbiology. 2018;**16**(3):143-155. DOI: 10.1038/nrmicro.2017.157

[16] Ling Z, Kong J, Liu F, Zhu H, Chen X, Wang Y, et al. Molecular analysis of the diversity of vaginal microbiota associated with bacterial vaginosis. BMC Genomics. 2010;**11**:488. DOI: 10.1186/1471-2164-11-488

[17] Voravuthikunchai SP, Bilasoi S, Supamala O. Antagonistic activity against pathogenic bacteria by human vaginal lactobacilli. Anaerobe. 2006;**12**(5-6):221-226. DOI: 10.1016/j.anaerobe.2006.06.003

[18] Ravel J, Gajer P, Abdo Z, Schneider GM, Koenig SS, McCulle SL, et al. Vaginal microbiome of reproductive-age women. Proceedings of the National Academy of Sciences of the United States of America. 2011;**108**(Suppl 1):4680-4687. DOI: 10.1016/j.anaerobe.2006.06.003

[19] Franasiak JM, Scott RT. Reproductive tract microbiome in assisted reproductive technologies. Fertility and Sterility. 2015;**104**(6):1364-1371. DOI: 10.1016/j.fertnstert.2015.10.012

[20] Li JJ, Yi S, Wei L. Ocular microbiota and intraocular inflammation. Frontiers in Immunology. 2020;**11**:609765. DOI: 10.3389/fimmu.2020.609765

[21] Qin J, Li R, Raes J, Arumugam M, Burgdorf KS, Manichanh C, et al. A human gut microbial gene catalogue established by metagenomic sequencing. Nature. 2010;**464**(7285):59-65. DOI: 10.1038/nature08821

[22] Joseph J, Loscalzo J. Nutri(meta) genetics and cardiovascular disease: novel concepts in the interaction of diet and genomic variation. Current Atherosclerosis Reports. 2015;**17**(5):505. DOI: 10.1007/s11883-015-0505-x

[23] Novakovic M, Rout A, Kingsley T, Kirchoff R, Singh A, Verma V, et al. Role of gut microbiota in cardiovascular diseases. World Journal of Cardiology. 2020;**12**(4):110-122. DOI: 10.4330/wjc.v12.i4.110

[24] Badal VD, Vaccariello ED, Murray ER, Yu KE, Knight R, Jeste DV, et al. The gut microbiome, aging, and longevity: A systematic review. Nutrients. 2020;**12**(12):3759. DOI: 10.3390/nu12123759

[25] Tuikhar N, Keisam S, Labala RK, Imrat RP, Arunkumar MC, et al. Comparative analysis of the gut microbiota in centenarians and young adults shows a common signature across genotypically non-related populations. Mechanisms of Ageing and Development. 2019;**179**:23-35. DOI: 10.1016/j.mad.2019.02.001

[26] Salazar N, Arboleya S, Fernández-Navarro T, de Los Reyes-Gavilán CG, Gonzalez S, Gueimonde M. Age-associated changes in gut microbiota and dietary components related with the immune system in adulthood and old age: A cross-sectional study. Nutrients. 2019;**11**(8). DOI: 10.3390/nu11081765

[27] David LA, Maurice CF, Carmody RN, Gootenberg DB, Button JE, Wolfe BE, et al. Diet rapidly and reproducibly alters the human gut microbiome. Nature. 2014;**505**(7484):559-563. DOI: 10.1038/nature12820

[28] De Filippo C, Cavalieri D, Di Paola M, Ramazzotti M, Poullet JB, Massart S, et al. Impact of diet in shaping gut microbiota revealed by a comparative study in children from Europe and rural Africa. Proceedings of the National Academy of Sciences of the United States of America. 2010;**107**(33):14691-14696. DOI: 10.1073/pnas.1005963107

[29] Schnorr SL, Candela M, Rampelli S, Centanni M, Consolandi C, Basaglia G, et al. Gut microbiome of the Hadza hunter-gatherers. Nature Communications. 2014;**5**:3654. DOI: 10.1038/ncomms4654

[30] Guo X, Huang C, Xu J, Xu H, Liu L, Zhao H, et al. Gut microbiota is a potential biomarker in inflammatory bowel disease. Frontiers in Nutrition. 2021;**8**:818902. DOI: 10.3389/fnut.2021.818902

[31] Antoniussen CS, Rasmussen HH, Holst M, Lauridsen C. Reducing disease activity of inflammatory bowel disease by consumption of plant-based foods and nutrients. Frontiers in Nutrition. 2021;**8**:733433. DOI: 10.3389/fnut.2021.733433

[32] Zuo T, Ng SC. The gut microbiota in the pathogenesis and therapeutics of inflammatory bowel disease. Frontiers in Microbiology. 2018;**9**:2247. DOI: 10.3389/fmicb.2018.02247

[33] Silva FA, Rodrigues BL, Ayrizono ML, Leal RF. The immunological basis of inflammatory bowel disease. Gastroenterology Research and Practice. 2016;**2016**:2097274. DOI: 10.1155/2016/2097274

[34] Santana PT, Rosas SLB, Ribeiro BE, Marinho Y, de Souza HSP. Dysbiosis in inflammatory bowel disease: Pathogenic role and potential therapeutic targets. International Journal of Molecular Sciences. 2022;**23**(7):3464. DOI: 10.3390/ijms23073464

[35] Sultan S, El-Mowafy M, Elgaml A, Ahmed TAE, Hassan H, Mottawea W. Metabolic influences of gut microbiota dysbiosis on inflammatory bowel disease. Frontiers in Physiology. 2021;**12**:715506. DOI: 10.3389/fphys.2021.715506

[36] Guzzo GL, Andrews JM, Weyrich LS. The neglected gut microbiome: Fungi, protozoa, and bacteriophages in inflammatory bowel disease. Inflammatory Bowel Diseases. 2022;**28**(7):1112-1122. DOI: 10.1093/ibd/izab343

[37] Jarmakiewicz-Czaja S, Zielińska M, Sokal A, Filip R. Genetic and epigenetic etiology of inflammatory bowel disease: An update. Genes. 2022;**13**(12):2388. DOI: 10.3390/genes13122388

[38] Tavakoli P, Vollmer-Conna U, Hadzi-Pavlovic D, Grimm MC. A Review of inflammatory bowel disease: A model of microbial, immune and neuropsychological integration. Public Health Reviews. 2021;**42**:1603990. DOI: 10.3389/phrs.2021.1603990

[39] Hisamatsu T, Kanai T, Mikami Y, Yoneno K, Matsuoka K, Hibi T. Immune aspects of the pathogenesis of inflammatory bowel disease. Pharmacology & Therapeutics. 2013;**137**(3):283-297. DOI: 10.1016/j.pharmthera.2012.10.008

[40] Shepherd FR, McLaren JE. T Cell immunity to bacterial pathogens: Mechanisms of immune control and bacterial evasion. International Journal of Molecular Sciences. 2020;**21**(17). DOI: 10.3390/ijms21176144

[41] Atarashi K, Tanoue T, Oshima K, Suda W, Nagano Y, Nishikawa H, et al. Treg induction by a rationally selected mixture of Clostridia strains from the human microbiota. Nature. 2013;**500**(7461):232-236. DOI: 10.1038/nature12331

[42] Halfvarson J, Brislawn CJ, Lamendella R, Vázquez-Baeza Y, Walters WA, Bramer LM, et al. Dynamics of the human gut microbiome in inflammatory bowel disease. Nature Microbiology. 2017;**2**:17004. DOI: 10.1038/nmicrobiol.2017.4

[43] Yilmaz B, Spalinger MR, Biedermann L, Franc Y, Fournier N, Rossel J-B, et al. The presence of genetic risk variants within PTPN2 and PTPN22 is associated with intestinal microbiota alterations in Swiss IBD cohort patients. PLoS One. 2018;**13**(7):e0199664. DOI: 10.1371/journal.pone.0199664

[44] Li E, Zhang Y, Tian X, Wang X, Gathungu G, Wolber A, et al. Influence of Crohn's disease related polymorphisms in innate immune function on ileal microbiome. PLoS One. 2019;**14**(2):e0213108. DOI: 10.1371/journal.pone.0213108

[45] Alshehri D, Saadah O, Mosli M, Edris S, Alhindi R, Bahieldin A. Dysbiosis of gut microbiota in inflammatory bowel disease: Current therapies and potential for microbiota-modulating therapeutic approaches. Bosnian Journal of Basic Medical Sciences. 2021;**21**(3):270-283. DOI: 10.17305/bjbms.2020.5016

[46] Torun A, Hupalowska A, Trzonkowski P, Kierkus J, Pyrzynska B. Intestinal microbiota in common chronic inflammatory disorders affecting children. Frontiers in Immunology. 2021;**12**:642166. DOI: 10.3389/fimmu.2021.642166

[47] Morgan XC, Tickle TL, Sokol H, Gevers D, Devaney KL, Ward DV, et al. Dysfunction of the intestinal microbiome in inflammatory bowel disease and treatment. Genome Biology. 2012;**13**(9):R79. DOI: 10.1186/gb-2012-13-9-r79

[48] Banfi D, Moro E, Bosi A, Bistoletti M, Cerantola S, Crema F, et al. Impact of microbial metabolites on microbiota-gut-brain axis in inflammatory bowel disease. International Journal of Molecular Sciences. 2021;**22**(4):1623. DOI: 10.3390/ijms22041623

[49] Yang M, Gu Y, Li L, Liu T, Song X, Sun Y, et al. Bile acid–gut microbiota axis in inflammatory bowel disease: From bench to bedside. Nutrients. 2021;**13**(9):3143. DOI: 10.3390/nu13093143

[50] Akram W, Garud N, Joshi R. Role of inulin as prebiotics on inflammatory bowel disease. Drug Discoveries & Therapeutics. 2019;**13**(1):1-8. DOI: 10.5582/ddt.2019.01000

[51] Sartor RB, Wu GD. Roles for intestinal bacteria, viruses, and fungi in pathogenesis of inflammatory bowel diseases and therapeutic approaches. Gastroenterology. 2017;**152**(2):327-39.e4. DOI: 10.1053/j.gastro.2016.10.012

[52] Mu C, Zhu W. Antibiotic effects on gut microbiota, metabolism, and beyond. Applied Microbiology and Biotechnology. 2019;**103**(23):9277-9285. DOI: 10.1007/s00253-019-10165-x

[53] Stojek M, Jabłońska A, Adrych K. The role of fecal microbiota transplantation in the treatment of inflammatory bowel disease. Journal of Clinical Medicine. 2021;**10**(18):4055. DOI: 10.3390/jcm10184055

[54] Sokol H, Landman C, Seksik P, Berard L, Montil M, Nion-Larmurier I, et al. Fecal microbiota transplantation to maintain remission in Crohn's disease: A pilot randomized controlled study. Microbiome. 2020;**8**(1):12. DOI: 10.1186/s40168-020-0792-5

[55] Paramsothy S, Paramsothy R, Rubin DT, Kamm MA, Kaakoush NO, Mitchell HM, et al. Faecal microbiota transplantation for inflammatory bowel disease: A systematic review and meta-analysis. Journal of Crohn's and Colitis. 2017;**11**(10):1180-1199. DOI: 10.1093/ecco-jcc/jjx063

[56] Li Q, Ding X, Liu K, Marcella C, Liu X, Zhang T, et al. Fecal Microbiota transplantation for ulcerative colitis: The optimum timing and gut microbiota as predictors for long-term clinical outcomes. Clinical and Translational Gastroenterology. 2020;**11**(8):e00224. DOI: 10.14309/ctg.0000000000000224

[57] Kelly CR, Fischer M, Allegretti JR, LaPlante K, Stewart DB, Limketkai BN, et al. ACG Clinical guidelines: Prevention, Diagnosis, and Treatment of Clostridioides difficile Infections. The American Journal of Gastroenterology. 2021;**116**(6):1124-1147. DOI: 10.14309/ajg.0000000000001278

[58] Chicco F, Magrì S, Cingolani A, Paduano D, Pesenti M, Zara F, et al. Multidimensional impact of mediterranean diet on IBD patients. Inflammatory Bowel Diseases. 2021;**27**(1):1-9. DOI: 10.1093/ibd/izaa097

[59] Gill PA, Inniss S, Kumagai T, Rahman FZ, Smith AM. The role of diet and gut microbiota in regulating gastrointestinal and inflammatory disease. Frontiers in Immunology. 2022;**13**:866059. DOI: 10.3389/fimmu.2022.866059

[60] Rapozo DC, Bernardazzi C, de Souza HS. Diet and microbiota in inflammatory bowel disease: The gut in disharmony. World Journal of Gastroenterology. 2017;**23**(12):2124-2140. DOI: 10.3748/wjg.v23.i12.2124

[61] Peppas S, Pansieri C, Piovani D, Danese S, Peyrin-Biroulet L, Tsantes AG, et al. The brain-gut axis: Psychological functioning and inflammatory bowel diseases. Journal of Clinical Medicine. 2021;**10**(3):377. DOI: 10.3390/jcm10030377

[62] Park S, Zhang T. A positive association of overactivated immunity with metabolic syndrome risk and mitigation of its association by a plant-based diet and physical activity in a large cohort study. Nutrients. 2021;**13**(7):2308. DOI: 10.3390/nu13072308

[63] Bhatia M. Inflammatory response on the pancreatic acinar cell injury. Scandinavian Journal of Surgery. 2005;**94**(2):97-102. DOI: 10.1177/145749690509400203

[64] Heckler M, Hackert T, Hu K, Halloran C, Büchler M, Neoptolemos J. Severe acute pancreatitis: surgical indications and treatment. Langenbeck's Archives of Surgery. 2021;**406**:521-535. DOI: 10.1007/s00423-020-01944-6

[65] Bhatia M. Acute pancreatitis as a model of SIRS. FBL. 2009;**14**(6):2042-2050. DOI: 10.2741/3362

[66] Carden DL, Granger DN. Pathophysiology of ischaemia-reperfusion injury. The Journal of Pathology. 2000;**190**(3):255-266. DOI: 10.1002/(SICI)1096-9896(200002)190:3<255::AID-PATH526>3.0.CO;2-6

[67] Bhatia M, Wong FL, Cao Y, Lau HY, Huang J, Puneet P, et al. Pathophysiology of acute pancreatitis. Pancreatology. 2005;**5**(2-3):132-144. DOI: 10.1159/000085265

[68] Thoeni RF. The revised Atlanta classification of acute pancreatitis: Its importance for the radiologist and its effect on treatment. Radiology. 2012;**262**(3):751-764. DOI: 10.1148/radiol.11110947

[69] Clemente JC, Manasson J, Scher JU. The role of the gut microbiome in systemic inflammatory disease. BMJ. 2018;**360**:j5145. DOI: 10.1136/bmj.j5145

[70] Liu H, Li W, Wang X, Li J, Yu W. Early gut mucosal dysfunction in patients

with acute pancreatitis. Pancreas. 2008;**36**(2):192-196. DOI: 10.1097/MPA.0b013e31815a399f

[71] Fishman JE, Levy G, Alli V, Zheng X, Mole DJ, Deitch EA. The intestinal mucus layer is a critical component of the gut barrier that is damaged during acute pancreatitis. Shock. 2014;**42**(3):264-270. DOI: 10.1097/shk.0000000000000209

[72] Capurso G, Zerboni G, Signoretti M, Valente R, Stigliano S, Piciucchi M, et al. Role of the gut barrier in acute pancreatitis. Journal of Clinical Gastroenterology. 2012;**46**(Suppl):S46-S51. DOI: 10.1097/MCG.0b013e3182652096

[73] Pietrzak B, Tomela K, Olejnik-Schmidt A, Mackiewicz A, Schmidt M. Secretory IgA in intestinal mucosal secretions as an adaptive barrier against microbial cells. International Journal of Molecular Sciences. 2020;**21**(23):9254. DOI: 10.3390/ijms21239254

[74] Bunker JJ, Flynn TM, Koval JC, Shaw DG, Meisel M, McDonald BD, et al. Innate and adaptive humoral responses coat distinct commensal bacteria with immunoglobulin A. Immunity. 2015;**43**(3):541-553. DOI: 10.1016/j.immuni.2015.08.007

[75] Yu S, Xiong Y, Xu J, Liang X, Fu Y, Liu D, et al. Identification of dysfunctional gut microbiota through rectal swab in patients with different severity of acute pancreatitis. Digestive Diseases and Sciences. 2020;**65**(11):3223-3237. DOI: 10.1007/s10620-020-06061-4

[76] Tan C, Ling Z, Huang Y, Cao Y, Liu Q, Cai T, et al. Dysbiosis of intestinal microbiota associated with inflammation involved in the progression of acute pancreatitis. Pancreas. 2015;**44**(6):868-875. DOI: 10.1097/MPA.0000000000000355

[77] Zhu Y, He C, Li X, Cai Y, Hu J, Liao Y, et al. Gut microbiota dysbiosis worsens the severity of acute pancreatitis in patients and mice. Journal of Gastroenterology. 2019;**54**(4):347-358. DOI: 10.1007/s00535-018-1529-0

[78] Cho I, Blaser MJ. The human microbiome: At the interface of health and disease. Nature Reviews. Genetics. 2012;**13**(4):260-270. DOI: 10.1038/nrg3182

[79] Parada Venegas D, De la Fuente MK, Landskron G, González MJ, Quera R, Dijkstra G, et al. Short chain fatty acids (SCFAs)-mediated gut epithelial and immune regulation and its relevance for inflammatory bowel diseases. Frontiers in Immunology. 2019;**10**:277. DOI: 10.3389/fimmu.2019.00277

[80] Li XY, He C, Zhu Y, Lu NH. Role of gut microbiota on intestinal barrier function in acute pancreatitis. World Journal of Gastroenterology. 2020;**26**(18):2187-2193. DOI: 10.3748/wjg.v26.i18.2187

[81] Li M, Liang P, Li Z, Wang Y, Zhang G, Gao H, et al. Fecal microbiota transplantation and bacterial consortium transplantation have comparable effects on the re-establishment of mucosal barrier function in mice with intestinal dysbiosis. Frontiers in Microbiology. 2015;**6**:692. DOI: 10.3389/fmicb.2015.00692

[82] Ding L, He C, Li X, Huang X, Lei Y, Ke H, et al. Efficacy and safety of faecal microbiota transplantation for acute pancreatitis: A randomised, controlled study. Frontiers in Medicine (Lausanne). 2021;**8**:772454. DOI: 10.3389/fmed.2021.772454

[83] Majumder S, Chari ST. Chronic pancreatitis. Lancet.

2016;**387**(10031):1957-1966. DOI: 10.1016/s0140-6736(16)00097-0

[84] Pitchumoni C. Interdependence of nutrition and exocrine pancreatic function. In: Vay Liang W. Go, et al., editors. The Pancreas: Biology, Pathobiology, and Disease. Second ed. New York: Raven Press Ltd; 1993. DOI: 10.1007/978-3-642-79167-3_48

[85] Pietzner M, Budde K, Rühlemann M, Völzke H, Homuth G, Weiss FU, et al. Exocrine pancreatic function modulates plasma metabolites through changes in gut microbiota composition. The Journal of Clinical Endocrinology & Metabolism. 2021;**106**(5):e2290-e22e8. DOI: 10.1210/clinem/dgaa961

[86] Frost F, Weiss FU, Sendler M, Kacprowski T, Rühlemann M, Bang C, et al. The gut microbiome in patients with chronic pancreatitis is characterized by significant dysbiosis and overgrowth by opportunistic pathogens. Clinical and Translational Gastroenterology. 2020;**11**(9):e00232. DOI: 10.14309/ctg.0000000000000232

[87] Akshintala VS, Talukdar R, Singh VK, Goggins M. The gut microbiome in pancreatic disease. Clinical Gastroenterology and Hepatology. 2019;**17**(2):290-295. DOI: 10.1016/j.cgh.2018.08.045

[88] Capurso G, Signoretti M, Archibugi L, Stigliano S, Delle FG. Systematic review and meta-analysis: Small intestinal bacterial overgrowth in chronic pancreatitis. United European Gastroenterology Journal. 2016;**4**(5):697-705. DOI: 10.1177/2050640616630117

[89] Ní Chonchubhair HM, Bashir Y, Dobson M, Ryan BM, Duggan SN, Conlon KC. The prevalence of small intestinal bacterial overgrowth in non-surgical patients with chronic pancreatitis and pancreatic exocrine insufficiency (PEI). Pancreatology. 2018;**18**(4):379-385. DOI: 10.1016/j.pan.2018.02.010

[90] Talukdar R, Jandhyala SM, Reddy R, Arutla M, Reddy D. Altered gut microbiota in patients with chronic pancreatitis is associated with gut barrier dysfunction and metabolic abnormalities. Clinical Gastroenterology and Hepatology. 2017;**15**:153. DOI: 10.1016/j.cgh.2016.09.023

[91] Morgan E, Arnold M, Gini A, Lorenzoni V, Cabasag CJ, Laversanne M, et al. Global burden of colorectal cancer in 2020 and 2040: Incidence and mortality estimates from GLOBOCAN. Gut. 2023;**72**(2):338. DOI: 10.1136/gutjnl-2022-327736

[92] Sánchez-Alcoholado L, Ramos-Molina B, Otero A, Laborda-Illanes A, Ordóñez R, Medina JA, et al. The role of the gut microbiome in colorectal cancer development and therapy response. Cancers (Basel). 2020;**12**(6):1406. DOI: 10.3390/cancers12061406

[93] Lichtenstein P, Holm NV, Verkasalo PK, Iliadou A, Kaprio J, Koskenvuo M, et al. Environmental and heritable factors in the causation of cancer--analyses of cohorts of twins from Sweden, Denmark, and Finland. The New England Journal of Medicine. 2000;**343**(2):78-85. DOI: 10.1056/nejm200007133430201

[94] Czene K, Lichtenstein P, Hemminki K. Environmental and heritable causes of cancer among 9.6 million individuals in the Swedish Family-Cancer Database. International Journal of Cancer. 2002;**99**(2):260-266. DOI: 10.1002/ijc.10332

[95] Rattray NJW, Charkoftaki G, Rattray Z, Hansen JE, Vasiliou V,

Johnson CH. Environmental influences in the etiology of colorectal cancer: The premise of metabolomics. Current Pharmacology Reports. 2017;**3**(3):114-125. DOI: 10.1007/s40495-017-0088-z

[96] Laqueur GL, McDaniel EG, Matsumoto H. Tumor induction in germfree rats with methylazoxymethanol (MAM) and synthetic MAM acetate. Journal of the National Cancer Institute. 1967;**39**(2):355-371. DOI: 10.1093/jnci/39.2.355

[97] Reddy BS, Narisawa T, Wright P, Vukusich D, Weisburger JH, Wynder EL. Colon carcinogenesis with azoxymethane and dimethylhydrazine in germ-free rats. Cancer Research. 1975;**35**(2):287-290

[98] Reddy BS, Narisawa T, Weisburger JH. Colon carcinogenesis in germ-free rats with intrarectal 1,2-dimethylhydrazine and subcutaneous azoxymethane. Cancer Research. 1976;**36**(8):2874-2876

[99] Wong SH, Yu J. Gut microbiota in colorectal cancer: Mechanisms of action and clinical applications. Nature Reviews Gastroenterology & Hepatology. 2019;**16**(11):690-704. DOI: 10.1038/s41575-019-0209-8

[100] Cheng Y, Ling Z, Li L. The intestinal microbiota and colorectal cancer. Frontiers in Immunology. 2020;**11**:615056. DOI: 10.3389/fimmu.2020.615056

[101] Saffarian A, Mulet C, Regnault B, Amiot A, Tran-Van-Nhieu J, Ravel J, et al. Crypt- and mucosa-associated core microbiotas in humans and their alteration in colon cancer patients. MBio. 2019;**10**(4):e01315-19. DOI: 10.1128/mBio.01315-19

[102] Chen W, Liu F, Ling Z, Tong X, Xiang C. Human intestinal lumen and mucosa-associated microbiota in patients with colorectal cancer. PLoS One. 2012;**7**(6):e39743. DOI: 10.1371/journal.pone.0039743

[103] Chung L, Thiele Orberg E, Geis AL, Chan JL, Fu K, DeStefano Shields CE, et al. Bacteroides fragilis toxin coordinates a pro-carcinogenic inflammatory cascade via targeting of colonic epithelial cells. Cell Host & Microbe. 2018;**23**(2):203-14.e5. DOI: 10.1016/j.chom.2018.01.007

[104] Dai Z, Coker OO, Nakatsu G, Wu WKK, Zhao L, Chen Z, et al. Multi-cohort analysis of colorectal cancer metagenome identified altered bacteria across populations and universal bacterial markers. Microbiome. 2018;**6**(1):70. DOI: 10.1186/s40168-018-0451-2

[105] Wirbel J, Pyl PT, Kartal E, Zych K, Kashani A, Milanese A, et al. Meta-analysis of fecal metagenomes reveals global microbial signatures that are specific for colorectal cancer. Nature Medicine. 2019;**25**(4):679-689. DOI: 10.1038/s41591-019-0406-6

[106] Thomas AM, Manghi P, Asnicar F, Pasolli E, Armanini F, Zolfo M, et al. Metagenomic analysis of colorectal cancer datasets identifies cross-cohort microbial diagnostic signatures and a link with choline degradation. Nature Medicine. 2019;**25**(4):667-678. DOI: 10.1038/s41591-019-0405-7

[107] Bashir A, Miskeen AY, Bhat A, Fazili KM, Ganai BA. Fusobacterium nucleatum: An emerging bug in colorectal tumorigenesis. European Journal of Cancer Prevention. 2015;**24**(5):373-385. DOI: 10.1097/cej.0000000000000116

[108] Mima K, Nishihara R, Qian ZR, Cao Y, Sukawa Y, Nowak JA, et al.

Fusobacterium nucleatum in colorectal carcinoma tissue and patient prognosis. Gut. 2016;**65**(12):1973-1980. DOI: 10.1136/gutjnl-2015-310101

[109] Wei Z, Cao S, Liu S, Yao Z, Sun T, Li Y, et al. Could gut microbiota serve as prognostic biomarker associated with colorectal cancer patients' survival? A pilot study on relevant mechanism. Oncotarget. 2016;**7**(29):46158-46172. DOI: 10.18632/oncotarget.10064

[110] Lo C-H, Wu D-C, Jao S-W, Wu C-C, Lin C-Y, Chuang C-H, et al. Enrichment of Prevotella intermedia in human colorectal cancer and its additive effects with Fusobacterium nucleatum on the malignant transformation of colorectal adenomas. Journal of Biomedical Science. 2022;**29**(1):88. DOI: 10.1186/s12929-022-00869-0

[111] Wang T, Cai G, Qiu Y, Fei N, Zhang M, Pang X, et al. Structural segregation of gut microbiota between colorectal cancer patients and healthy volunteers. The ISME Journal. 2012;**6**(2):320-329. DOI: 10.1038/ismej.2011.109

[112] Molska M, Reguła J. Potential mechanisms of probiotics action in the prevention and treatment of colorectal cancer. Nutrients. 2019;**11**(10). DOI: 10.3390/nu11102453

[113] Imen K, Meenakshi M, Alaoui-Jamali MA, Prakash S. In-Vitro characterization of the anti-cancer activity of the probiotic bacterium lactobacillus fermentum NCIMB 5221 and potential against colorectal cancer. Journal of Cancer Science & Therapy. 2015;**07**:224-235. DOI: 10.4172/1948-5956.1000354

[114] van Munster IP, Tangerman A, Nagengast FM. Effect of resistant starch on colonic fermentation, bile acid metabolism, and mucosal proliferation. Digestive Diseases and Sciences. 1994;**39**(4):834-842. DOI: 10.1007/bf02087431

[115] Dronamraju SS, Coxhead JM, Kelly SB, Burn J, Mathers JC. Cell kinetics and gene expression changes in colorectal cancer patients given resistant starch: A randomised controlled trial. Gut. 2009;**58**(3):413-420. DOI: 10.1136/gut.2008.162933

[116] Rafter J, Bennett M, Caderni G, Clune Y, Hughes R, Karlsson PC, et al. Dietary synbiotics reduce cancer risk factors in polypectomized and colon cancer patients. The American Journal of Clinical Nutrition. 2007;**85**(2):488-496. DOI: 10.1093/ajcn/85.2.488

[117] Nakatsu G, Zhou H, Wu WKK, Wong SH, Coker OO, Dai Z, et al. Alterations in enteric virome are associated with colorectal cancer and survival outcomes. Gastroenterology. 2018;**155**(2):529-41.e5. DOI: 10.1053/j.gastro.2018.04.018

[118] Hannigan GD, Duhaime MB, MTt R, Koumpouras CC, Schloss PD. Diagnostic potential and interactive dynamics of the colorectal cancer virome. MBio. 2018;**9**(6):e02248-18. DOI: 10.1128/mBio.02248-18

[119] Luan C, Xie L, Yang X, Miao H, Lv N, Zhang R, et al. Dysbiosis of fungal microbiota in the intestinal mucosa of patients with colorectal adenomas. Scientific Reports. 2015;**5**:7980. DOI: 10.1038/srep07980

[120] Coker OO, Nakatsu G, Dai RZ, Wu WKK, Wong SH, Ng SC, et al. Enteric fungal microbiota dysbiosis and ecological alterations in colorectal cancer. Gut. 2019;**68**(4):654-662. DOI: 10.1136/gutjnl-2018-317178

[121] Kostic AD, Chun E, Robertson L, Glickman JN, Gallini CA,

Michaud M, et al. Fusobacterium nucleatum potentiates intestinal tumorigenesis and modulates the tumor-immune microenvironment. Cell Host & Microbe. 2013;**14**(2):207-215. DOI: 10.1016/j.chom.2013.07.007

[122] Long X, Wong CC, Tong L, Chu ESH, Ho Szeto C, Go MYY, et al. Peptostreptococcus anaerobius promotes colorectal carcinogenesis and modulates tumour immunity. Nature Microbiology. 2019;**4**(12):2319-2330. DOI: 10.1038/s41564-019-0541-3

[123] Zaharuddin L, Mokhtar NM, Muhammad Nawawi KN, Raja Ali RA. A randomized double-blind placebo-controlled trial of probiotics in post-surgical colorectal cancer. BMC Gastroenterology. 2019;**19**(1):131. DOI: 10.1186/s12876-019-1047-4

[124] Ohara T, Yoshino K, Kitajima M. Possibility of preventing colorectal carcinogenesis with probiotics. Hepato-Gastroenterology. 2010;**57**(104):1411-1415

[125] Biarc J, Nguyen IS, Pini A, Gossé F, Richert S, Thiersé D, et al. Carcinogenic properties of proteins with pro-inflammatory activity from Streptococcus infantarius (formerly S.bovis). Carcinogenesis. 2004;**25**(8):1477-1484. DOI: 10.1093/carcin/bgh091

[126] Rubinstein MR, Wang X, Liu W, Hao Y, Cai G, Han YW. Fusobacterium nucleatum promotes colorectal carcinogenesis by modulating E-cadherin/β-catenin signaling via its FadA adhesin. Cell Host & Microbe. 2013;**14**(2):195-206. DOI: 10.1016/j.chom.2013.07.012

[127] Gur C, Ibrahim Y, Isaacson B, Yamin R, Abed J, Gamliel M, et al. Binding of the Fap2 protein of Fusobacterium nucleatum to human inhibitory receptor TIGIT protects tumors from immune cell attack. Immunity. 2015;**42**(2):344-355. DOI: 10.1016/j.immuni.2015.01.010

[128] Cremonesi E, Governa V, Garzon JFG, Mele V, Amicarella F, Muraro MG, et al. Gut microbiota modulate T cell trafficking into human colorectal cancer. Gut. 2018;**67**(11):1984. DOI: 10.1136/gutjnl-2016-313498

[129] Arthur JC, Gharaibeh RZ, Mühlbauer M, Perez-Chanona E, Uronis JM, McCafferty J, et al. Microbial genomic analysis reveals the essential role of inflammation in bacteria-induced colorectal cancer. Nature Communications. 2014;**5**:4724. DOI: 10.1038/ncomms5724

[130] Cuevas-Ramos G, Petit CR, Marcq I, Boury M, Oswald E, Nougayrède JP. Escherichia coli induces DNA damage in vivo and triggers genomic instability in mammalian cells. Proceedings of the National Academy of Sciences of the United States of America. 2010;**107**(25):11537-11542. DOI: 10.1073/pnas.1001261107

[131] Martin OCB, Bergonzini A, D'Amico F, Chen P, Shay JW, Dupuy J, et al. Infection with genotoxin-producing Salmonella enterica synergises with loss of the tumour suppressor APC in promoting genomic instability via the PI3K pathway in colonic epithelial cells. Cellular Microbiology. 2019;**21**(12):e13099. DOI: 10.1111/cmi.13099

[132] Singh N, Gurav A, Sivaprakasam S, Brady E, Padia R, Shi H, et al. Activation of Gpr109a, receptor for niacin and the commensal metabolite butyrate, suppresses colonic inflammation and carcinogenesis. Immunity. 2014;**40**(1):128-139. DOI: 10.1016/j.immuni.2013.12.007

[133] Collins D, Hogan AM, Winter DC. Microbial and viral pathogens in colorectal cancer. The Lancet Oncology. 2011;**12**(5):504-512. DOI: 10.1016/S1470-2045(10)70186-8

[134] Furusawa Y, Obata Y, Fukuda S, Endo TA, Nakato G, Takahashi D, et al. Commensal microbe-derived butyrate induces the differentiation of colonic regulatory T cells. Nature. 2013;**504**(7480):446-450. DOI: 10.1038/nature12721

[135] Buda A, Qualtrough D, Jepson MA, Martines D, Paraskeva C, Pignatelli M. Butyrate downregulates $\alpha_2\beta_1$ integrin: A possible role in the induction of apoptosis in colorectal cancer cell lines. Gut. 2003;**52**(5):729. DOI: 10.1136/gut.52.5.729

[136] Boleij A, Hechenbleikner EM, Goodwin AC, Badani R, Stein EM, Lazarev MG, et al. The bacteroides fragilis toxin gene is prevalent in the colon mucosa of colorectal cancer patients. Clinical Infectious Diseases. 2015;**60**(2):208-215. DOI: 10.1093/cid/ciu787

[137] Wu S, Rhee K-J, Albesiano E, Rabizadeh S, Wu X, Yen H-R, et al. A human colonic commensal promotes colon tumorigenesis via activation of T helper type 17 T cell responses. Nature Medicine. 2009;**15**(9):1016-1022. DOI: 10.1038/nm.2015

[138] Kortylewski M, Xin H, Kujawski M, Lee H, Liu Y, Harris T, et al. Regulation of the IL-23 and IL-12 balance by Stat3 signaling in the tumor microenvironment. Cancer Cell. 2009;**15**(2):114-123. DOI: 10.1016/j.ccr.2008.12.018

[139] Wang K, Kim MK, Di Caro G, Wong J, Shalapour S, Wan J, et al. Interleukin-17 receptor a signaling in transformed enterocytes promotes early colorectal tumorigenesis. Immunity. 2014;**41**(6):1052-1063. DOI: 10.1016/j.immuni.2014.11.009

[140] Scudamore CL, Jepson MA, Hirst BH, Miller HR. The rat mucosal mast cell chymase, RMCP-II, alters epithelial cell monolayer permeability in association with altered distribution of the tight junction proteins ZO-1 and occludin. European Journal of Cell Biology. 1998;**75**(4):321-330. DOI: 10.1016/s0171-9335(98)80065-4

[141] Zhang DM, Jiao RQ, Kong LD. High dietary fructose: Direct or indirect dangerous factors disturbing tissue and organ functions. Nutrients. 2017;**9**(4):335. DOI: 10.3390/nu9040335

[142] Cretoiu D, Ionescu RF, Enache RM, Cretoiu SM, Voinea SC. Gut microbiome, functional food, atherosclerosis, and vascular calcifications-is there a missing link? Microorganisms. 2021;**9**(9):1913. DOI: 10.3390/microorganisms9091913

[143] Lusis AJ. Atherosclerosis. Nature. 2000;**407**(6801):233-241. DOI: 10.1038/35025203

[144] Rosenfeld ME, Campbell LA. Pathogens and atherosclerosis: Update on the potential contribution of multiple infectious organisms to the pathogenesis of atherosclerosis. Thrombosis and Haemostasis. 2011;**106**(5):858-867. DOI: 10.1160/th11-06-0392

[145] Jonsson AL, Bäckhed F. Role of gut microbiota in atherosclerosis. Nature Reviews. Cardiology. 2017;**14**(2):79-87. DOI: 10.1038/nrcardio.2016.183

[146] Pastori D, Carnevale R, Nocella C, Novo M, Santulli M, Cammisotto V, et al. Gut-derived serum lipopolysaccharide is associated with enhanced risk of major adverse cardiovascular

events in atrial fibrillation: Effect of adherence to Mediterranean diet. Journal of the American Heart Association;**6**(6):e005784. DOI: 10.1161/JAHA.117.005784

[147] Yamashita T, Yoshida N, Emoto T, Saito Y, Hirata KI. Two gut microbiota-derived toxins are closely associated with cardiovascular diseases: A review. Toxins (Basel). 2021;**13**(5):297. DOI: 10.3390/toxins13050297

[148] Yoshida N, Yamashita T, Kishino S, Watanabe H, Sasaki K, Sasaki D, et al. A possible beneficial effect of Bacteroides on faecal lipopolysaccharide activity and cardiovascular diseases. Scientific Reports. 2020;**10**(1):13009. DOI: 10.1038/s41598-020-69983-z

[149] Ding L, Chang M, Guo Y, Zhang L, Xue C, Yanagita T, et al. Trimethylamine-N-oxide (TMAO)-induced atherosclerosis is associated with bile acid metabolism. Lipids in Health and Disease. 2018;**17**(1):286. DOI: 10.1186/s12944-018-0939-6

[150] Witkowski M, Weeks TL, Hazen SL. Gut microbiota and cardiovascular disease. Circulation Research. 2020;**127**:553-570. DOI: 10.3390/microorganisms9091913

[151] Trøseid M, Ueland T, Hov JR, Svardal A, Gregersen I, Dahl CP, et al. Microbiota-dependent metabolite trimethylamine-N-oxide is associated with disease severity and survival of patients with chronic heart failure. Journal of Internal Medicine. 2015;**277**(6):717-726. DOI: 10.1111/joim.12328

[152] Tang WHW, Li DY, Hazen SL. Dietary metabolism, the gut microbiome, and heart failure. Nature Reviews. Cardiology. 2019;**16**(3):137-154. DOI: 10.1038/s41569-018-0108-7

[153] Mutalub YB, Abdulwahab M, Mohammed A, Yahkub AM, Al-Mhanna SB, Yusof W, et al. Gut microbiota modulation as a novel therapeutic strategy in cardiometabolic diseases. Food. 2022;**11**(17):2575. DOI: 10.3390/foods11172575

[154] Kummen M, Mayerhofer CCK, Vestad B, Broch K, Awoyemi A, Storm-Larsen C, et al. Gut microbiota signature in heart failure defined from profiling of 2 independent cohorts. Journal of the American College of Cardiology. 2018;**71**(10):1184-1186. DOI: 10.1016/j.jacc.2017.12.057

[155] Pasini E, Aquilani R, Testa C, Baiardi P, Angioletti S, Boschi F, et al. Pathogenic gut flora in patients with chronic heart failure. JACC Heart Failure. 2016;**4**(3):220-227. DOI: 10.1016/j.jchf.2015.10.009

[156] Ionescu RF, Boroghina SC, Cretoiu SM. Is there a link between the gut microbiome and arterial hypertension. Journal of Hypertension Research. 2021;**7**:12-17

[157] Miura K, Stamler J, Nakagawa H, Elliott P, Ueshima H, Chan Q, et al. Relationship of dietary linoleic acid to blood pressure. The international study of macro-micronutrients and blood pressure study [corrected]. Hypertension. 2008;**52**(2):408-414. DOI: 10.1161/hypertensionaha.108.112383

[158] Tsukamoto I, Sugawara S. Low levels of linoleic acid and α-linolenic acid and high levels of arachidonic acid in plasma phospholipids are associated with hypertension. Biomedical Reports. 2018;**8**(1):69-76. DOI: 10.3892/br.2017.1015

[159] Djoussé L, Arnett DK, Pankow JS, Hopkins PN, Province MA, Ellison RC.

Dietary linolenic acid is associated with a lower prevalence of hypertension in the NHLBI family heart study. Hypertension. 2005;**45**(3):368-373. DOI: 10.1161/01.HYP.0000154679.41568.e6

[160] Sun S, Lulla A, Sioda M, Winglee K, Wu MC, Jacobs DR Jr, et al. Gut microbiota composition and blood pressure. Hypertension. 2019;**73**(5):998-1006. DOI: 10.1161/hypertensionaha.118.12109

[161] Jin M, Qian Z, Yin J, Xu W, Zhou X. The role of intestinal microbiota in cardiovascular disease. Journal of Cellular and Molecular Medicine. 2019;**23**(4):2343-2350. DOI: 10.1111/jcmm.14195

[162] Pluznick JL. Microbial short-chain fatty acids and blood pressure regulation. Current Hypertension Reports. 2017;**19**(4):25. DOI: 10.1007/s11906-017-0722-5

[163] Li J, Zhao F, Wang Y, Chen J, Tao J, Tian G, et al. Gut microbiota dysbiosis contributes to the development of hypertension. Microbiome. 2017;**5**(1):14. DOI: 10.1186/s40168-016-0222-x

[164] Lu D, Zou X, Zhang H. The relationship between atrial fibrillation and intestinal flora with its metabolites. Frontiers in Cardiovascular Medicine. 2022;**9**:948755. DOI: 10.3389/fcvm.2022.948755

[165] Wang L, Wang S, Zhang Q, He C, Fu C, Wei Q. The role of the gut microbiota in health and cardiovascular diseases. Molecular Biomedicine. 2022;**3**(1):30. DOI: 10.1186/s43556-022-00091-2

[166] Drapkina OM, Yafarova AA, Kaburova AN, Kiselev AR. Targeting gut microbiota as a novel strategy for prevention and treatment of hypertension, atrial fibrillation and heart failure: Current knowledge and future perspectives. Biomedicine. 2022;**10**(8):2019. DOI: 10.3390/biomedicines10082019

[167] Zhang J, Zuo K, Fang C, Yin X, Liu X, Zhong J, et al. Altered synthesis of genes associated with short-chain fatty acids in the gut of patients with atrial fibrillation. BMC Genomics. 2021;**22**(1):634. DOI: 10.1186/s12864-021-07944-0

[168] Ballini A, Scacco S, Boccellino M, Santacroce L, Arrigoni R. Microbiota and obesity: Where are we now? Biology (Basel). 2020;**9**(12):415. DOI: 10.3390/biology9120415

[169] Ley RE, Bäckhed F, Turnbaugh P, Lozupone CA, Knight RD, Gordon JI. Obesity alters gut microbial ecology. Proceedings of the National Academy of Sciences of the United States of America. 2005;**102**(31):11070-11075. DOI: 10.1073/pnas.0504978102

[170] Ahmad A, Riaz S, Tanveer M. Obesity and gut microbiota. In: Effect of Microbiota on Health and Disease. London: IntechOpen; 2022. DOI: 10.5772/intechopen.105397

[171] Ojeda P, Bobe A, Dolan K, Leone V, Martinez K. Nutritional modulation of gut microbiota - the impact on metabolic disease pathophysiology. The Journal of Nutritional Biochemistry. 2016;**28**:191-200. DOI: 10.1016/j.jnutbio.2015.08.013

[172] Jumpertz R, Le DS, Turnbaugh PJ, Trinidad C, Bogardus C, Gordon JI, et al. Energy-balance studies reveal associations between gut microbes, caloric load, and nutrient absorption in humans. The American Journal of Clinical Nutrition. 2011;**94**(1):58-65. DOI: 10.3945/ajcn.110.010132

[173] Kalliomäki M, Collado MC, Salminen S, Isolauri E. Early differences

in fecal microbiota composition in children may predict overweight. The American Journal of Clinical Nutrition. 2008;**87**(3):534-538. DOI: 10.1093/ajcn/87.3.534

[174] Di Domenico M, Pinto F, Quagliuolo L, Contaldo M, Settembre G, Romano A, et al. The role of oxidative stress and hormones in controlling obesity. Frontiers in Endocrinology (Lausanne). 2019;**10**:540. DOI: 10.3389/fendo.2019.00540

[175] Turnbaugh PJ, Bäckhed F, Fulton L, Gordon JI. Diet-induced obesity is linked to marked but reversible alterations in the mouse distal gut microbiome. Cell Host & Microbe. 2008;**3**(4):213-223. DOI: 10.1016/j.chom.2008.02.015

[176] Davis CD. The gut microbiome and its role in obesity. Nutrition Today. 2016;**51**(4):167-174. DOI: 10.1097/nt.0000000000000167

[177] Turnbaugh PJ, Ridaura VK, Faith JJ, Rey FE, Knight R, Gordon JI. The effect of diet on the human gut microbiome: A metagenomic analysis in humanized gnotobiotic mice. Science Translational Medicine. 2009;**1**(6):6ra14. DOI: 10.1126/scitranslmed.3000322

[178] Wu GD, Chen J, Hoffmann C, Bittinger K, Chen YY, Keilbaugh SA, et al. Linking long-term dietary patterns with gut microbial enterotypes. Science. 2011;**334**(6052):105-108. DOI: 10.1126/science.1208344

[179] Chen J, Thomsen M, Vitetta L. Interaction of gut microbiota with dysregulation of bile acids in the pathogenesis of nonalcoholic fatty liver disease and potential therapeutic implications of probiotics. Journal of Cellular Biochemistry. 2019;**120**(3):2713-2720. DOI: 10.1002/jcb.27635

[180] Pols TW, Nomura M, Harach T, Lo Sasso G, Oosterveer MH, Thomas C, et al. TGR5 activation inhibits atherosclerosis by reducing macrophage inflammation and lipid loading. Cell Metabolism. 2011;**14**(6):747-757. DOI: 10.1016/j.cmet.2011.11.006

[181] Maruvada P, Leone V, Kaplan LM, Chang EB. The human microbiome and obesity: Moving beyond associations. Cell Host & Microbe. 2017;**22**(5):589-599. DOI: 10.1016/j.chom.2017.10.005

[182] Chassaing B, Ley RE, Gewirtz AT. Intestinal epithelial cell toll-like receptor 5 regulates the intestinal microbiota to prevent low-grade inflammation and metabolic syndrome in mice. Gastroenterology. 2014;**147**(6):1363-77.e17. DOI: 10.1053/j.gastro.2014.08.033

[183] Sonnenburg ED, Smits SA, Tikhonov M, Higginbottom SK, Wingreen NS, Sonnenburg JL. Diet-induced extinctions in the gut microbiota compound over generations. Nature. 2016;**529**(7585):212-215. DOI: 10.1038/nature16504

[184] Helmink BA, Khan MAW, Hermann A, Gopalakrishnan V, Wargo JA. The microbiome, cancer, and cancer therapy. Nature Medicine. 2019;**25**(3):377-388. DOI: 10.1038/s41591-019-0377-7

[185] Murphy EF, Cotter PD, Healy S, Marques TM, O'Sullivan O, Fouhy F, et al. Composition and energy harvesting capacity of the gut microbiota: relationship to diet, obesity and time in mouse models. Gut. 2010;**59**(12):1635-1642. DOI: 10.1136/gut.2010.215665

[186] Petersen C, Bell R, Klag KA, Lee SH, Soto R, Ghazaryan A, et al. T cell-mediated regulation of the microbiota protects against obesity. Science.

2019;**365**(6451):eaat9351. DOI: 10.1126/science.aat9351

[187] den Besten G, Bleeker A, Gerding A, van Eunen K, Havinga R, van Dijk TH, et al. Short-chain fatty acids protect against high-fat diet-induced obesity via a PPARγ-dependent switch from lipogenesis to fat oxidation. Diabetes. 2015;**64**(7):2398-2408. DOI: 10.2337/db14-1213

[188] Wlodarska M, Thaiss CA, Nowarski R, Henao-Mejia J, Zhang JP, Brown EM, et al. NLRP6 inflammasome orchestrates the colonic host-microbial interface by regulating goblet cell mucus secretion. Cell. 2014;**156**(5):1045-1059. DOI: 10.1016/j.cell.2014.01.026

[189] Cani PD, Delzenne NM. The gut microbiome as therapeutic target. Pharmacology & Therapeutics. 2011;**130**(2):202-212. DOI: 10.1016/j.pharmthera.2011.01.012

[190] Turnbaugh PJ, Ley RE, Mahowald MA, Magrini V, Mardis ER, Gordon JI. An obesity-associated gut microbiome with increased capacity for energy harvest. Nature. 2006;**444**(7122):1027-1031. DOI: 10.1038/nature05414

[191] Le Chatelier E, Nielsen T, Qin J, Prifti E, Hildebrand F, Falony G, et al. Richness of human gut microbiome correlates with metabolic markers. Nature. 2013;**500**(7464):541-546. DOI: 10.1038/nature12506

[192] Shajib MS, Khan WI. The role of serotonin and its receptors in activation of immune responses and inflammation. Acta Physiologica (Oxford, England). 2015;**213**(3):561-574. DOI: 10.1111/apha.12430

[193] Sandhu KV, Sherwin E, Schellekens H, Stanton C, Dinan TG, Cryan JF. Feeding the microbiota-gut-brain axis: Diet, microbiome, and neuropsychiatry. Translational Research. 2017;**179**:223-244. DOI: 10.1016/j.trsl.2016.10.002

[194] Delzenne NM, Cani PD, Daubioul C, Neyrinck AM. Impact of inulin and oligofructose on gastrointestinal peptides. The British Journal of Nutrition. 2005;**93**(Suppl 1):S157-S161. DOI: 10.1079/bjn20041342

[195] Torres-Fuentes C, Schellekens H, Dinan TG, Cryan JF. A natural solution for obesity: Bioactives for the prevention and treatment of weight gain. A review. Nutritional Neuroscience. 2015;**18**(2):49-65. DOI: 10.1179/1476830513y.0000000099

[196] Cox LM, Blaser MJ. Antibiotics in early life and obesity. Nature Reviews Endocrinology. 2015;**11**(3):182-190. DOI: 10.1038/nrendo.2014.210

[197] Salazar J, Angarita L, Morillo V, Navarro C, Martínez MS, Chacín M, et al. Microbiota and diabetes mellitus: Role of lipid mediators. Nutrients. 2020;**12**(10):3039. DOI: 10.3390/nu12103039

[198] Schwartz SS, Epstein S, Corkey BE, Grant SF, Gavin JR 3rd, Aguilar RB. The time is right for a new classification system for diabetes: Rationale and implications of the β-cell-centric classification schema. Diabetes Care. 2016;**39**(2):179-186. DOI: 10.2337/dc15-1585

[199] Zozulinska D, Wierusz-Wysocka B. Type 2 diabetes mellitus as inflammatory disease. Diabetes Research and Clinical Practice. 2006;**74**(2):98-107. DOI: 10.1016/j.diabres.2006.06.007

[200] Roohi A, Tabrizi M, Abbasi F, Ataie-Jafari A, Nikbin B, Larijani B,

et al. Serum IL-17, IL-23, and TGF-β levels in type 1 and type 2 diabetic patients and age-matched healthy controls. BioMed Research International. 2014;**2014**:718946. DOI: 10.1155/2014/718946

[201] Abdel-Moneim A, Bakery HH, Allam G. The potential pathogenic role of IL-17/Th17 cells in both type 1 and type 2 diabetes mellitus. Biomedicine & Pharmacotherapy. 2018;**101**:287-292. DOI: 10.1016/j.biopha.2018.02.103

[202] Zhang L, Chu J, Hao W, Zhang J, Li H, Yang C, et al. Gut microbiota and type 2 diabetes mellitus: Association, mechanism, and translational applications. Mediators of Inflammation. 2021;**2021**:5110276. DOI: 10.1155/2021/5110276

[203] Huang X, Yan D, Xu M, Li F, Ren M, Zhang J, et al. Interactive association of lipopolysaccharide and free fatty acid with the prevalence of type 2 diabetes: A community-based cross-sectional study. Journal of Diabetes Investigation. 2019;**10**(6):1438-1446. DOI: 10.1111/jdi.13056

[204] Gomes JMG, Costa JA, Alfenas RCG. Metabolic endotoxemia and diabetes mellitus: A systematic review. Metabolism. 2017;**68**:133-144. DOI: 10.1016/j.metabol.2016.12.009

[205] Matheus VA, Monteiro L, Oliveira RB, Maschio DA, Collares-Buzato CB. Butyrate reduces high-fat diet-induced metabolic alterations, hepatic steatosis and pancreatic beta cell and intestinal barrier dysfunctions in prediabetic mice. Experimental Biology and Medicine (Maywood NJ). 2017;**242**(12):1214-1226. DOI: 10.1177/1535370217708188

[206] Larsen N, Vogensen FK, van den Berg FW, Nielsen DS, Andreasen AS, Pedersen BK, et al. Gut microbiota in human adults with type 2 diabetes differs from non-diabetic adults. PLoS One. 2010;**5**(2):e9085. DOI: 10.1371/journal.pone.0009085

[207] Endesfelder D, Engel M, Davis-Richardson AG, Ardissone AN, Achenbach P, Hummel S, et al. Towards a functional hypothesis relating anti-islet cell autoimmunity to the dietary impact on microbial communities and butyrate production. Microbiome. 2016;**4**:17. DOI: 10.1186/s40168-016-0163-4

[208] Murri M, Leiva I, Gomez-Zumaquero JM, Tinahones FJ, Cardona F, Soriguer F, et al. Gut microbiota in children with type 1 diabetes differs from that in healthy children: A case-control study. BMC Medicine. 2013;**11**:46. DOI: 10.1186/1741-7015-11-46

[209] Jandhyala SM, Madhulika A, Deepika G, Rao GV, Reddy DN, Subramanyam C, et al. Altered intestinal microbiota in patients with chronic pancreatitis: Implications in diabetes and metabolic abnormalities. Scientific Reports. 2017;7:43640. DOI: 10.1038/srep43640

[210] Remely M, Aumueller E, Merold C, Dworzak S, Hippe B, Zanner J, et al. Effects of short chain fatty acid producing bacteria on epigenetic regulation of FFAR3 in type 2 diabetes and obesity. Gene. 2014;**537**(1):85-92. DOI: 10.1016/j.gene.2013.11.081

[211] Gurung M, Li Z, You H, Rodrigues R, Jump DB, Morgun A, et al. Role of gut microbiota in type 2 diabetes pathophysiology. eBioMedicine. 2020;**51**:102590. DOI: 10.1016/j.ebiom.2019.11.051

[212] Ionescu R, Enache R, Cretoiu S, Bogdan G. Gut microbiome changes

in gestational diabetes. International Journal of Molecular Sciences. 2022;**23**:12839. DOI: 10.3390/ijms232112839

[213] Rahat-Rozenbloom S, Fernandes J, Cheng J, Wolever TMS. Acute increases in serum colonic short-chain fatty acids elicited by inulin do not increase GLP-1 or PYY responses but may reduce ghrelin in lean and overweight humans. European Journal of Clinical Nutrition. 2017;**71**(8):953-958. DOI: 10.1038/ejcn.2016.249

[214] Duran ALC, Medina MFD, Valdivieso MRA, Dunn MAE, Torres WPR, Barrera LNA, et al. Terapia incretinomimética: evidencia clínica de la eficacia de los agonistas del GLP-1R y sus efectos cardio-protectores. Revista Latinoamericana de Hipertensión. 2018;**13**(4):400-415

[215] Grasset E, Puel A, Charpentier J, Collet X, Christensen JE, Tercé F, et al. A specific gut microbiota dysbiosis of type 2 diabetic mice induces GLP-1 resistance through an enteric NO-dependent and gut-brain axis mechanism. Cell Metabolism. 2017;**25**(5):1075-90.e5. DOI: 10.1016/j.cmet.2017.04.013

[216] Perry RJ, Peng L, Barry NA, Cline GW, Zhang D, Cardone RL, et al. Acetate mediates a microbiome-brain-β-cell axis to promote metabolic syndrome. Nature. 2016;**534**(7606):213-217. DOI: 10.1038/nature18309

[217] Zhang S, Cai Y, Meng C, Ding X, Huang J, Luo X, et al. The role of the microbiome in diabetes mellitus. Diabetes Research and Clinical Practice. 2021;**172**:108645. DOI: 10.1016/j.diabres.2020.108645

[218] De Pessemier B, Grine L, Debaere M, Maes A, Paetzold B, Callewaert C. Gut-skin axis: Current Knowledge of the Interrelationship between Microbial Dysbiosis and Skin Conditions. Microorganisms. 2021;**9**(2):353. DOI: 10.3390/microorganisms9020353

[219] Ellis SR, Nguyen M, Vaughn AR, Notay M, Burney WA, Sandhu S, et al. The skin and gut microbiome and its role in common dermatologic conditions. Microorganisms. 2019;**7**(11):550. DOI: 10.3390/microorganisms7110550

[220] Coates M, Lee MJ, Norton D, MacLeod AS. The skin and intestinal microbiota and their specific innate immune systems. Frontiers in Immunology. 2019;**10**:2950. DOI: 10.3389/fimmu.2019.02950

[221] Nast A, Spuls PI, van der Kraaij G, Gisondi P, Paul C, Ormerod AD, et al. European S3-guideline on the systemic treatment of psoriasis vulgaris - update apremilast and secukinumab - EDF in cooperation with EADV and IPC. Journal of the European Academy of Dermatology and Venereology. 2017;**31**(12):1951-1963. DOI: 10.1111/jdv.14454

[222] Zhang X, Shi L, Sun T, Guo K, Geng S. Dysbiosis of gut microbiota and its correlation with dysregulation of cytokines in psoriasis patients. BMC Microbiology. 2021;**21**(1):78. DOI: 10.1186/s12866-021-02125-1

[223] Tan L, Zhao S, Zhu W, Wu L, Li J, Shen M, et al. The Akkermansia muciniphila is a gut microbiota signature in psoriasis. Experimental Dermatology. 2018;**27**(2):144-149. DOI: 10.1111/exd.13463

[224] Hidalgo-Cantabrana C, Gómez J, Delgado S, Requena-López S, Queiro-Silva R, Margolles A, et al. Gut microbiota dysbiosis in a cohort of

patients with psoriasis. British Journal of Dermatology. 2019;**181**(6):1287-1295. DOI: 10.1111/bjd.17931

[225] Scher JU, Ubeda C, Artacho A, Attur M, Isaac S, Reddy SM, et al. Decreased bacterial diversity characterizes the altered gut microbiota in patients with psoriatic arthritis, resembling dysbiosis in inflammatory bowel disease. Arthritis & Rheumatology. 2015;**67**(1):128-139. DOI: 10.1002/art.38892

[226] West CE, Rydén P, Lundin D, Engstrand L, Tulic MK, Prescott SL. Gut microbiome and innate immune response patterns in IgE-associated eczema. Clinical and Experimental Allergy. 2015;**45**(9):1419-1429. DOI: 10.1111/cea.12566

[227] Abrahamsson TR, Jakobsson HE, Andersson AF, Björkstén B, Engstrand L, Jenmalm MC. Low diversity of the gut microbiota in infants with atopic eczema. The Journal of Allergy and Clinical Immunology. 2012;**129**(2):434-40, 440.e1-2. DOI: 10.1016/j.jaci.2011.10.025

[228] Sator PG, Schmidt JB, Hönigsmann H. Comparison of epidermal hydration and skin surface lipids in healthy individuals and in patients with atopic dermatitis. Journal of the American Academy of Dermatology. 2003;**48**(3):352-358. DOI: 10.1067/mjd.2003.105

[229] Nylund L, Nermes M, Isolauri E, Salminen S, de Vos WM, Satokari R. Severity of atopic disease inversely correlates with intestinal microbiota diversity and butyrate-producing bacteria. Allergy. 2015;**70**(2):241-244. DOI: 10.1111/all.12549

[230] McCarthy S, Barrett M, Kirthi S, Pellanda P, Vlckova K, Tobin A-M, et al. Altered skin and gut microbiome in hidradenitis suppurativa. Journal of Investigative Dermatology. 2022;**142**(2):459-68.e15. DOI: 10.1016/j.jid.2021.05.036

[231] Kam S, Collard M, Lam J, Alani RM. Gut microbiome perturbations in patients with hidradenitis suppurativa: A case series. Journal of Investigative Dermatology. 2021;**141**(1):225-8.e2. DOI: 10.1016/j.jid.2020.04.017

[232] Lam SY, Radjabzadeh D, Eppinga H, Nossent YRA, van der Zee HH, Kraaij R, et al. A microbiome study to explore the gut-skin axis in hidradenitis suppurativa. Journal of Dermatological Science. 2021;**101**(3):218-220. DOI: 10.1016/j.jdermsci.2020.12.008